LASERS IN GYNECOLOGY

LASERS IN GYNECOLOGY

David S. McLaughlin, M.D.

Indianapolis Fertility Center
Indianapolis, Indiana

WITH 28 CONTRIBUTORS

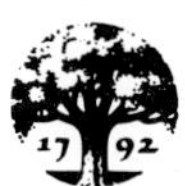

J.B. LIPPINCOTT
Philadelphia

Grand Rapids • New York • St. Louis • San Francisco
London • Sydney • Tokyo

Acquisitions Editor: Lisa McAllister
Coordinating Editorial Assistant: Paula M. Callaghan
Project Editor: Melissa McElroy
Indexer: Lillian Rodberg
Designer: Doug Smock
Production Manager: Helen Ewan
Production Coordinator: Kathryn Rule
Compositor: Bi-Comp, Incorporated
Printer/Binder: Arcata Graphics/Halliday

6 5 4 3 2 1

Library of Congress Cataloging-in-Publication Data

Lasers in gynecology/[edited by] David S. McLaughlin: with 28 contributors.
　　p. cm.
　ISBN 0-397-50986-3
　1. Generative organs, Female—laser surgery. I. McLaughlin, David S.
　[DNLM: 1. Genital Diseases, Female—therapy. 2. Genitalia, Female—surgery. 3. Laser Surgery.
　4. Lasers—therapeutic use. WP 660 L3435]
　RG104.L38　1991
　618.1′059—dc20
　DNLM/DLC　　　　　　　　　　　　　　　　　　　　　　　　　　　　90-5632
　for Library of Congress　　　　　　　　　　　　　　　　　　　　　　　　CIP

CONTRIBUTORS

Gregory T. Absten
Laser Consultant, Advanced Laser Services Corp., Grove City, Ohio

Randle S. Corfman, Ph.D., M.D.
Assistant Professor, Department of Obstetrics and Gynecology, Mayo Medical School, Director, Assisted Reproductive Technologies, Mayo Clinic, Rochester, Minnesota

James F. Daniell, M.D.
Clinical Associate Professor, Department of Obstetrics and Gynecology, Vanderbilt University School of Medicine, Attending Physician, Westside Hospital, Nashville, Tennessee

Gordon D. Davis, M.D.
Director of Laser Surgery, Phoenix Integrated Residency, Obstetrics and Gynecology, Maricopa Medical Center, Attending Physician, St. Joseph Medical Center and Hospital, Attending Physician, Department of Obstetrics and Gynecology, Good Samaritan Medical Center and Hospital, Phoenix, Arizona

Michael P. Diamond, M.D.
Assistant Professor, Division of Reproductive Endocrinology, Department of Obstetrics and Gynecology, Yale University School of Medicine, New Haven, Connecticut

James H. Dorsey, M.D.

Chairman, Department of Gynecology, Greater Baltimore Medical Center, Assistant Professor, Johns Hopkins University School of Medicine, Baltimore, Maryland

Joseph R. Feste, M.D.

Clinical Associate Professor, Department of Obstetrics and Gynecology, Baylor College of Medicine, Clinical Associate Professor, Department of Obstetrics and Gynecology, University of Texas Health Science Center, Houston, Texas

John C. Fisher, Sc.D.

Formerly Visiting Associate Professor, Laser Medicine and Surgery, University of Cincinnati School of Medicine, Cincinnati, Ohio, Consultant in Laser Medicine and Surgery, St. Luke's Medical Center, Milwaukee, Wisconsin, Member, Medical Staff, St. Barnabas Medical Center, Livingston, New Jersey

Milton H. Goldrath, M.D.

Associate Professor, Department of OB-GYN, Wayne State University School of Medicine, Section Chief of Gynecology, Sinai Hospital of Detroit, Southfield, Michigan

Mitchell D. Greenberg, M.D.

Clinical Coordinator, Richard Reid Foundation for Cervical Cancer Research, Southfield, Michigan

Leonard I. Grossweiner, Ph.D.

Professor of Physics, Illinois Institute of Technology, Chicago, Illinois, Research Director, Wenske Laser Center, Ravenwood Hospital Medical Center, Chicago, Illinois

John D. Harryman, M.H.A.

Executive Director, Humana Women's Hospital–Indianapolis, Indianapolis, Indiana

William M. Jamieson, M.D.

Clinical Associate Professor, Department of Obstetrics and Gynecology, University of Cincinnati College of Medicine, Director of Gynecologic Laser Education, Christ Hospital, Cincinnati, Ohio

William R. Keye, Jr., M.D.

Chief, Division of Reproductive Endocrinology, Department of Obstetrics and Gynecology, William Beaumont Hospital, Royal Oak, Michigan

Rocco V. Lobraico, M.D.
Clinical Professor Emeritus, Department of Obstetrics and Gynecology, College of Medicine, Chicago, Illinois, Medical Director, Wenske Laser Center, Ravenswood Hospital Medical Center, Chicago, Illinois

Jack M. Lomano, M.D.
Clinical Associate Professor, Department of Obstetrics and Gynecology, Ohio State University School of Medicine, Director, Education and Development, Grant Laser Center, Grant Hospital Medical Center, Columbus, Ohio

Carolyn J. Mackety, R.N., M.A.
Nursing Administrator, Surgical Services, Medical Center Hospital of Vermont, Burlington, Vermont

Barbara E. Marlay, R.N.
Medical Photographer, Ocean Grove, New Jersey

John L. Marlow, M.D.
Assistant Professor, Department of OB–GYN, George Washington University School of Medicine, Assistant Clinical Professor, Department of OB–GYN, Georgetown University School of Medicine, Director of Continuing Medical Education, Columbia Hospital for Women Medical Center, Washington, D.C.

Dan C. Martin, M.D.
Reproductive Surgeon, Baptist Memorial Hospital, Memphis, Tennesse, Clinical Assistant Professor, University of Tennessee, Memphis, Memphis, Tennessee

David S. McLaughlin, M.D.
Reproductive Surgeon, Humana Women's Hospital, Associate Director, Indianapolis Fertility Center, Pregnancy Initiation Center, Indianapolis, Indiana

Richard Reid, M.D.
Assistant Professor, Department of Obstetrics and Gynecology, Wayne State University Medical School, Director, Genital Dysplasia Clinic, Sinai Hospital, Detroit, Michigan

Mary Ann Riopelle, B.A.
Research Associate, St. Joseph's Hospital, London, Ontario, Canada

Helmut F. Schellhas, M.D.
Clinical Professor, University of Cincinnati Medical Center, Cincinnati, Ohio

Gerald J. Shirk, M.D.
Director of Laser Research, St. Luke's Hospital, Cedar Rapids, Iowa

Jose E. Torres, M.D.

Professor, Department of Obstetrics and Gynecology, Louisiana State University Medical School, New Orleans, Louisiana

Jay W. Williams, M.H.A.

Executive Director and CEO, Humana Hospital—Overland Park, Overland Park, Kansas

V. Cecil Wright, M.D.

Clinical Professor of Obstetrics and Gynecology, University of Western Ontario, Director of Abnormal Pap Smear Clinic, Chairman, Laser Committee, St. Joseph's Hospital, London, Ontario, Canada

PREFACE

Although lasers have been widely used and accepted in several surgical and medical specialties, it has taken nearly 2 decades for lasers to become routinely integrated into gynecologic practice. Healthy skepticism has finally been replaced by widespread acceptance and even enthusiasm for this new treatment modality. Lasers are currently used in gynecology in two ways: (1) externally—freehand or in conjunction with the colposcope to treat benign, premalignant, or viral diseases of the vulva, vagina, or cervix; or (2) intra-abdominally—freehand or in conjunction with an operating microscope or endoscope (laparoscope or hysteroscope) to treat adhesive disease, myomas, tubal disease, ovarian cysts, and ablate endometrial glands.

The CO_2 laser remains the most commonly used wavelength in gynecology; however, physicians have recently begun to use lasers delivered through fiberoptic bundles (Nd:YAG, Argon, and KTP) for specific indications because of the ease of delivering the laser's energy to targeted tissue. Further research should develop newer methods of delivery and indications (*e.g.* photodynamic therapy).

This text is designed as a primer for gynecologists new to this treatment modality, and as a reference for more experienced gynecologic laser surgeons. It is intended to help readers glean pertinent information to help them evaluate the appropriate place of laser therapy in their gynecologic practice. Each type of laser used in gynecology is discussed in conjunction with specific indications and delivery systems; laser physics and safety are emphasized. New indications and delivery modes are presented along with a perspective on laser therapy related to current operative techniques.

Hopefully, this text will enlighten readers enough to stimulate their interests and to seek further information and surgical skills. The novice should feel free to consult other physicians who have already gained these skills, either in the local hospital setting, or in preceptorships, to maximize his or her potential.

As a member of the Gynecologic Practice Committee of the American College of Obstetrics and Gynecology during the inception of lasers in gynecology in the fall of 1980, I have enjoyed watching the evolution of laser therapy in gynecology, particularly for fertility-promoting procedures. Beginning with an initial handful of early investigators, safe gynecologic laser therapy has been taught to a multitude of gynecologists. It is my sincere hope that as others improve upon the use of lasers, the integration of this technique into the mainstream of gynecologic practice will help to alleviate pain and suffering for many women, while allowing them to achieve or preserve their reproductive potential.

ACKNOWLEDGMENTS

My initial interest in gynecologic lasers was piqued more than a decade ago while serving as a junior fellow member of the American College of Obstetrics and Gynecology–Gynecologic Practice Committee. Drs. Kermit Krantz and Ervin Nichols charged me with the task of writing the ACOG Physician's Statements on microsurgery and laser surgery based on available data. Microsurgery appeared to be efficacious for tubal reanastomosis; however, there was a dearth of published articles on the use of lasers in gynecology. While researching the application of this new modality, I met other laser physicians, particularly Drs. Joe Bellina, Mickey Baggish, Jim Daniell, Bud Keye, and Cecil Wright, as well as many of the laser pioneers who contributed chapters to this book. As a result, in 1981 I became one of a handful of gynecologic surgeons using the carbon dioxide laser for intra–abdominal reproductive surgery. While pioneering intra–abdominal laser techniques to preserve or enhance reproductive potential, I was stimulated to develop new intra–abdominal laser instruments, photodocument new laser techniques, and publish new intra–abdominal laser applications by Jim and Bob Marlay, Elissa Debarone, and my wife, Barb. I am eternally grateful for the support and encouragement given to me by them, which allowed me to fully develop my interest in reproductive surgery. *Lasers in Gynecology* was written with the assistance of Humana, Inc., and with the efforts of Jay Williams and John Harryman at Humana Women's Hospital-Indianapolis. Editorial assistance was provided by Elissa DeBarone, Ph.D. and manuscript preparation accomplished by Becky Staley and Cheryl Gaines. Most of all, I am greatly indebted to all contributing authors who have been willing to take time out of their busy schedules to share their expertise in order to help others learn the applications of lasers in gynecologic surgery.

CONTENTS

LASERS IN GYNECOLOGY

Part One

THE BASICS

1

History of the Laser

Jose E. Torres

The theoretical basis for the development of light amplification by the stimulated emission of radiation, or *laser,* as it is known by its acronym, can be traced back to the early years of this century.

In 1900, Max Planck[20] proposed a theory that described energy as traveling in discrete packets (later developed as the quantum theory) rather than by wave phenomena. He subsequently predicted that the energy of an oscillator was equal to the frequency of radiation in cycles per second times a constant, which was later calculated to be $6.6262 \times 10(-27)$ erg seconds (Planck's constant).

A few years later, Niels Bohr[5] postulated that atoms had a planetary structure (*i.e.,* a central positive nucleus and a series of shells or orbits) that would be occupied by "planetary" electrons. Electrons having orbits farther away from the proton would have higher energy states while those closer would have lower energy states. Thus, when an electron dropped from an outer orbit to an inner orbit (lower energy state), it emitted a photon (Planck's packet) of energy, and if a photon of energy was absorbed, the electron would move to an orbit farther away from the nucleus, corresponding to its new higher energy state.

Based on the work of Planck and Bohr, Albert Einstein[7] developed the concepts of absorption, spontaneous emission, and stimulated emission of energy that would serve as the basis for the development of the laser.

In 1954, Gordon and co-workers[12] developed the fundamental concept of population inversion necessary to sustain stimulated emission of energy. They were able to force a beam of excited (higher energy state) molecules to emit a photon of energy of the same (coherence) frequency (wavelength). By continuing to inject the beam of excited molecules into the cavity (resonator), they were able to achieve amplification of a coherent wavelength produced by the stimulated emission of radiation, or as they named the process, microwave amplification by stimulated emission of radiation, also known by its acronym, *maser.*

Shortly thereafter, Schawlow and Townes[22] outlined the principles for the development of a maser in the optical region of the electromagnetic spectrum, postulating that by placing two parallel flat mirrors at either end of a resonator (optical) cavity, amplification of the coherent radiation would be achieved. In 1960, Maiman[17] announced the development of the first working model of an optical maser (laser) using the stimulated emission of radiation by a ruby crystal generating a beam of light with a wavelength of 0.69 μm. The duration of this beam of light was only of the order of milliseconds, and therefore the beam could only be generated in a pulsed mode. After Maiman's announcement, a flurry of activity ensued to find other materials that would be able to generate laser light and produce it in a continuous form, not just in pulses.[21]

There followed in rapid succession publications by Javan and associates[14] on the helium–neon laser, Snitzer[23] and Johnson and colleagues[15] on the neodymium ion laser, Patel[18] on the CO_2 laser, and Gordon and co-workers[11] on the argon laser. Thus, the lasers that are currently used in surgery had been described by 1964. However, because much of the early laser research was developed for use in the communications industry, several years elapsed before laser delivery systems were developed for medical use.[8]

The first lasers to be evaluated in medicine were the ruby (0.69-μm wavelength) and the neodymium (1.06-μm wavelength) lasers, which have very small absorption coefficients in nonpigmented tissues. Therefore, in order to destroy experimental tumors using lasers of these wavelengths, it became necessary to develop and deliver to the tumors very high energies at very high power densities. The interaction of such high power densities of these wavelengths with tissues led to mechanical tissue disruption and cavitation at some distance from the point of impact. Additionally, when laser light of these wavelengths was shot into experimental tumors, it was discovered that the mechanical tissue disruption caused viable tumor cells to be scattered into adjacent tissue and the environment near the impact site. These findings quickly stopped further investigations into the use of lasers for treatment of neoplasias. However, the very poor absorption of laser energy of these wavelengths by water and the excellent absorption by pigments quickly led to the investigation of the role of the ruby and argon lasers in ophthalmology. These two lasers were found to effect photocoagulation and have become important surgical tools for ophthalmologists.

Yahr and Strully,[26] working in Polanyi's laboratory at the American Optical Corporation, used a focused CO_2 laser beam on a laboratory animal and discovered that the CO_2 laser had surgical potential. In subsequent experiments, they determined the hemostatic properties of the CO_2 laser as well. This exciting discovery led Stellar and colleagues[23] to develop a CO_2 laser system for use in surgery. An articulated arm was subsequently developed to deliver the laser beam, as well as a hand piece with a lens in order to focus the beam. With the development of this free-hand delivery system of the CO_2 laser beam, surgical research by Gonzalez and associates,[10] at the University of Minnesota, revealed the ability of the beam to vaporize superficial tissue without causing deeper damage (as had been encountered with the ruby laser) and also demonstrated the hemostatic action of the CO_2 laser in tissue.

Other delivery systems were researched by Bredemeier.* These allowed for the development of endoscopic laser surgery and microscopic laser surgery with the use of his micromanipulator.

Jako,[13] after extensive CO_2 laser animal research, along with Strong[24] published the first clinical application of the CO_2 laser by reporting his experience in laryngeal surgery using this new modality.

The initial use of the CO_2 laser in gynecology was for ablating cervical erosions, reported by Kaplan and colleagues,[16] in Israel. Bellina,[3] in New Orleans, used the CO_2 laser to eradicate cervical intraepithelial neoplasia.

The first generation of CO_2 laser delivery systems had fixed focal distances[19]; thus, in order to decrease the power density, one had to defocus the beam by moving the delivery system away from the target tissue. This technique worked well when using the hand-held piece but was inadequate when using delivery systems attached to an operating microscope or colposcope, as defocusing the laser beam also caused the viewing optics to be out of focus. A major step forward in the field of microsurgery was the development of a defocusing mechanism for the laser beam that was independent of the optical lens. This device enabled gynecological laser surgeons to visualize the target tissue at all times and allowed them the ability to rapidly change the spot diameter of the laser beam and, thus, the power density delivered to the target tissue.

Experience was gained using the CO_2 laser in the lower genital tract. Attention was then directed to its use in the abdomen.[2,4] As noted in other chapters in this book, much progress and success have been achieved with the CO_2, Nd:YAG, argon, and KTP lasers in the management of infertility and endometriosis using open laparotomy or laparoscopy techniques. The need to decrease thermal damage for tubal surgery led to the development of superpulsing delivery systems, which also enable surgeons to perform vulvar surgery and prevent deep dermal destruction that might necessitate the use of skin grafts.[23]

Although the CO_2 laser has been the workhorse of gynecological laser surgery, exciting work published by Goldrath and colleagues,[9] who used a Nd:YAG laser fiber delivered through a hysteroscope, has opened new vistas in gynecological laser surgery.

As a gynecological oncologist, the author is excited about the future use of lasers for the exploration and extension of the work by Dougherty[6] and extended by R. Lobraico (personal communication, 1987) using photoradiation therapy. The possibility of using this form of laser surgery to treat disseminated ovarian carcinoma without damaging adjacent normal tissue is within our grasp.

We have just begun to investigate the potential applications of lasers in gynecology, and the contributors to other chapters in this book will enlarge on these possibilities. Sophisticated delivery systems, fiberoptics to permit the use of increasing numbers of wavelengths, and tumor-specific dyes that absorb selected wavelengths all have been developed since Schawlow and Townes introduced the first optical maser (laser) more than 30 years ago.

---

* *Bredemeier HC: Laser accessory for surgical application—U.S. Patent No. 3,659,613 (1972). Stereo laser endoscope—Patent Pending (1973).*

REFERENCES

1. Andrews AH, Polanyi TG (eds): Microscopic and Endoscopic Surgery with the CO_2 Laser. Littleton, John Wright PSG, 1982
2. Baggish MS (ed): Basic and Advanced Laser Surgery in Gynecology. Norwalk, Appleton-Century-Crofts, 1985
3. Bellina JH: Gynecology and the laser. Contemporary Obstetrics and Gynecology 4:24, 1974
4. Bellina JH, Bandieramonte G: Principles and Practice of Gynecologic Laser Surgery. New York, Plenum Publishing, 1984
5. Bohr N: On the constitution of atoms and molecules. Philosophical Magazine 26:476, 1913
6. Dougherty TJ: An overview of the status of photoradiation therapy. Clayton Foundation Symposium on Porphyrin Localization and Treatment of Tumors. Santa Barbara, 1983
7. Einstein A: Quantum Theorie der Strahlung. Physikalische Zeitschrift 18:121, 1917
8. Goldman L, Rockwell RJ Jr: Lasers in Medicine. New York, Gordon and Breach Science Publishers, 1971
9. Goldrath MH, Fuller TA, Segal S: Laser photovaporization of the endometrium for the treatment of menorrhagia. Am J Obstet Gynecol 140:14, 1981
10. Gonzalez R, Edlich RF, Bredemeier HC et al: Rapid control of massive hepatic hemorrhages by laser radiation. Surg Gynecol Obstet 131:198, 1970
11. Gordon EI, Labuda EF, Bridges WB: Continuous visible laser action in singly ionized argon, krypton and xenon. Applied Physics Letters 4:178, 1964
12. Gordon JP, Zeiger HJ, Townes CH: Molecular microwave oscillator and new hyperfine structure in the microwave spectrum of NH3. Physical Review 95:282, 1954
13. Jako GJ: Laser surgery of the vocal cords. An experimental study with CO_2 laser on dogs. Laryngoscope 82:2204, 1971
14. Javan A, Bennett WB Jr, Herriott TR: Population inversion and continuous optical maser oscillation in a gas discharge containing a He–Ne mixture. Physical Review Letters 6:106, 1961
15. Johnson LF, Boyd GD, Nassau K: Continuous operation of the CaWO4: Trivalent neodymium optical maser at room temperature. J Opt Soc Am 52:608, 1962
16. Kaplan I, Goldman J, Ger R: The treatment of erosions of the uterine cervix by means of the CO_2 laser. Obstet Gynecol 41:795, 1973
17. Maiman TH: Stimulated optical radiation in ruby. Nature 187:493, 1960
18. Patel CKN: Continuous wave laser action on vibrational rotational transitions of CO_2. Physical Review 136:1187, 1964
19. Patel CKN: High power carbon dioxide lasers. Sci Am 219:22, 1968
20. Planck M: Uber eine Verbesserung der Wien'schen Spektralgleichung. Verhand lungen der Deutschen Physilealischen gesellschaft 2:202, 1900
21. Schawlow AL: Advances in optical masers. Sci Am 209:34, 1963
22. Schawlow AL, Townes CH: Infrared and optical masers. Physical Review 112:1940, 1958
23. Snitzer E: Optical maser action of Nd3+ in crown glass. Physical Review Letters 7:444, 1961
24. Stellar S, Polanyi TG, Bredemeier HC: Lasers in surgery. In Wolbarsht M (ed): Laser Applications in Medicine and Biology, Vol 2. New York, Plenum Publishing,
25. Strong MS, Jako GJ: Laser surgery in the larynx, early clinical experience with continuous CO_2 laser. Am Otol Rhinol Laryngol 81:791, 1972
26. Yahr WZ, Strully KJ: Blood vessel anastomosis by laser and other biomedical applications. Journal of the Association for the Advancement of Medical Instrumentation 1:28, 1966

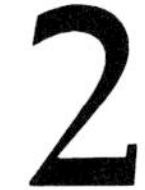# Basic Laser Physics
for the Gynecologist

Gregory T. Absten

The applications of lasers in medicine have expanded prolifically in the past several years. As surgical instruments, lasers rely primarily on their precise heating effect on tissue to cut, vaporize, or coagulate.

An introduction to biophysical principles of laser use enables physicians to employ lasers in various surgical procedures safely and effectively once the basic mechanisms of action are understood. The laser is an instrument—not a technique.

LIGHT

". . . and God said: 'Let there be light' "

In the beginning, everything existed as energy, which then condensed into solid matter to make up our universe. Everything is energy in one form or another, and light may be the purest form of energy. Light exhibits properties of both waves and particles (photons). In order to better understand the electromagnetic spectrum and unique characteristics of lasers, we can look at the wave characteristics of light.

Light is an electromagnetic wave like radio waves, but with a much shorter wavelength (Fig. 2–1). Our eyes are capable of sensing electromagnetic waves within only a short range of the spectrum, from about 385 to 760 nm. Like water waves, light waves exhibit characteristic amplitude, wavelength, frequency, and velocity.

Wavelength of lasers is important to us because it describes the color of light that the laser emits, such as green, red, or infrared. The special safety glasses required when using some lasers are also labeled according to the wavelengths of

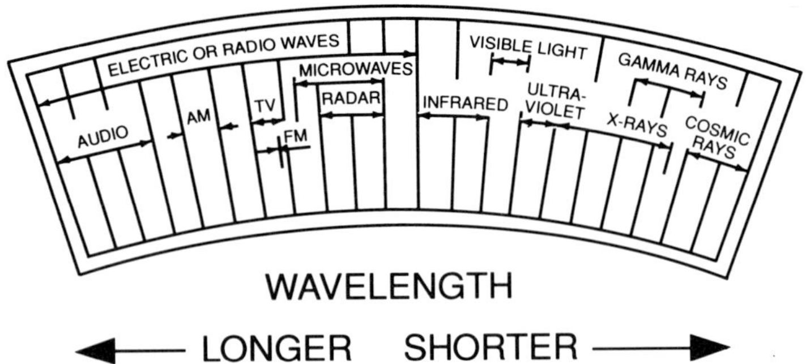

FIGURE 2–1. Light waves consist of medium to shorter wavelengths of the electromagnetic spectrum. They consist of infrared, visible, and ultraviolet light.

protection offered. Therefore, it is important for operators to know the wavelength of each laser. Shorter wavelengths are found toward the blue end of the spectrum and longer wavelengths toward the red.

Waves are said to be in *phase* when the peaks and troughs of opposing wave patterns correspond. They are out of phase when the peak of one wave corresponds to the trough of another, resulting in a diminished amplitude where they meet—a "flat spot" in the wave pattern (Fig. 2–2).

The *velocity* of a wave describes how rapidly it travels. The velocity of light is constant, slightly greater than 186,000 miles per second. Nothing travels faster than light.

Because the velocity (speed) of a light wave is constant, when wavelengths are shorter, more waves pass a point in a given period of time. The *frequency* of the wave

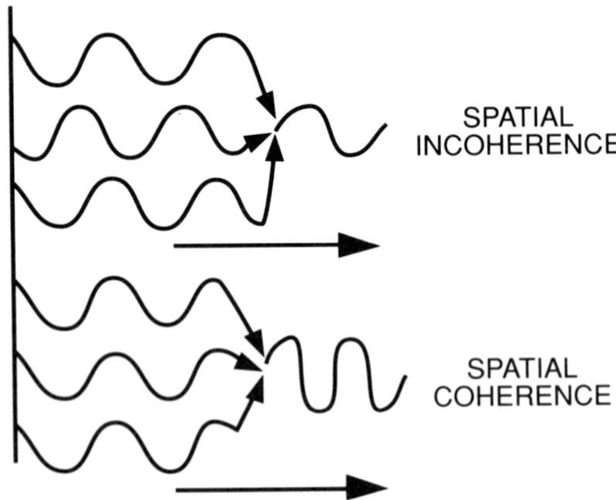

FIGURE 2–2. Spatial incoherence occurs when light waves are out of phase resulting in diminished amplitude. In phase light waves, spatial coherence results in amplification of amplitude.

is thus described. The relationship between wavelength (color) and frequency is, therefore, inverse—the higher the frequency, the shorter the wavelength. The wavelength of a laser is usually referred to (in nanometers, one billionth of a meter) rather than the laser's frequency.

One specific type of medical laser is *frequency doubled, (i.e.,* the KTP laser), a concept that will be discussed at greater length later. Because of the inverse relationship between frequency and wavelength, if the frequency is doubled, the wavelength must be halved. With the KTP laser, the wavelength of 1064 nm (near-infrared) Nd : YAG laser is halved to 532 nm (green).

The *amplitude* of a light wave is much like that of a water wave in that it determines the amount of power contained in the wave. For example, a 10-foot wave in the surf is obviously more powerful than a 3-foot wave on the beach. With light, power defines its brightness. A 100-watt light bulb is brighter than a 40-watt one. The power of a laser is set by the user as the number of watts delivered. Watts are the rate, or speed, of energy delivery—not the total energy delivered. These energy concepts are critical for optimal use of a laser and will be discussed further later.

LASER

Laser light differs from ordinary light in somewhat the same way that music differs from noise. Both are sounds, but the musical sounds are more organized than noise. Laser light is made up of the same basic particles of light (photons) as ordinary light, but the wave patterns of the photons in laser light exhibit a much higher degree of organization.

Stimulated emission describes the mechanism by which laser light is emitted from matter. Radiation in this context only means light and not ionizing radiation commonly associated with x-rays. A radiant body shines, or emits light. Ordinary light is emitted through the process of spontaneous emission.

Laser is a quality of light rather than the machine that emits it. Lasers may emit any color, high or low power, and may be virtually any size from a transistor to a 12-story-high chemical laser, which may one day orbit the earth.

LASER VERSUS ORDINARY LIGHT EMISSION

Everything that can be seen, felt, or touched—all physical matter—is basically electronic in nature. Light is emitted as an energy by-product of these electronic forces within matter. Laser light is more highly organized than regular light. Light may be emitted anytime an electric charge is accelerated or deflected. The first step in emission of a laser, or any other light source, is to energize and excite the medium that emits the light. With lasers this is called pumping the medium.

The emission of light may be illustrated in the simplified case of an atom. Electrons in the atom occupy certain discrete energy levels or orbits and are not free to occupy states between these levels. When the energy level of this type of system is changed, the electrons move up or down to new orbital levels in order to accommodate the energy surplus or deficit. When energy is added, the transition is upward; when energy is emitted, the change is downward.

When an atom or molecule absorbs energy and moves to a higher electron orbit, it almost immediately falls to the previous resting orbital level and emits excess energy in the process. With light, the surplus energy is emitted as a photon. The energy of the photon determines its color (by wavelength) and is simply the difference in energy levels between the higher and lower orbital levels. The frequency of the light (and hence its wavelength) may be determined by the equation n = TE/h, where h is Planck's constant, equal to $6.62 \times 10(-34)$ joule-seconds, and TE equals the transition energy between the orbital levels. In effect, this makes atoms and molecules electronic instruments that may be tuned to play certain colors of light on demand.

In a conventional light source, many atoms or molecules may spontaneously undergo orbital decay randomly. Many energy transitions occur, and the resulting white light (from multiple colors) is emitted out of phase and in all directions. As when taking the lid off a popcorn popper, the "kernels" of light come flying out in all directions at different times. This is ordinary incoherent light produced through *spontaneous emission* (Fig. 2–3A).

In a laser, excitation of the medium causes more atoms to exist in the excited state than in the resting state. This is called *population inversion* and is a requirement for lasing to occur. Media that have longer spontaneous lifetimes (electrons stay excited longer) are more suitable as continuous-wave lasers like carbon dioxide (CO_2) and argon. Those whose spontaneous lifetimes are very short tend to be high-frequency pulsed lasers like excimers or gold vapor lasers.

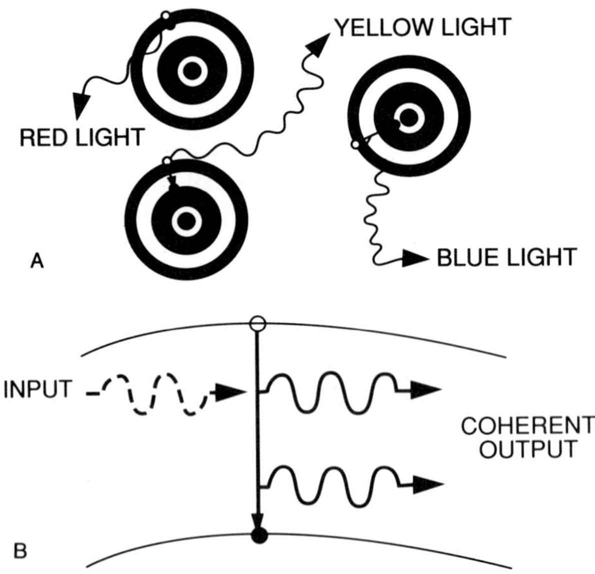

FIGURE 2–3. (*A*) Ordinary incoherent white light is produced from spontaneous emission. (*B*) Laser light is produced by synchronized coherent light.

Stimulated emission of light is the mechanism that makes laser light unique. As one atom in an excited medium spontaneously emits a photon of the appropriate wavelength, it travels down the laser tube, further stimulating each atom in its path to emit an additional photon of identical wavelength (color) traveling in the same direction. These ghostlike particles of light merge to travel together in time and space. This synchronization of direction, color, and waves results in a *coherent* wave output (Fig. 2–3B).

Every substance has the theoretical potential to emit light and therefore to be made into a laser. Different materials emit characteristic colors and have inherent tendencies to emit in either rapid bursts (pulsed systems) or steady output (continuous wave) configurations. The laser is usually named after the medium used to emit the light (Fig. 2–4). Various colors, power outputs, and pulsing characteristics are used for different surgical tasks.

The laser tube is designed to amplify the output from this process of stimulated emission. Facing mirrors are situated at each end of the laser tube, causing the waves of emitted light to be reflected back and forth through the laser medium situated between them. Each wave of light stimulates additional atoms in the laser medium, resulting in increased amplitude (power and brightness) of the light. The front mirror is only partially reflective to allow a small percentage of the light to leak out the end. This emitted light is the laser beam.

LASERS — LIGHT PRODUCED		
CARBON DIOXIDE	INFRARED	10600 nm
ARGON	BLUE GREEN	488 nm 515 nm
Nd:YAG	NEAR - INFRARED NEAR - INFRARED	1064 nm 1318 nm
KTP (POTASSIUM TITANYL PHOSPHATE)	GREEN	532 nm
KRYPTON	RED YELLOW GREEN	647 nm 568 nm 531 nm
RUBY	DEEP RED	694 nm
HELIUM NEON	RED	632 nm
GOLD VAPOR	RED	632 nm
COPPER VAPOR	GREEN YELLOW	510 nm 578 nm
DYE LASER	VARIABLE WITH DYES	
	RED YELLOW YELLOW GREEN	632 nm 577 nm 585 nm 504 nm
ERBIUM: YAG	MID-INFRARED	2930 nm
HOLMIUM: YAG	MID-INFRARED	2060 nm
EXCIMERS: ArF KrCl KrF XeCl XeF	ULTRAVIOLET	 193 nm 222 nm 248 nm 308 nm 351 nm

FIGURE 2–4. Different colors are produced by different lasers, named after the medium used to emit the light.

When the beam is emitted, it is delivered through an articulated arm or a flexible fiber. The articulated arms are hollow tubes that transmit the beam. Knuckles at joints contain mirrors to allow some degree of mobility for these small robotlike arms. CO_2 lasers are delivered by these arms because the wavelength will not pass through conventional fibers. Flexible fibers are used with the argon, Nd:YAG, and KTP lasers, thus facilitating endoscopic procedures.

UNIQUE QUALITIES OF LASER LIGHT

Laser light is different from ordinary light because it is *coherent, collimated, and monochromatic.* Not all of these characteristics are important for the current surgical applications of lasers. However, a basic understanding of these properties enables one to better understand developing diagnostic and interventional applications of lasers (see Fig. 2–4).

Coherence of laser light refers to the synchronization and phasing of the wave patterns of light. Many other non-laser light sources are coherent, but only for extremely short distances; the laser retains its coherence over longer distances. This property is not very important for current surgical applications that rely on heating of tissues. However, coherence does add mathematical order to the light and allows it to be used as a sensing and diagnostic probe. Combined with the pure colors, coherence allows the creation of three-dimensional holograms. Endoscopic holography allows pathology to be determined with no actual tissue ever being taken. Fibers and light probes may be used to measure temperature, pressure, sound, and blood flow.

Monochromaticity describes the ability of the laser to emit pure, narrow bandwidth colors of light. Many lasers produce multiple colors of light, such as argon and krypton, which together emit greens, blues, oranges, yellows, and reds. Each laser is still considered monochromatic because the individual color is very pure, separated distinctly from neighboring colors. This is unlike multichromatic light sources such as light bulbs, which emit a broad spectrum of colors with continuous overlap resulting in white light.

The pure color aspect of the laser is only marginally important in the surgical techniques of cutting, vaporizing, or coagulating, because it is heat that determines the surgical effect. Color indirectly affects heat production because the color of the beam and of the tissue determines the amount of light absorbed and, therefore, heat generation. There is considerable overlap in the surgical applications of many lasers because power, intensities, and exposure may be manipulated to easily overwhelm the color selectivity effect on absorption. Nevertheless, many current and developing applications rely on the color specificity of certain lasers to affect the target tissue while sparing adjacent normal tissues of different colors—for example, dye laser applications in both ophthalmology and dermatology. Argon and KTP lasers may also be used as color-selective photocoagulators for endometrial implants in gynecology.

Photodynamic therapy is a developing medical area of photopharmacology that uses the pure colors of laser light in combination with light-sensitive drugs. Its most common current use is for detection and treatment of cancers as an adjunct to radiation therapy, chemotherapy, or surgery. A patient is given a systemic injection of the light-sensitizing drug about 3 days before a procedure. All cells usually take up the drug initially, but only the abnormal target cells retain it. By itself the drug is latent, but when excited by various colors of light (which may be provided by laser), the drug either causes the cancer cells to fluoresce as a diagnostic aid or to die from toxic products from intracellular photochemistry, depending on the colors and intensities of light. Adjacent healthy cells are unharmed, and there is no upper limit of allowable dosage. The laser light is not hot and causes no thermal effects. It is simply used as a bright, monochromatic light source to initiate photochemistry within the cells.

Collimation of the laser beam is the most important characteristic for current conventional surgical applications. Collimation means that the laser beam stays together as a tight beam of parallel light and does not appreciably diverge as it travels from its source. Because most laser surgical applications rely on heat generation, collimation becomes critical for two reasons.

First of all, collimation retains the power of the beam all along its path (which is not true for divergent light sources, such as light bulbs). These divergent sources lose their power (intensity) with the square of the distance from the source. Collimation with the laser means that almost all of the power generated within the head of the laser is available to the delivery system or in the surgical field.

Second, collimation allows the beam to be focused to very small spots. Focusing intensifies the effects of the beam in much the same way that a magnifying glass may be used to focus sunlight and burn objects. This ability to intensify the brightness (later referred to as power density) of the beam is the single most important aspect of a laser for surgical use. The ability to focus the incident power into small spots also allows transmission of virtually all the generated power through narrow fibers to remote endoscopic locations by such lasers as the argon, KTP, and Nd:YAG.

ENERGY CONCEPTS

Power of a laser is defined as the rate of energy delivery and is measured in *watts*. One watt equals 1 joule per second. Power is sometimes mistakenly thought to relate to eye–hand coordination and thus to controllability of the rate of tissue vaporization.

Surgical control, coordination, and tissue effects are more directly related to *power density,* or irradiance. This is the single most important factor in the safe, effective use of any laser. Power density describes how the power output of the beam is concentrated on the tissue. The same amount of power set on the machine has very little effect when spread over a large surface area and, conversely, an intense effect when concentrated within small spot diameters.

Power density is the combined effect of both power in watts and spot size, as follows:

$$\text{Power density (watts/cm}_2) = \frac{\text{watts}}{\text{spot size } (\pi r^2)}$$

$$r = \text{radius of spot in centimeters}$$

Power density may be estimated if desired using a rougher, but quicker calculation, as follows:

$$\frac{\text{Watts}}{\text{D}^2}$$

$$\text{D} = \text{diameter in centimeters}$$

Laser vaporization is similar to using a paintbrush to paint tissue. One can effectively change the size of the paintbrush (spot size) without changing the required eye-hand coordination by varying the power. The larger the spot, the greater the power required to maintain the same power density.

For example:

$$1900 \text{ watts/cm}^2 = \frac{10 \text{ watts}}{0.6\text{-mm spot}} \quad \text{or} \quad \frac{60 \text{ watts}}{2.0\text{-mm spot}}$$

Larger spots are usually desirable when vaporizing (debulking) tissue. Laser incision of tissues requires using the smallest spot possible. Because the spot size is fixed at the smallest setting, power in watts directly controls the speed and required coordination for the incision. In this case, laser power is similar to the accelerator on a car; the higher the power, the quicker the incision. In the case of vaporizations, because of a variable spot size, power is not the direct determinant of the rate of vaporization.

Most laparoscope couplers for CO_2 lasers emit a fixed spot size. The lack of a variable spot size in the coupler also equates power with speed and coordination.

Focusing hand pieces allow the beam to converge to a focal point and then defocus. Varying the distance from the end of the hand piece to the tissue changes the incident spot size and hence power density.

Laser micromanipulators attached to microscopes usually incorporate a defocusing device that, when turned, changes the spot size and thus the power density.

Fibers (used on argon, KTP, and Nd:YAG lasers) allow the beam to diverge at a 10- to 15-degree angle once it is emitted from the tip of the naked fiber so that the beam is no longer collimated (Fig. 2–5). This divergence results in the smallest spot occurring at the tip of the fiber and continuously enlarging as the fiber tip is moved away from the target, as when the nozzle of a garden hose is set to spray. The power density therefore decreases exponentially with the distance from the tip. Close to the tip one may incise, a little farther away vaporize, and back farther coagulate tissue protein. All of these tissue effects may be observed within about an inch of the fiber tip.

The total energy within the beam is expressed in joules. It is obvious that the longer the beam is applied at any given power, the greater will be the delivered energy:

$$\text{Energy (joules)} = \text{power (watts)} \times \text{time (seconds)}$$

Joules may quantitate the total dosage of delivered light; it does not delineate laser intensity as does power density. A large total energy of light delivered over a

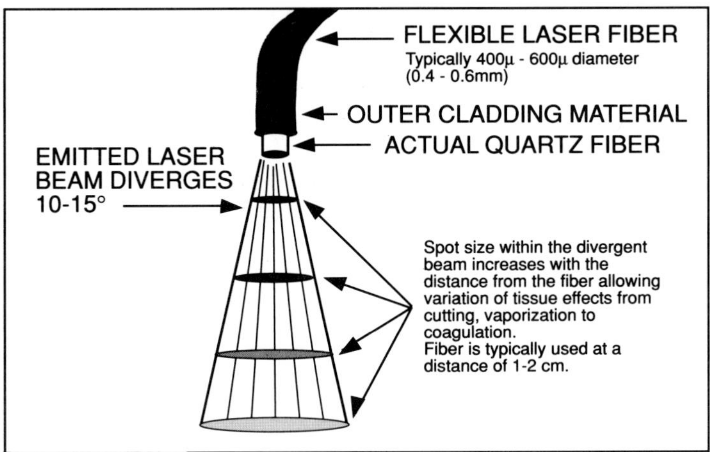

FIGURE 2–5. Loss of collimation occurs as the laser beam diverges at a 10 to 15 degree angle from the quartz fiber. Thus, the spot size progressively enlarges the further the laser travels from the fiber tip.

very large surface area may have little tissue effect. Conversely, the same amount of total energy applied to a small area may produce intense tissue effects. This is the concept of fluence.

Fluence combines the concepts of power density and total energy; it is expressed in joules/cm^2. The greater the fluence, the more rapid is the tissue effect, whereas the thermal effect is confined to the immediate target. The lower the fluence, the slower the effect while allowing thermal tissue injury to occur in a wider zone around the immediate target. Limiting the exposure time of any laser in any one spot is a learned technique critical to maintaining thermal precision.

Most laser surgery is a visual exercise. One need not be overwhelmed by all the laser physics calculations, because in reality the adjustment of laser parameters is all relative. Once the appropriate hands-on training is obtained, after acquiring an understanding of the underlying laser surgery principles, a laser surgeon can easily recognize the desired tissue effects and change settings as needed.

PRINCIPLES OF SURGICAL TISSUE EFFECTS

Surgical lasers rely primarily on thermal effects in tissue to cause incisions, vaporization, or coagulation. At sufficiently high power densities, phenomena begin to occur that are not simple linear extrapolations of thermal effects. These are conveniently referred to as nonlinear laser effects, which are primarily a spark and sonic "snap" that may be created with high-intensity light. In medicine, these effects are used in ophthalmology and urology but do not really apply to gynecological laser use. Our discussion is therefore limited to the usual linear thermal effects of the laser.

HEAT IS HEAT—HOT IS HOT

Cutting, vaporizing, and coagulating tissue all are caused by heating the tissue. Figure 2–6 describes the effects on soft tissue as the temperature increases. Lasers offer advantages over other heat sources because of precision, surgical access, or selectivity. One unique characteristic of lasers while vaporizing is their ability to mold and sculpt tissue as desired. Although frequently advantageous, lasers are not always the only surgical alternative to cutting or coagulating tissue. If tissue temperatures significantly exceed the boiling point of water, at the point of impact, tissue explodes and emits steam and particles. At a small point, an incision is created; at larger spots, tissue debulking occurs. At lower temperatures, protein coagulation and desiccation may occur. It is helpful to quickly review the mechanisms of tissue heating employed by both laser and electrosurgery.

Light heats tissue indirectly through absorption. When light is absorbed in tissue, its energy is converted into heat, much the same way that microwave vibrations in water generate heat when food is heated in a microwave oven. An induced heating effect results. Heat is heat, and the various wavelengths and delivery techniques determine how well this heat may be localized. Absorptive heating is commonly noted when one leaves a car with black leather seats sitting in a hot parking lot all day. Sunlight is highly absorbed by the dark material, converting the light into heat.

Electrosurgical instruments (bipolar and monopolar) also generate heat in tissue indirectly through resistive heating of the tissue (Fig. 2–7). Whenever an electrical current meets resistance, heat is generated as a by-product. The filament in a light bulb resists the flow of current and consequently becomes hot and radiates light. Tissue acts as a resistor to the flow of current from the electrosurgical generator and becomes hot in the process through ohmic heating (heat generated by resistance). The results are the same. Heat is heat. Tissue is vaporized, desiccated, or coagulated. Although needle-point cautery provides a high degree of precision through electrical stimulation, a questionable zone of damage results in surrounding sensitive areas.

The term *electrocautery* has been used very loosely. Unlike electrosurgery, in which electrical current heats tissue through resistive heating, true electrocautery involves no current passing through tissue. Instead, the electrical current is confined to the surgical element generating high temperatures at the tip. This is a true hot cautery, and it causes tissue vaporization or desiccation through the direct application of a hot element. Heat is still heat, whether directly applied or induced.

	Visual Change	Biological Change
100°C	———————— SMOKE PLUME	VAPORIZATION, CARBONIZATION
90-100°C	———— PUCKERING ——	DRYING
65-90°C	—— WHITE/GREY ————	PROTEIN DENATURIZATION
60-65°C	— BLANCHING ————————	COAGULATION
37-60°C	NONE ————————————	WARMING, WELDING

FIGURE 2–6. Different soft tissue effects occur as the laser energy is absorbed and the tissue is heated.

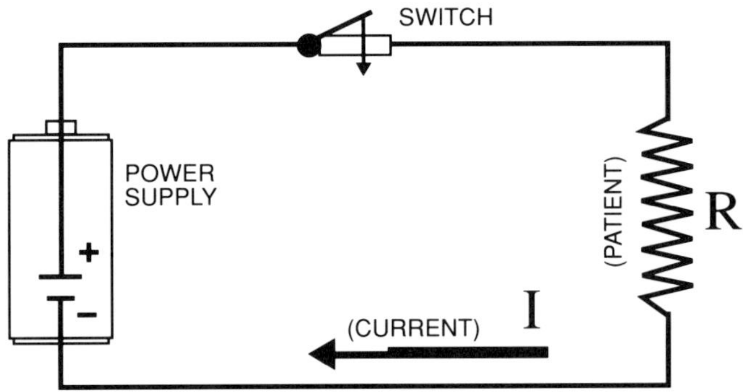

FIGURE 2–7. Tissue heating occurs as heat is generated from electrosurgical instruments due to tissue resistance to the electrical current.

Some laser delivery systems have attached elements to the fiber tips, which serve as hot tips because they are able to generate and sustain higher temperatures more quickly. This method has been used by vascular surgeons to recanalize vessels. When the laser is fired directly into the metal tip, it becomes very hot and causes tissue vaporization on contact. With this system, the laser is simply used as an energy source to produce the high temperatures of the metal probe.

Another laser system in gynecology uses a sapphire tip attached to the fiber of the Nd:YAG laser. Although any fiberoptic laser could be used with these probes, they have been developed specifically for use with Nd:YAG lasers. The predominant mechanism of action of these probes is direct heating of the sapphire tip.

Sapphire tips are used laparoscopically to enhance the fine cutting and vaporization effects of the Nd:YAG laser, which would otherwise cause more diffuse tissue coagulation. These probes must be held in contact with tissue, and they burn up if fired for more than a few seconds off tissue. Various sizes and shapes of probes are available to cause chiseling, cutting, vaporization, and coagulation when using very low power settings of the Nd:YAG laser.

Some controversy exists about whether the tissue effects are due to pure heating of the element or to high power density laser light exiting the tip of the probes. Several characteristics of the sapphire tips seem to point to the direct heating effect and are briefly described here:

1. A lag time exists between the beginning of lasing and the onset of tissue effects. This allows for the heat to build up in the probe.
2. "Virgin," clean probes must develop a slight blackening or discoloration of the material before the probe will work. The high power density theory would point to a better effect with a clean probe (like a clean lens). The discoloration allows better absorption of the light by the probe and better internal heat generation. Dirty lenses absorb energy and become hot.
3. The lateral extent of tissue coagulation is not determined by the power of the laser. Power determines only how quickly the probe

works. Direct heating of the element provides an explanation for both of these characteristics.

4. Probes burn up quickly when they are not in contact with tissue when fired. The excess heat generated has no tissue heat sink to dissipate it and melts as a consequence.
5. Cutting occurs more quickly if the laser continues to function while the probe is momentarily lifted for another pass of the incision. On contact, the rate of cutting is slightly higher than after its temperature stabilizes in the tissue.
6. The probes may actually be seen to glow with heat as they are being used. The Nd:YAG light is invisible.
7. A change in power and time, maintaining total energy density, does not produce the same tissue effects. Fifty watts at 0.1 second produces no effect, whereas 5 watts for 1 second will produce an effect. This indicates the lag time required for the probe to build up heat. (Note: Probes are not normally intended for use at powers as high as 50 watts. Consult the manufacturer.)
8. A fluid drip, cooling off the fiber, dampens the rate at which the probes work. Fluid acts as a heat sink on the hot sapphire probe.

Regardless of the mechanism of action, the results are the same. Sapphire tips greatly expand the conventional uses of the Nd:YAG laser by enabling fine cutting and tissue vaporization in addition to the deep coagulation achieved with the Nd:YAG laser light through a naked fiber.

LASER-TISSUE EFFECTS

The wavelength (color) of the laser is important only in determining how efficiently the transformation of light into heat energy occurs by absorption. In order for the light to generate heat, it must be absorbed. If it is reflected from or transmitted through tissue, little heating occurs. Scattering results in absorption over a larger volume of tissue so that the heating effects are more diffuse.

By combining effects, specific lasers may be exploited to obtain highly selective results. An argon or KTP laser may be shined on a small endometrial implant located just beneath the rather transparent peritoneum. At appropriate power settings, the laser light shines through the peritoneal membrane with no damage (similar to light shining through a window pane) and is absorbed by the dark implant below.

Figure 2–8 compares the relative effects of tissue absorption of the CO_2, argon (or KTP), and Nd:YAG lasers. These effects may blend together by changing power, power densities, pulsing characteristics, and delivery systems.

Several parameters may be controlled to facilitate delivery of laser energy to tissue. These include power (watts), total energy delivered (watts and time), power density (varying with the size of spot used to intensify the light), the color of the light, and the color and vascularity of the tissue.

Understanding how to control these laser parameters is important. Use of a magnifying glass to focus sunlight and create a burn is a good analogy. The brighter

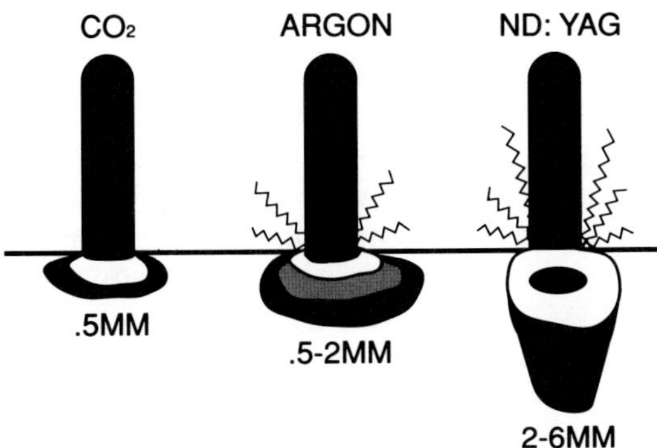

FIGURE 2–8. Unique tissue effects occur following application of CO_2, Argon, and Nd : YAG laser energy due to different tissue absorption of each wavelength.

the sunlight (power), the more it burns. The smaller the spot created by the glass (power density), the hotter it burns. The longer the sun is focused in one place (total energy), the more extensively it burns. The wetter the object that is to be burned (vascularity), the longer it takes to create the same effect. A surgeon has control over a combination of three parameters—power, time, and spot size—to create the desired effect.

The CO_2 laser wavelength (10,600 nm) is the most highly absorbed by water, and therefore by soft tissue, and causes the most intense heating effects by cutting and vaporizing. Hemostasis is a by-product of the heat of vaporization because it seals small vessels, but it is not bloodless. Correct technique in adjusting for the appropriate scoop-shaped geometry of the impact crater is one of the best ways to assure reasonable hemostasis. The CO_2 laser is excellent when debulking tissue in a no-touch, atraumatic, hemostatic, precise fashion—particularly in conjunction with a colposcope or microscope. Lateral heat damage from the side of the incision or crater, when used properly, may be limited to 0.5 mm or less. The CO_2 laser may be used with a hand piece, laparoscope, or microscope, but the beam is not transmitted through conventional fibers. The laser energy also is not transmitted through blood or water (which are excellent backstops) so that it may *not* be used through solutions, such as in operative hysteroscopy. Medical CO_2 laser units are available from 20 to 100 watts of power. The higher the power one can afford the better, but 50 to 60 watts is sufficient for almost all applications.

Waveguide delivery systems are available now for CO_2 laser laparoscopy. Without the waveguides, the CO_2 laser beam must be introduced through a special laser laparoscope by a laser coupler cube that attaches to the laparoscope. The beam is then directed straight through the operating channel of the scope in a line-of-sight fashion. This is satisfactory, but problems reoccur with aligning the beam through the channel. Waveguides are hollow, slender tubes that may be passed through the operating channel of any laparoscope. The laser beam is focused into this tube and, by glancing off the inner reflective lining, is directed out the distal end. This technique reduces the alignment problems of rigid coupler cubes and allows the output from the waveguide to be closely directed to the target. Although these waveguides are helpful for laser laparoscopy, because they are rigid, they are not true CO_2 laser fibers.

There are three classic physics mistakes to avoid when using the CO_2 lasers. The first mistake is using a higher power density than can be controlled. Lack of control results not from too high a power, but from too small a spot for the power used. The consequences are penetration of tissue or cutting too deeply. Avoid this mistake by starting at low power densities and working up as experience allows—provided that no charring occurs. When making incisions with a fine spot, the power of the laser becomes the speed control.

The second mistake is spending excessive time on tissue as a result of using very low powers, causing significant heat buildup and injury to adjacent tissue. It is avoided by using higher powers or by pulsing, using short pulses. The short pulses avoid the excessive damage from the power while gaining surgical control over the beam.

The third mistake involves repeated lasing over char previously created by the laser. This increases the surface temperatures from just over 100°C for the first pass, to over 1500°C when lasing through the char. On skin this would cause significant heat spread and scarring. Power densities should be sufficient to preclude the buildup of char. Any accumulated char may be wiped away with a moist sponge before lasing the same area. Lasing through char does offer excellent hemostasis because of the high temperature, and in some situations it may be warranted, such as when debulking an isolated vascular tumor or cutting a vascular organ. However, heat damage to adjacent tissue may be substantial, and extensive charring should not be created if preservation of adjacent or underlying tissue is desired.

The blue-green beam of the argon and the green beam of the KTP are used through slender, flexible fibers, as is the Nd:YAG laser. Fiberoptic delivery is a definite asset for laser laparoscopy. The argon and KTP lasers transmit through clear fluid so that copious irrigation may be used. These colored beams of light are absorbed better by red or very dark pigmented tissue such as that found in endometrial implants.

Argon (488 and 515 nm) and KTP (532 nm) lasers are generally considered superficial photocoagulators (0.5 to 2 mm) but will vaporize tissue at sufficient power densities and may be used to cut if the tip of the fiber is drawn along the tissue. This feature makes them versatile laparoscopic tools. No smoke is produced when tissue is photocoagulated, so that visibility is preserved and the pneumoperitoneum is easier to maintain. There are some differences in the absorption of argon and KTP wavelengths by hemoglobin. The argon is also continuous wave, whereas the KTP laser is a high-frequency pulsed system, but for almost all clinical situations the tissue effects between them are indiscernible. Power outputs range from 12 to 16 watts with these units. The low-powered (3 to 5 watts) ophthalmic intraoperative argon lasers are not adequate for gynecological use.

Nd:YAG lasers (1064 nm) are also delivered fiberoptically, and medical units are available from 40 to 100 watts. Again, the higher the power, the better, but about 60 watts is sufficient for almost all gynecological applications. This laser is a solid crystal of yttrium-aluminum-garnet (YAG) that contains a dopant of the rare-earth element of neodymium (Nd), which actually makes the light. Other medical lasers using the YAG crystal to hold various dopants are being developed; these include the erbium (Er) YAG and holmium (Ho) YAG lasers, each with a different wavelength and tissue effect.

A slightly different wavelength of the Nd:YAG laser (1318 nm) called a harmonic of the YAG is being investigated for use in operative tissue fusion (welding). Milliwatt CO_2 lasers have previously been used for this.

When applied through a bare fiber, the Nd:YAG causes deep tissue coagulation because of its high degree of scatter. Protein coagulation of 4 to 6 mm may be accomplished, if so desired. Limiting the delivered energy to about 20 watts for 1 to 3 seconds produces only 1 or 2 mm of coagulation. The Nd:YAG laser is more highly absorbed by dark tissues and may also be transmitted through fluid. Its primary use in gynecology has been for photocoagulation of the endometrium in endometrial ablation as a treatment for unresponsive menorrhagia. For this indication, deep coagulation is desirable. Argon and KTP lasers have also been used for endometrial ablation, but their superficial depths of coagulation may make results suboptimal.

With the advent of the contact sapphire tips, the Nd:YAG laser has gained wider use in operative laparoscopy. Various probe shapes and sizes are available to attach to the fibers to allow for precise cutting, vaporization, or coagulation of tissue without the extensive coagulation damage that may otherwise result after application of the Nd:YAG laser. The thermal use of the probes limits lateral damage to less than 0.5 mm in most instances for cutting and to about 2 mm when vaporizing.

PULSING OF LASER AS A SURGICAL CONTROL TECHNIQUE

As previously discussed, lasers are generally designed to operate in a continuous-wave or high-frequency pulsed configuration. These characteristics are inherent in the active medium used and in the design of the laser, over which the user has no control. The CO_2, argon, and Nd:YAG lasers used in gynecology all operate in the continuous-wave mode. The KTP laser is a high-frequency pulsed system, although to the unaided eye it appears to be a continuous beam. All of these lasers may be controlled with various pulsing techniques that are used as methods of surgical control over the beam, although pulsing usually is applied to the CO_2 laser. The argon, KTP, and Nd:YAG lasers may be placed in a pulsed mode also, but these are all exclusively the gated pulses. Discussion of Q-switching and mode-locking techniques used to create sparks is also omitted because these are not currently applicable to gynecology.

Medical lasers offer a choice of operating modes to include continuous and pulsed modes. Many CO_2 lasers additionally offer a superpulse mode. It is important to remember that these terms such as *pulsing* are used loosely when describing a control setting and often do not fit the correct technical definition.

Continuous wave refers to a steady-state power output from the laser. Most medical laser systems work in this mode, even when set to a pulse of around 0.1 second. This term also sometimes refers to a mode in which the laser beam is emitted for the entire time that the foot pedal is depressed—such as with the KTP laser or a CO_2 laser used in a continuous superpulse. Technically, the latter application is incorrect because a series of true pulses may also be emitted in this manner, but it is a common expression for laser operation and should be noted. The foot pedal control of the laser may be pumped to achieve a pulsing effect, though it will not be as consistent as with the gated pulse.

Gated pulse (Fig. 2–9) is most commonly referred to as simply *pulse*. This feature is merely a timer for a continuous-wave beam and is seen on the four common medical lasers we have discussed. True laser pulses, which are different, may also be emitted in this timed fashion. The differentiating characteristic of a gated pulse is that the peak power output of the pulses is no higher than it would be if the laser were emitted in a continuous fashion.

Most of the CO_2 lasers offer an option for a repeat pulse. This is simply the gated pulse that continues to be emitted at short intervals as long as the foot pedal is depressed. This is a very useful feature on CO_2 lasers, and models that allow varying the speed of the repeat rate are the most versatile.

A true laser pulse is able to compress the power output of the laser tube and deliver very high peak powers of energy during the pulse, but it cannot maintain these high powers in a steady state. A 504-nm dye laser may be pulsed in microseconds to deliver 40 kilowatts of peak power to fragment kidney stones in laser lithotripsy. Even though the peak power is very high, it is not sustained, and the total delivered energy will only amount to 10 to 60 millijoules. With current gynecological lasers, the user has no control nor options for use of these true pulses so that the information is presented only to differentiate a true laser pulse from a timed pulse of a continuous wave.

Superpulse (Fig. 2–10) is found on many CO_2 lasers and is called various names by manufacturers, such as superpulse, varipulse, megapulse, and so on. This is a true pulse on CO_2 lasers, usually producing a train of pulses from 250 to 500 watts maximum per pulse at a rate of 300 to 1000 times per second (hertz). This rate is so fast that it looks continuous, but the pulsing may be picked up as an audible buzz as the focused beam hits its target. Again, the total delivered energy is not as high as the

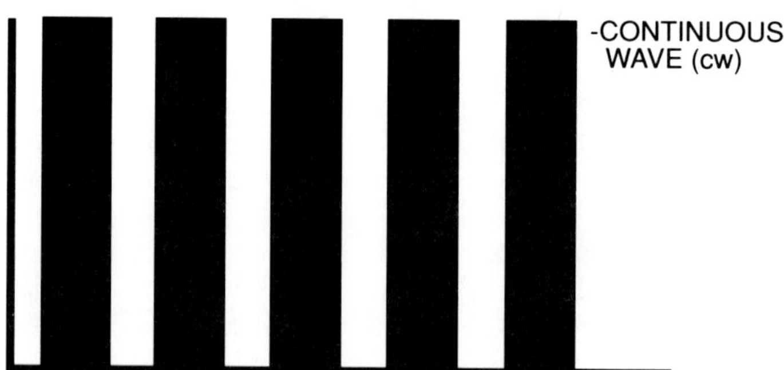

FIGURE 2–9. Gated pulses are simply a continuous wave (CW) beam interrupted by a timer. Maximum pulse powers are no higher than that attainable in CW mode and pulse width are typically from .05 seconds up to 0.5 seconds.

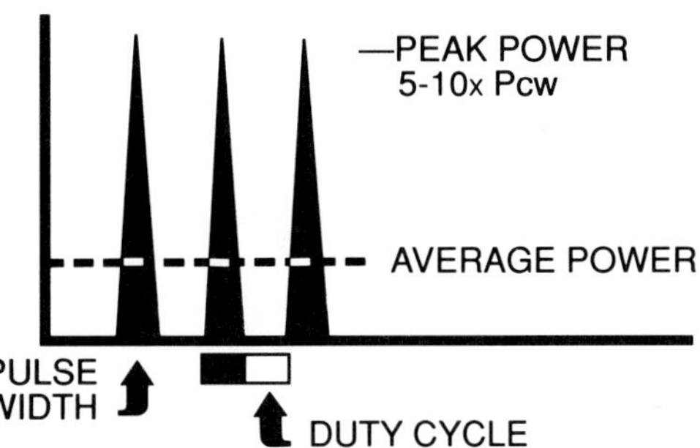

FIGURE 2–10. Superpulse is a true pulse on CO_2 lasers, producing 250 to 500 watts peak power at 300 to 1000 times per second. The average power is much lower due to the time the laser energy is off of the tissue (duty cycle). Due to the rapidity of the pulses, the laser energy appears to be applied continuously.

500-watt pulses might imply. On CO_2 lasers, this will be read out as the average power of the beam rather than joules energy, and the maximum average power in superpulse will always be substantially lower than the maximum power available in continuous mode. Superpulse allows for cleaner cutting of tissues, resulting in less charring. It is a cooler use of the heat energy to obtain cutting or vaporization. The user has the option of selecting the superpulse mode on many models and can additionally choose its parameters on some.

A *chopped wave* (Fig. 2–11) could be described as a cross between a continuous wave and a superpulse. It cycles on and off at such a rapid rate that it looks continuous to the eye, but it is actually a series of pulses. It was originally designed as an engineering technique to keep the physical size of the laser head small while still gaining a high power output for that size. The peak powers of the pulses on the chopped wave are not nearly as high as that of superpulse, perhaps achieving only 1.5 times the normal continuous–wave output on the pulse, but the chopped wave is able to maintain higher average powers and therefore greater speed than the superpulse. This modality is designed into the initial manufacture of the laser, and the

FIGURE 2–11. A chopped wave, designed into the initial manufacture of a particular laser, operates continuously with no external control by the operator. Pulses are of greater power than the maximum available in continuous wave (CW). Pulses are fast enough that they appear to be a continuous beam.

operator has no control to choose or delete this mode. It operates this way at all times.

An understanding of laser biophysics is actually only an understanding of the fundamental mechanisms by which lasers perform surgical tasks. An understanding of these basic principles will help one make the transition from marginal to effective use of various surgical lasers.

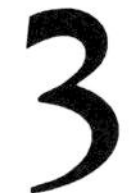 **3**

The Safe Use of Lasers in Gynecology

John C. Fisher

Like many devices used in surgery and therapy, lasers have the potential to cause serious injuries to patients and medical personnel.[4,11] Such injuries can be fatal, and the author estimates that as many as 35 patients may have died of laser-induced trauma during the past 18 years. Virtually all of the laser-related fatalities have resulted from burns of the respiratory tract or from perforation of the great cardio-pulmonary blood vessels. Exact numbers are difficult to acquire because medical personnel and hospital authorities are understandably reluctant to discuss such matters for public record. The author's estimate is based on firsthand knowledge and on information confidentially reported, as well as a digest of unconfirmed but probably reliable anecdotes heard during his 12 years of extensive involvement in the use of lasers in all parts of the human body.[2,3]

Many nonfatal injuries, ranging in severity from trivial to highly morbid, have been caused by lasers in hospitals, outpatient clinics, and physicians' offices. Some of these have permanently impaired the victims, who are usually patients, but most have not been serious. Numbers of victims are, again, difficult to estimate, except by multiplying the reported injuries by some factor, greater than unity, based on experience. Since 1970, the total number of nonfatal laser injuries of all degrees of severity to patients and attending personnel is probably less than 3000.

When compared with the number of all medical or surgical procedures performed with lasers during the past 18 years, which now exceeds 1 million, the total of all laser accidents is relatively small. The overall rate is probably less than 0.5%. Although this figure is not a cause for complacency, neither is it a cause for alarm. It is comparable to or lower than the morbidity (all complications) of diagnostic coronary angiography.

DEFINITION OF RISK

For the purposes of this discussion, it is useful to define the term *risk*. Risk can be defined as the arithmetic product of an accident's probability and the severity of its consequences to the victim, measured on a scale from 0 to 10, with 10 being the highest risk. On this scale, we can rank the possible laser accidents into categories of risk as follows:

1.	Burns from laser-ignited combustion	10
2.	Accidental trauma to unintended targets	6
3.	Inappropriate or unskilled use of lasers	5
4.	Delayed morbid sequelae of laser treatment	2
5.	Malfunction of laser equipment	0.1

Fortunately for gynecologists, the life-threatening kinds of accidents listed in the foregoing table are largely confined to laser surgery in the airway, where endotracheal tubes and flexible bronchoscopes are often used in an oxygen-rich atmosphere and can be ignited by the beam of a carbon dioxide (CO_2) or Nd : YAG laser, and where the beam can perforate the trachea, bronchi, and great vessels. The laser hazards faced by gynecologists are usually of much lower risk.

SPECIFIC HAZARDS IN GYNECOLOGY

The five categories tabulated earlier will be discussed as they relate specifically to the use of lasers in gynecology, including a general analysis of surgical laser hazards in other specialties.

Burns from Laser-Ignited Combustion

In this category, the major hazards, in order of declining risk, are as follows:

- **A.** Ignition of rectal gas.
- **B.** Ignition of sterile drapes or pads.
- **C.** Vaporization or combustion of surgical preparatory liquids or diagnostic solutions, such as povidone-iodine, acetic acid, Schiller's stain, and toluidine blue.
- **D.** Ignition of plastic vaginal specula.

Rectal gas is mostly air ingested with food, but it sometimes contains enough methane to be combustible in room air. When using the CO_2 laser for vaginal, vulvar, or perianal lesions, gynecologists are well advised to ensure that the patient's lower bowel has been evacuated naturally or by enema just before surgery and that her anus has been plugged with a piece of wet cotton. Otherwise, incandescent particles of tissue vaporized by the laser beam can ignite gas expelled from the patient's rectum.

Sterile drapes and pads around the surgical site should be soaked in normal saline or sterile water, and *kept wet* during the procedure to avoid ignition by the laser beam. The beams of argon-ion and Nd : YAG lasers are less likely to ignite white cotton pledgets than is the beam of a CO_2 laser, but they can ignite dry materials of darker colors, including dried bloodstains. It is wise to keep on hand a large bowl of sterile saline or water to douse the fire if drapes or pads should be ignited. A CO_2 fire extinguisher is very useful to have at hand in a laser operating room. It is preferable to the dry-chemical type of extinguisher, because the CO_2 gas dissipates into the air after first forming a layer of ice crystals where the jet strikes the burning material, rather than leaving behind a layer of dry chemical, which might contaminate an open laser wound.

Alcohol should never be used for preparing the surgical area, because the rays of the CO_2 laser can ignite it. Nonflammable liquid preparations should be allowed to dry on the surgical site before the laser is fired, because these liquids can be vaporized by the laser beam. Although they do not burn, their hot vapors can be chemically active and cause injuries to skin and eyes. Plastic vaginal specula are unnecessary and should not be used.

Accidental Trauma to Unintended Targets

The following kinds of injury to unintended targets within the body can occur. They are listed below in order of declining risk:

    A. Perforation of the large and small bowel.
    B. Perforation of the urinary bladder.
    C. Puncture of the vaginal wall.
    D. Thermal injury to any abdominal organ by scattered, reflected, or direct laser rays, especially those of the Nd:YAG laser.
    E. Puncture of the abdominal blood vessels.
    F. Perforation of the uterine wall.
    G. Injuries to the eyes.
    H. Injuries to the epidermis.

A, B, C, D, and E above are most likely to occur when a laser (CO_2, Nd:YAG, or argon–ion) is used within the peritoneal cavity, particularly through a laparoscope, which affords a limited field of view and poor perception of depth. Beam-absorbing backstops should be used, and the laser beam fired in short bursts. Adequate smoke evacuation should be used at all times, especially when the laser beam is delivered laparoscopically.

Because of its shallow extinction depth and lack of scattering, the CO_2 laser is the safest choice for laparoscopic procedures, despite the fact that the beams of visible and near-infrared lasers can be delivered through flexible optical fibers, and the CO_2 laser beam must be delivered either through a rigid laparoscope or through a hollow reflective waveguide. The argon–ion, Nd:YAG, and frequency-doubled (KTP) Nd:YAG lasers have been used with laparoscopes because their rays can easily be transmitted by quartz fibers. However, their absorption by tissue is color selective, and their reflection from first surfaces can be a large fraction of the total radiant power. Furthermore, the scattering of the laser light in soft tissue can be copious, especially with the Nd:YAG laser.

If carefully used, the argon–ion or the KTP laser is safe for ablation of darkly pigmented lesions such as endometriomas, but it can be dangerous if used too aggressively on lightly pigmented tissue. The Nd:YAG laser beam, if delivered from a fiber not touching the tissue, is hazardous for intra-abdominal use, although it can be safe for ablation of the endometrial lining of the uterus. If the Nd:YAG is delivered through flexible quartz fibers fitted with sapphire tips placed in contact with the tissue, it can be used for laparoscopic surgery, but care must be exercised. Multiple-puncture laparoscopy gives a more comprehensive view of the target area and better manipulative control of the treated organs that can be achieved with a single puncture. Adequate evacuation of smoke, particularly with the CO_2 laser, is mandatory for clear visualization of the surgical site. Special evacuation systems that have been devised either remove the smoke only during firing of the laser or continuously recirculate the CO_2 insufflating gas so as to avoid deflating the abdomen.

For coagulation of the uterine endometrium to relieve intractable menorrhagia, the Nd:YAG laser is the best choice. Noncontact delivery affords a larger beam-impact area at the uterine surface than does a contact probe, but the former requires a higher power in the laser beam to achieve the requisite power density at the endometrium. The major hazard here is hypervolemia caused by absorption of the uterine-distention liquid through open veins. Early users of this technique, pioneered by Goldrath and colleagues,[7] used a solution of high-molecular-weight dextran, but it caramelized from the heat produced by the laser beam. Normal saline is now used by most gynecologists who perform this procedure. In order to avoid accumulation of excess water in a patient's circulatory system, it is advisable to use a closed system in which the cervix acts as a seal to prevent leakage of the saline around the barrel of the hysteroscope, while the distending liquid flows into the uterus through one tube and out through another. This system allows continuous monitoring of the volume flowing in and the somewhat lower volume flowing out. With careful technique, less than 50 ml will be absorbed by the patient during a complete endometrial ablation. In some cases, the liquid uptake has been several liters during a procedure, which can lead to cardiac and respiratory complications.

The consequences of visceral puncture by a laser beam are serious and include peritonitis and hemorrhage. Such sequelae are easier to deal with if the surgery is being performed through an open laparotomy than through a laparoscope. In all cases, however, perforation can be avoided by proper choice of laser and use of an appropriate technique. It is imperative that the gynecological laser surgeon *pay constant attention, use short, intermittent laser shots, and not be overly aggressive.*

Perforation of a major abdominal artery or vein during laser surgery is simply inexcusable. Knowledge of anatomy and constant attention to the surgical site will prevent such an occurrence during use of the CO_2 laser, where, to quote the familiar teaching maxim, *what you see is what you get.* However, with the argon-ion, KTP, and Nd:YAG lasers, whose absorption in soft tissue is color dependent and whose scattering may be extensive, injury can occur to organs distal and lateral to the primary impact point of the laser beam. With such lasers, gynecologists will do well to remember that *what you don't see can hurt you.* For example, in some reported cases, the rays of a Nd:YAG laser, delivered via a noncontacting fiber through a cystoscope to a bladder-wall tumor, have caused severe burns of the bowel without perforating the bladder wall.

Although accidental laser injuries to eyes of patients who are not being treated for eye conditions are serious and often irreparable, their probability in gynecological laser surgery is very low, thus yielding a low risk as demonstrated by clinical experience. However, this hazard is always present. Good operating room practice dictates that *everyone in a laser operating room should wear protective glasses, goggles, or face shields.* Warning signs should be posted outside the operating room to keep unauthorized people out during laser procedures. Protective eye wear must be appropriate for the wavelength to be attenuated and should provide protection against rays entering from the sides, the cheeks, and the eyebrows. The optical density, which is the power of 10 by which the transmitted power density is attenuated, should be marked on the frame or bows, together with the wavelength that is screened out. For example, an optical density of six at 1060 means that the rays of a Nd:YAG laser will be reduced in intensity to $1/1,000,000$ (1×10^{-6}) in passing through the glasses. For general use, an optical density of six is required.

It must always be remembered that *commonly available protective eye wear will not afford protection against the beam of a laser at its focal point for more than a few seconds at most.* This eye wear is designed to shield the wearer's eyes against diffused, scattered, reflected, or divergent rays of a laser. In this regard it should be noted that glass is more durable than plastic for extended exposures. At surgical power densities, which may exceed $1,000,000$ watts/cm^2 at the focal point, no transparent material that strongly absorbs the laser rays will restrict puncture indefinitely.

The rays of the CO_2 laser, at 10,600 nm, are strongly attenuated by any glass or plastic through which the wearer can see in normal visible illumination. This is not true of the rays of visible and near-infrared lasers, however. For these lasers, the protective eye wear often has a distinct color or tint (blue or green for Nd:YAG and orange for argon-ion and KTP). However, the color of the material is not a reliable guide to its attenuation at a particular wavelength. The wearer should always check the legend on the glasses for wavelength and optical density before relying on them to protect his or her eyes.

Suitable protective glasses and goggles are available from several manufacturers. Laser Peripherals and Glendale Protective Technologies* offer reliable products in the United States. Laser Peripherals will furnish protective laser glasses with side and eyebrow shields, ground to the user's corrective prescription. This is a considerable advantage as compared with wearing goggles over corrective glasses.

A gynecological patient is rarely at risk from the direct laser beam, but her eyes should be protected, nevertheless. If she is conscious during the procedure, her eyes should be covered by the same glasses or goggles used by the gynecologist and medical personnel. If she is anesthetized, her eyelids should be taped shut, covered with wet 4 $\times$ 4-inch cotton squares, and then by a double layer of rumpled, heavy-gauge aluminum foil taped in place.

Gynecologists and attending personnel may become lax about eye protection after long use of lasers without an accident. As in all aspects of human life, hazards lose their ability to frighten when they do not cause injuries. It is tempting to dispense with protective eye wear, especially when the laser is being used through a laparoscope or a hysteroscope. The danger is still there, however; ignoring it can lead to accidental eye injury. The risk can be reduced to a low level by always

---

* *Laser Peripherals, 100 Station Street, Hingham, MA 02043. (617) 740-2934*
Glendale Protective Technologies, Inc., 130 Crossways Park Drive, Woodbury, NY 11797. (516) 921-5800

requiring protective glasses or goggles for everyone in the room and by training the laser nurse to disarm the laser routinely when it is not being actively used by the gynecologist.

Epidermal injuries from laser beams are rare, although the lay public thinks of lasers as ray guns that can vaporize objects in a flash. Because exposure of skin to a laser beam causes immediate pain, reflex action causes the victim to withdraw the exposed part from the beam unless he or she is anesthetized. This reflex minimizes the exposure. Furthermore, the healing of epidermal laser injuries is usually rapid and uncomplicated. The potential victims of such injuries are usually gynecologists and the attending personnel. The best defense against laser wounds to the skin of those other than the patient is an operating rule requiring that the laser be put into a standby condition when the gynecologist is engaged in other activities, like taking biopsies, suctioning, and so on.

Epidermal injury to patients when the laser (usually the CO_2) is used for ablation of vulvar or perianal lesions is chiefly the result of allowing the beam to penetrate too deeply, especially with condylomata, whose virus resides only in the epidermis. Ablating these warts below the papillary dermis may cause scarring and excessive postoperative pain. In any procedure in which the basal cell layer is ablated, there is a possibility of causing permanent vitiligo in patients with dark skin.

Inappropriate or Unskilled Use of Lasers

Although inappropriate or unskilled use of lasers seldom results in serious injuries, it can leave a patient unhappy about the outcome of the procedure, and resentful or even litigious toward the surgeon. Careless, improper use of lasers can negate the distinct advantages of this unique modality. Every laser gynecologist should thoroughly understand the biophysics of laser light and soft tissue at the wavelengths commonly used in surgery, apply the laser cautiously to the target, and carefully observe the results at every stage of the procedure. For gynecologists, the major hazards in this category are listed below in order of declining risk:

A. Treatment of a lesion of unknown cytology, histology, or spatial extent, especially if the lesion is not fully irradiable by the laser beam.

B. Excess thermal necrosis resulting from low power density or prolonged irradiation.

C. Failure to ablate cervical intraepithelial neoplasia (CIN) deeply enough to reach disease at the bottom of the cervical crypts (5.0 and 7.0 mm) or to destroy the entire transformation zone.

D. Excessive bleeding with the CO_2 laser caused by improper technique in excisional procedures on the cervix.

Biopsy specimens should routinely be taken before laser treatment and during and after laser ablation of malignant lesions. Small skin lesions should be *excised*, not vaporized, if there is any suspicion that they might be malignant. Although it is appropriate to use a laser as a surgical tool for debulking or excising a known invasive primary or a metastatic malignancy, the laser should not be considered as curative, and other appropriate adjunctive therapies should be employed as needed.

In noninvasive malignant tumors, it can be curative, if sequential biopsies reveal lateral and distal margins free of disease.

Excessive thermal necrosis, with the CO_2 laser, is avoidable by using power densities of at least 600 watts/cm^2 at the focal plane of the beam and by minimizing the duration of exposure. With the Nd : YAG laser, which is inherently a coagulative device unless its beam is delivered via a sapphire tip in contact with the tissue, the duration of each shot should not exceed 2 seconds, and adequate cooling intervals should be allowed between successive shots. The operating rule to remember is that *high power density in the laser beam and short exposures cause less thermal damage than low power densities and long exposures.* This is true for all types of lasers that destroy tissue by thermal mechanisms (*i.e.*, for all lasers other than the excimers). In general, when using a CO_2 laser, gynecologists should use the highest focal power density that they can control, within the limits of acquired mind–eye–hand coordination, without excessive destruction of tissue.

Most commercially available CO_2 lasers for surgery now offer a pulsed mode of operation, often called by the unfortunate name *superpulse,* which provides a rapid sequence of short pulses having high peak power and relatively long cooling periods between successive pulses. The purposes of superpulsing are two: (1) to reduce the time-rate of tissue destruction while still maintaining high power density at the target and (2) to minimize thermal damage to adjacent tissue.

At this late date in the clinical history of the CO_2 laser for treatment of CIN, there is no excuse for failing to remove the disease to a depth of 5 to 7 mm below the cervical tissue surface. Neither is there any excuse for failing to ablate the entire transformation zone. When the proper technique is used, the CO_2 laser can achieve cure rates greater than 95% for CIN III.[12]

Excessive or uncontrollable bleeding during excisional cervical procedures can be avoided in the great majority of cases if the following preoperative precautions are taken:

1. Know the patient's clinical history; if she has either an idiopathic (thrombocytopenia) or a drug-induced (*e.g.*, aspirin) coagulopathy, then postpone the surgery or be prepared to employ special hemostatic measures.
2. Peripherally inject the cervix with properly diluted vasopressin in appropriate quantity.
3. Place cervical sutures at the 3- and 9-o'clock positions.

If such measures are not taken and copious bleeding ensues, an inexperienced laser gynecologist may become panicky and misuse the laser while trying to achieve hemostasis. The CO_2 laser is not a good coagulator, and its rays will not penetrate flowing liquid blood. The blood must be removed from the surface by absorbent tamponade or suction, and the laser beam then defocused to reduce the power density until surface vaporization ceases, while the beam is "painted" randomly over the surface. Heat from the absorption of CO_2 laser rays close to the first surface is transmitted to the interior tissue only by thermal conduction, which can transfer only about 10 watts/cm^2. If the CO_2 laser cannot control the bleeding, it is necessary and appropriate to use electrocautery, more sutures, hemostats, or topically applied Monsel's solution (ferric subsulfate).

Delayed Sequelae of Laser Treatment

In this category the major problems, in order of declining risk, are as follows:

> **A.** Postoperative pain following vulvar ablation.
> **B.** Postoperative scarring, depilation, and vitiligo.
> **C.** Postoperative bleeding.

Postoperative pain following vulvar laser procedures is not uncommon, and its intensity and duration vary from one individual patient to another. Its occurrence is not entirely avoidable but can be minimized by proper technique in using the CO_2 laser. Superpulsing helps to avoid lateral thermal damage and excessive depth of ablation, especially when dealing with condylomata. During the first few days after a laser procedure on the vulva, sitz baths in ordinary tea (in which the beneficial ingredient is tannic acid) help greatly to alleviate the pain. Also very effective is the topical application of sterile extract of aloe vera in either a gel or an emollient ointment several times per day to the ablated area.

Superpulsing and careful attention to depth of ablation can minimize scarring, depilation, and vitiligo. Coaptation of the labia minora can be a problem after laser removal of condylomata and can be minimized by keeping the denuded labia apart during the healing process.

Postoperative bleeding is not often a problem if careful attention is paid to hemostasis during the laser procedure. It seldom requires emergency treatment. However, if the patient has an unsuspected coagulopathy, it can be serious, as mentioned earlier.

Malfunction of Laser Equipment

Malfunction of equipment is extremely rare in surgical lasers, but it can happen in several ways, the more frequent of which are as follows:

> **A.** The laser fires accidentally without pressure on the foot switch.
> **B.** The helium–neon aiming beam of a CO_2 or a Nd : YAG laser fails.
> **C.** The helium–neon aiming beam of a CO_2 laser is not aligned with the CO_2 laser beam.

The author is aware of only one instance when a laser fired itself accidentally without having the foot switch depressed. This happened in an outpatient surgical clinic in Texas when a CO_2 laser was being demonstrated to physicians who had registered for a laser course there. Fortunately, it did not cause a serious injury, but one of the operating room nurses was burned on the face by the errant beam. It could have resulted in severe trauma to her eye, however. This kind of accident is not totally preventable, even if each laser is thoroughly checked before each procedure. In the case cited, the problem was caused by a short-circuit in the footswitch. Statistically, such mishaps are exceeedingly uncommon.

Failure of a helium–neon aiming beam is not a common occurrence and is a problem only in the case of a CO_2 laser being used with a micromanipulator or with a rigid laparoscope. Only if the aiming beam fails immediately before firing the CO_2 laser is it a hazard. If the helium–neon beam is not on before the procedure begins, the surgeon should simply delay the surgery until the problem is corrected.

When the helium–neon beam is functioning but not aligned with the CO_2 laser beam—a condition that can and should be checked before surgery—it should be correctly aligned before the procedure begins. Many CO_2 lasers for surgery have a provision for this alignment to be done in the operating room. This is a problem only with a micromanipulator and surgical microscope or colposcope.

Other kinds of equipment malfunction can occur, such as failure of the cooling system or exhaustion of the laser gas in flowing-gas systems. The microprocessors now used in many surgical lasers can fail but are usually designed to fail in a noninjurious way. Most such failures, which are rare, result in nothing more serious than the interruption of the procedure. To avoid embarrassment and the possible litigation resulting from the interruption of a surgical procedure after a patient has been anesthetized, gynecologists should insist that all lasers to be used in a particular procedure, as well as their auxiliary devices, be thoroughly checked for proper operation before the patient is anesthetized.

The flexible quartz fibers used to transmit the beams of visible and near-infrared lasers (*e.g.*, the argon–ion, KTP, and Nd : YAG) deteriorate with prolonged use. This is evident from a gradual loss of transmittance, which can be detected by measuring the input and output power of the beam as it passes through the fiber. If the transmittance of a particular fiber falls below the manufacturer's specification, it should be replaced with a new one. With repeated flexing, a quartz fiber may eventually break, even though its external protective sheath usually remains intact. This situation can be dangerous, because the laser light escapes from the fiber at the site of the fracture and can cause injury to the medical personnel in the vicinity. A break in the fiber core is easy to detect by turning on the helium–neon aiming beam of a Nd : YAG laser (or by reducing the power of an argon–ion or KTP laser beam to a few milliwatts) and visually examining the whole length of the fiber for spots where the visible light is escaping. There is always enough light escaping radially from a normal, intact fiber to see with the unshielded eye when the power of the beam of a visible laser is in the order of a few watts. However, when only the aiming beam is turned on, the light leaking from the break is visible to the unshielded eye, even if no light is seen leaking radially along the length of the fiber.

SMOKE AND VAPOR FROM THE SURGICAL TARGET

Smoke and vapor from the surgical target were not discussed as risks at the start of this chapter because they affect the surgeon and the medical personnel rather than the patient. However, they are a matter of great concern to all those who use lasers in surgery, particularly the CO_2 laser, which generates the most copious smoke plumes during vaporization of human or animal tissue. The smoke plumes from surgical laser beams have three morbid properties:

1. They are malodorous.
2. They cause nausea and headaches after prolonged inhalation.
3. They contain particulate matter, which accumulates in the alveoli of the lungs of those who inhale the smoke.

The question of viability of tumor cells in the smoke plume of a CO_2 laser was carefully studied by J. W. Oosterhuis[10] in the Netherlands. He used an American Optical Model 100 CO_2 laser to vaporize tumors of the Cloudman S91 mouse melanoma from the bodies of mice. Although he detected morphologically normal cells in the plume captured close around the impact point of the laser beam on the tumor, attempts to culture these cells *in vitro* and to inoculate healthy mice with the cells extracted from the plume failed to demonstrate any viability whatever of these cells retrieved from the plume. Furthermore, to test the possibility that it was not the laser beam but rather the toxic products in the smoke that devitalized the tumor cells, he attempted to produce tumors in healthy mice by injecting mixtures of viable S91 cells and plume residues. The results of this test demonstrated that the smoke residues were not cytotoxic to the viable tumor cells. The trypan blue exclusion test was used to check the viability of the cells studied.

Though Oosterhuis's experiments demonstrated quite convincingly that no viable cells from the highly malignant Cloudman S91 mouse melanoma were to be found in the smoke plume of a continuous-wave CO_2 laser used to evaporate the tumors at power densities of hundreds or thousands of watts per square centimeter, they left unanswered the question of whether viable cells from such tumors would be found in the smoke plume from the Nd:YAG or argon-ion lasers used for vaporization. This question lingered in the minds of many laser surgeons for the next 12 years, but it never engendered a controversy or serious anxiety. Then, in late summer of 1987, a dermatologist at Northwestern University Medical School, Jerome M. Garden,[6] announced that he had found "intact and presumably viable" viral DNA in the smoke plume of a CO_2 laser used to ablate human mosaic and plantar warts. This announcement ignited near panic among physicians, nurses, and operating room supervisors around the country.

Garden's experiments were not performed with the thoroughness exhibited by Oosterhuis, and the tests did not take the logical step of examining the viability of the viral DNA of the human papillomavirus recovered from the plume. The author and Dr. Garden have discussed at some length the method used in his tests of last year. As a result of that discussion, this author feels strongly that it was irresponsible to publish such sensational statements without having determined whether an inoculum derived from the contents of the smoke plume would, in fact, produce new viral warts in previously uninfected sites of the same patient's body. In this opinion, the author concurs with such prominent laser gynecologists as V. Cecil Wright, Michael Baggish, Rocco V. Lobraico, and Joseph Bellina, each of whom has publicly expressed skepticism about the claim that the viral DNA recovered by Garden was viable.

Behind all of the uproar caused by Garden's report lies the fear that a patient harboring the virus of acquired immunodeficiency syndrome (AIDS) and undergoing laser surgery might be a source of AIDS infection to those in the operating room who inhale some of the smoke plume. Because of the almost total mortality from this disease, such concerns are valid. Pending resolution of the question of infectiousness of DNA recovered from smoke plumes of surgical lasers, the laser surgeon is well advised to ensure that adequate suction is always used during procedures with any laser.

Quite apart from the sensationalism set off by Garden's report, there are compelling reasons to avoid inhalation of laser-generated smoke. Among these are the following:

1. Of all particles in the smoke plume of a CO_2 laser, 77% are less than 1.1 micrometers.
2. In this range of sizes, the predominant sites of accumulation in the respiratory tract are the alveoli.
3. These particles accumulate in the alveoli and are not exhaled.
4. Significant mutagenicity of plume particles has been demonstrated.
5. Viruses, if they are present in smoke plumes, can attach to the particulates in the smoke.

Items 1 through 4 were conclusions of a study by Mihashi and colleagues[8] in Japan. Other investigators agreed.[1,5,9] This study showed also that a suction tip with a flow rate of 28 L/minute could remove 99% of the smoke when the tip was 1 cm or less from the laser-impact site; but when the tip was 2 cm away from the site, the collection efficiency declined to only 51%. A jet of cooling gas from a surgical hand piece or optical fiber can substantially reduce the collection efficiency.

Suction systems and smoke evacuators now available for laser surgery can filter out particles as small as 0.1 micrometer. One such system is manufactured by Stackhouse Associates, Inc., 150 Sierra Street, El Segundo, CA 90245 (213-322-6676). This firm was the first in the United States to make a surgical laser smoke evacuator commercially available. Other firms, such as Laser Accessories and Safety Equipment of Cincinnati, Ohio, also offer smoke evacuators for surgical lasers. Even if the surgery is performed in the operating room, the typical wall suction of the operating room is inadequate to handle the smoke plume from a CO_2 laser, and the particulates may quickly clog the system.

Viruses range in size from about 0.0015 to 0.02 micrometer and are difficult to filter out of otherwise clean air. However, in a smoke plume, these viruses usually attach to particulates of much larger diameter and can be filtered out by a system that traps particles of 0.1 micrometer.

CONCLUSION

Lasers are unique, versatile surgical tools that offer many advantages in gynecological surgery. When used carefully and intelligently, they are as safe as any surgical devices ever invented. However, they are not magical instruments. They require basic understanding of the interaction of light with living tissue, training in their proper use, and hands-on learning with experienced practitioners to develop the necessary skills. Gynecologists who heed the information given in this chapter can look forward to successful laser surgery for years to come.

REFERENCES

1. Bellina JH, Stjernholm RL, Kurpel JE: Analysis of plume emissions after papovavirus irradiation with the carbon-dioxide laser. J Reprod Med 27:268–270, 1982
2. Fisher JC: CO₂ lasers for gynecologic surgery: How safe are they? Contemp Ob/Gyn 21:3–11, 1983

3. Fisher JC: Principles of safety in laser surgery and therapy. In Baggish M (ed): Basic and Advanced Laser Surgery in Gynecology. Norwalk, Appleton-Century-Crofts, 1985
4. Fisher JC: Basic laser physics and interaction of laser light with soft tissue. In Sharpshay SM (ed): Endoscopic Laser Surgery Handbook. New York, Marcel Dekker, 1987
5. Freitag L, Chapman A, Sielczak M et al: Laser smoke effect on the bronchial system. Lasers Surg Med 7:283–288, 1987
6. Garden JM: Papillomavirus in the vapor of carbon dioxide laser-treated verrucae. JAMA 259:1199–1202. 1988.
7. Goldrath MH, Fuller TA, Segal S: Laser photovaporization of endometrium for the treatment of menorrhagia. Am J Obstet Gynecol 104:14, 1981
8. Mihashi S, Ueda S, Hirano M et al: Some problems about condensates induced by CO_2 laser irradiation. In Atsumi K (ed): Transactions of the 4th Congress of the International Society for Laser Surgery and Medicine. Tokyo, Intergroup Corp, 1981
9. Nezhat C, Winer WK, Nezhat F et al: Smoke from laser surgery: Is there a health hazard? Lasers Surg Med 7:376–382, 1987
10. Oosterhuis JW: Tumor Surgery with the CO_2 Laser: Studies with the Cloudman S91 Mouse Melanoma. Groningen, Netherlands, Veenstra-Visser, 1977
11. Sliney D, Wolbarsht M: Safety with lasers and other optical sources. New York, Plenum Publishing Corp, 1980
12. Wright VC: Laser surgery for the cervix and vagina. In Shapshay SM (ed): Endoscopic Laser Surgery Handbook. New York, Marcel Dekker, 1987

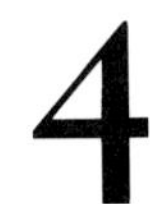

4

Photo Documentation for
the Gynecologic Laser Surgeon

David S. McLaughlin
John L. Marlow
Barbara E. Marlay

Visual images were first recorded by prehistoric humans on the walls of caves in Lascaux, France, as early as the year 15,000 B.C. The first known visual recording of a diseased state, human poliomyelitis, was drawn by early Egyptians. The first known photograph was taken by Niepce in 1826. Photography became reproducible when Daguerre improved the process in 1835. Medical photographs of surgery performed in the 1800s and of diseases that are now rare remain to help document the historical progression of medicine.[5,6] The single-lens reflex (SLR) camera was patented in 1888; however, it did not become commercially available until 1937. Fiberoptic technology, which developed in the mid 1960s, then enabled the practicality of endoscopic photography.[6]

WHY USE PHOTO DOCUMENTATION?

There are several reasons to document gynecologic surgery photographically (Table 4–1):

1. *Education.* Informing the patient or referring physician of the diagnosis established by laparoscopy, hysteroscopy, colposcopy, or microsurgery is helpful in selecting the appropriate therapy. Thirty-five-millimeter slides, prints, and videotapes help educate other physicians and allied health personnel, through lectures and publications, about what new therapies and techniques are available for contemporary treatment of gynecologic diseases.

TABLE 4–1
Reasons for Photographic Documentation in Gynecology

Education
Consultation
Evaluation of new treatment
Legal record

2. *Consultation.* Reviewing slides, prints, or videotapes with the consulting gynecologic oncologist or reproductive surgeon helps define the extent of disease and plan appropriate therapy without repeating another laparoscopy, hysteroscopy, or colposcopy. "A picture is worth a thousand words" is certainly applicable when comparing a visual image with most operative notes.
3. *When evaluating new surgical techniques and medical therapies.* Photographic documentation is helpful when evaluating new therapeutic modalities (*e.g.,* second-look laparoscopies after microlaser surgery or post-treatment Lupron therapy for endometriosis).
4. *Legal record.* Photographic documentation of a properly performed laparoscopic sterilization procedure that subsequently failed would be invaluable in defending a physician in a malpractice action. Peer review is also facilitated by reviewing visual as well as written records.

Photography requires no translation for foreign physicians, as it is essentially a universal medical language. It also historically records medicine's achievements to help bridge the gap between generations of physicians.[5]

MATERIALS AND METHODS

Several options are available to gynecological surgeons for photographic documentation, depending on the goals and objectives (Tables 4–2 and 4–3). Thirty-five-millimeter slides and prints are most suited for lectures and publications. Sixteen-

TABLE 4–2
Photographic Media Available

35-mm slides and prints (color or black and white)
16-mm movies
Video: videotape (½-inch or ¾-inch), hard copy (Polaprint or Mavigraph)

TABLE 4–3
Documentation Systems Used

Microscope, colposcope
Endoscope: laparoscope, hysteroscope
Second person for operating room procedures

millimeter movies produce the best animated visual images, but the equipment is cumbersome and now is infrequently used. Video cameras, on the other hand, have become almost standard in many operating rooms because of their ease of use and surgeons' familiarity with the medium. Hard copies of a still frame may be made from a picture of the video image (Polaprint) or from an electronically generated image (Mavigraph). The videotape or hard copy may be easily given to the patient or made a part of a patient's permanent record.

In assessing one's needs and defining one's goals, a basic understanding of photography is required.

PLANNING

Surgeons must anticipate the opportunity for filming by having a loaded camera and videotapes always available. Patient consent should be signed in the event that photography is undertaken during the procedure.[5]

Endoscopes

A 10-mm diagnostic laparoscope and a 5-mm diagnostic hysteroscope are basic requirements for successful gynecological endoscopic photography. The lenses should be optically brilliant to gather all the available light during photography of the pelvic or uterine cavity.[4] A telescopic heater (Fig. 4–1) to prevent condensation on the distal endoscopic lens is helpful as well.

35-mm Film

Tungsten film, ASA 160, is best for microscopic/colposcopic photography, whereas daylight film, ASA 200 or 400, is best for endoscopic photography.[2] Daylight film is color balanced for electronic flash and emphasizes the blue-light spectrum. The ASA (American Standards Association) or DIN (the German equivalent) number refers to the degree of light sensitivity of the film. Professional film usually gives the best results but needs to be stored at 55°F. It may be removed from the refrigerator one-half hour before use or from the freezer one hour before use. Amateur film, on the other hand, may be stored at room temperature and retains latent images longer before development. Negative color film allows for the development of both color prints and slides. The film expense may be reduced by bulk loading several rolls at a time. Because the cost of the film is the least expense incurred, it is important to take numerous pictures in order to obtain the best.[5]

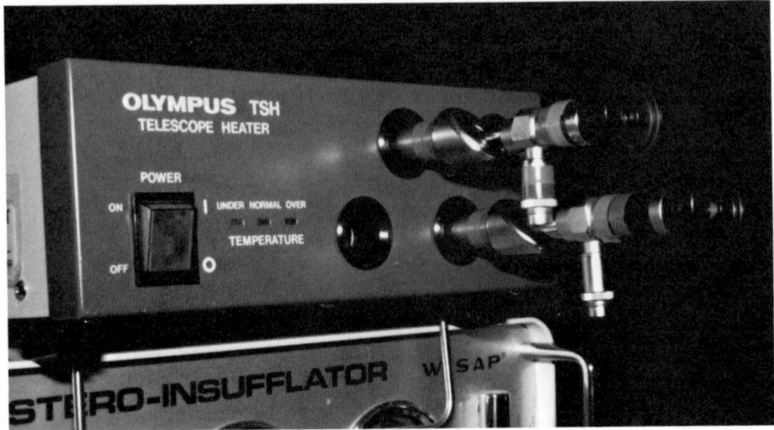

FIGURE 4–1. Olympus TSH telescopic heater helps prevent condensation on the distal lens.

Light

Success depends on an adequate light source, as failures are directly or indirectly attributable to inadequate light.[1-7] One may elect to use the automatic setting on the 35-mm camera with a high-intensity xenon light source, which is commonly used in conjunction with video recording.[1-3] Because of prolonged shutter time, blurred images may result if a small endoscope is used to photograph a dark image using slow film speed. For this reason, the authors prefer to use an external electronically generated flash fired through the fiberoptic light cable with the shutter speed regulated by the flash generated (Fig. 4–2). A brilliant fiberoptic cable with a minimum of broken fibers or a liquid light cable is essential.

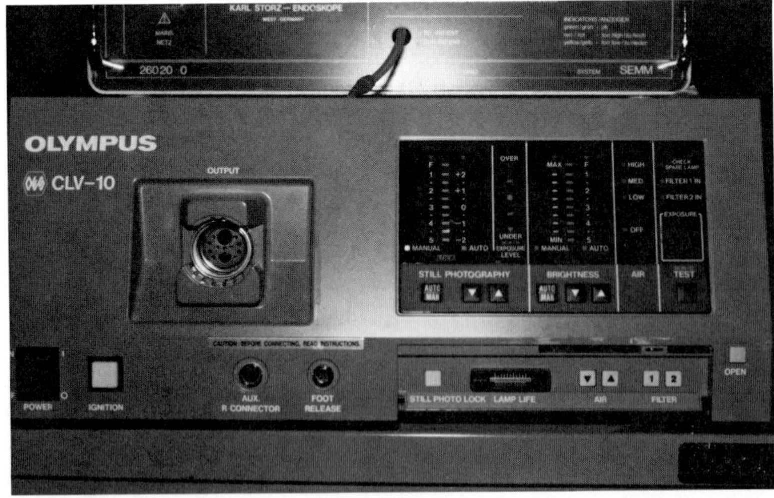

FIGURE 4–2. Olympus CLV-10 light source for video and still photography.

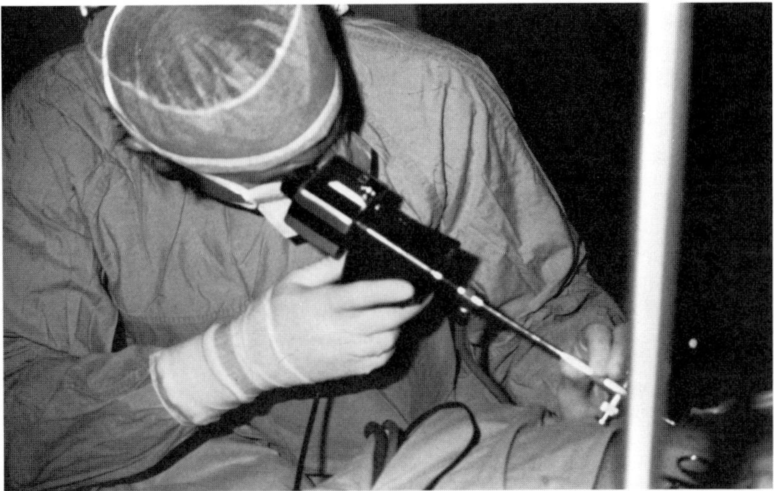

FIGURE 4–3. Olympus 8-mm camera.

35-mm Camera and Lens Systems

Endoscope

The lightest, simplest camera is desirable to facilitate endoscopic photography. Several years ago, Olympus introduced a small camera (Fig. 4–3) that was easy to use, but it produced too small a slide image and subsequently was abandoned. The Olympus OM-2N, with a feature called a Recordadataback and an automatic winding device (Auto-winder) was selected (Fig. 4–4). A clear focusing screen (Olympus

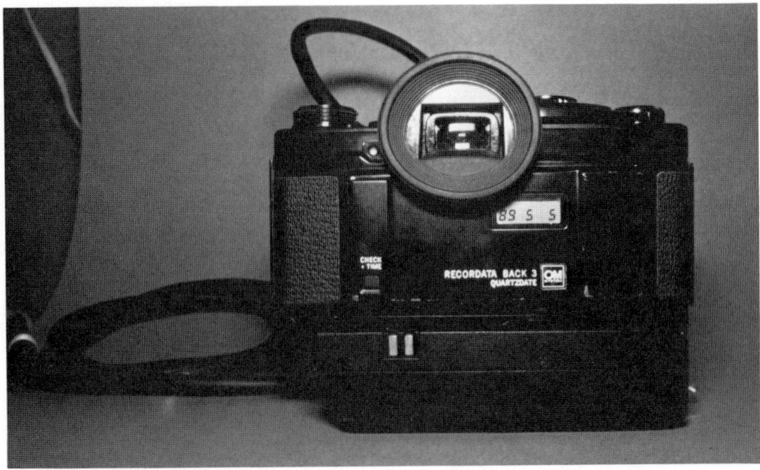

FIGURE 4–4. Olympus OM-2N camera with eyepiece, Auto-winder II, and Recordadataback.

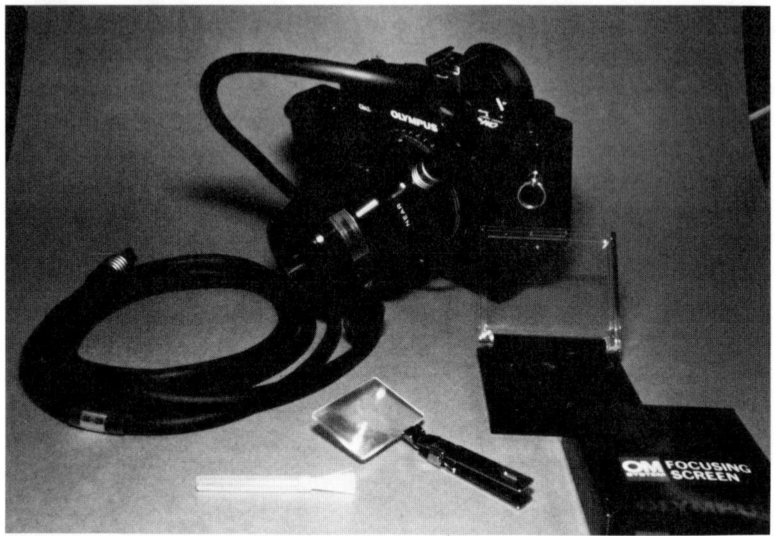

FIGURE 4–5. Clear-focusing screen kit seen with a camera and electronic sensing cord.

1-9) should be installed to facilitate appropriate focusing through the endoscope (Fig. 4–5). A circular rubber eyepiece helps keep external light out of a surgeon's eye when trying to focus precisely. The Olympus SLE-F and SLR-SM lenses, specifically designed for endoscopic photography, are used. When using the Olympus CLE-F or CLV-10 light sources, which have flash capability, the camera is set on manual with a time setting of 4, flash setting of FP, compensation dial of +2, Auto-

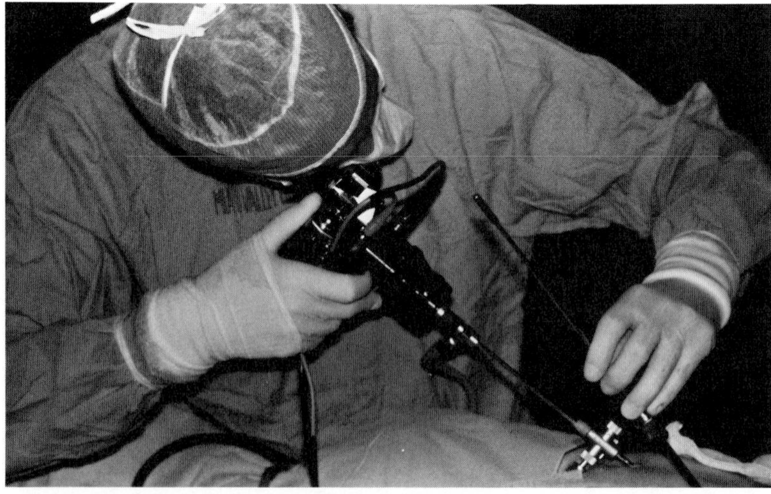

FIGURE 4–6. Camera attached to the laparoscope. Note the second glove used on the right hand to hold the nonsterile camera.

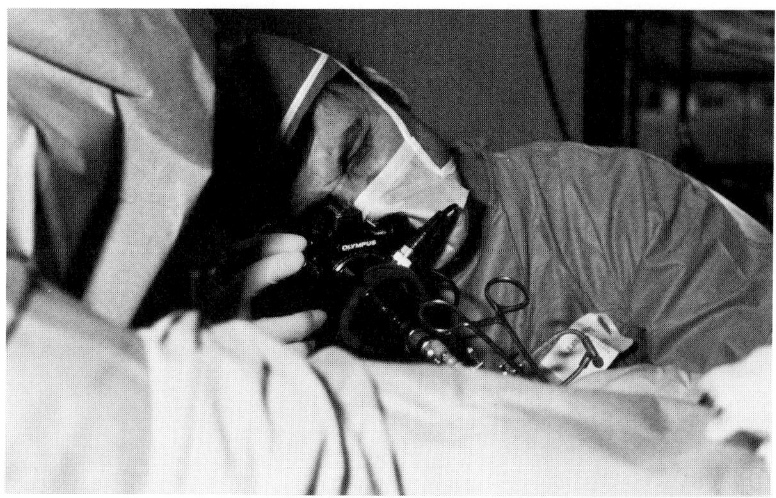

FIGURE 4–7. Camera used on the hysteroscope.

winder II–single, databack to the date or time of day, and ASA 200 slide film are used. The camera is usually handled with one hand, covered with a second sterile surgical glove (Figs. 4–6 and 4–7).

A newer, lighter system, the Olympus OM-88 (Fig. 4–8), was attached to the Storz variable-focus endoscopic lens (Fig. 4–9), through-the-lens (TTL) light metering to enable proper exposure. The camera has been specially modified with the insertion of a clear focusing screen to facilitate endoscopic photography. The vari-

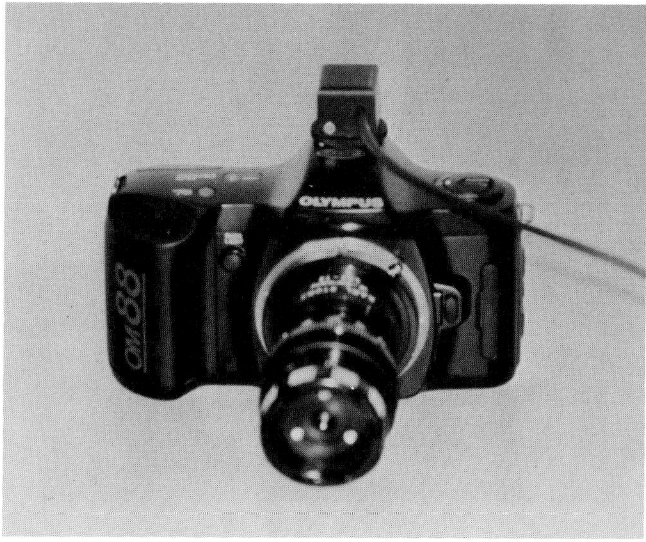

FIGURE 4–8. OM-88 endoscopic camera.

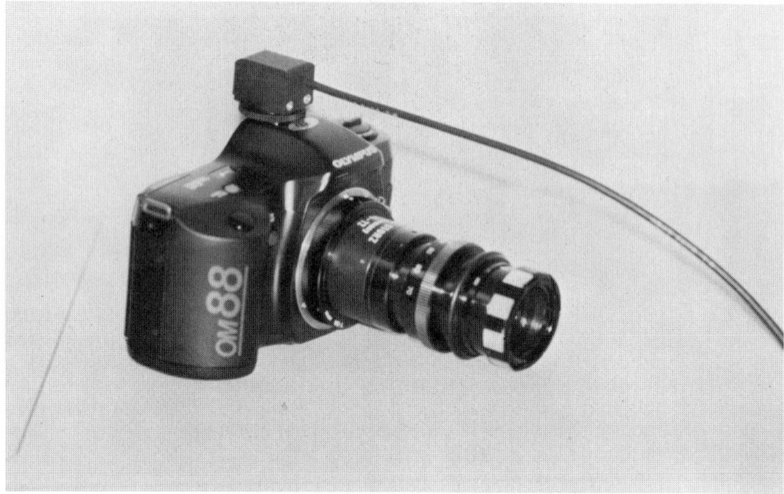

FIGURE 4–9. OM-88 camera. Note the variable-focus Storz lens.

able zoom lens produces different sizes of endoscopic images on the slide (Figs. 4–10 through 4–17). A disadvantage of the system is that no Recordadataback is currently available to record the date on the slide automatically. Both systems require the use of an electronic sensing cable joining the camera to the external flash generator. It is helpful for one of the operating room personnel to be familiar with endoscopic photography or to have a medical photographer available to assist (Figs. 4–18 through 4–20) and record appropriate data (Fig. 4–21).

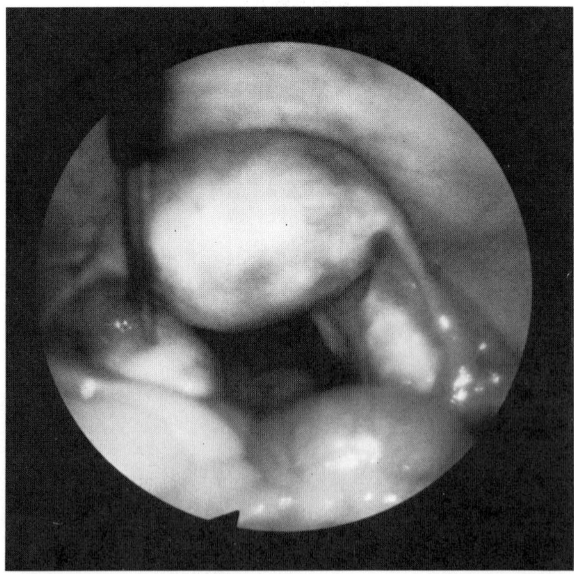

FIGURE 4–10. Laparoscopic view of the pelvis — 70 mm.

(text continued on page 50)

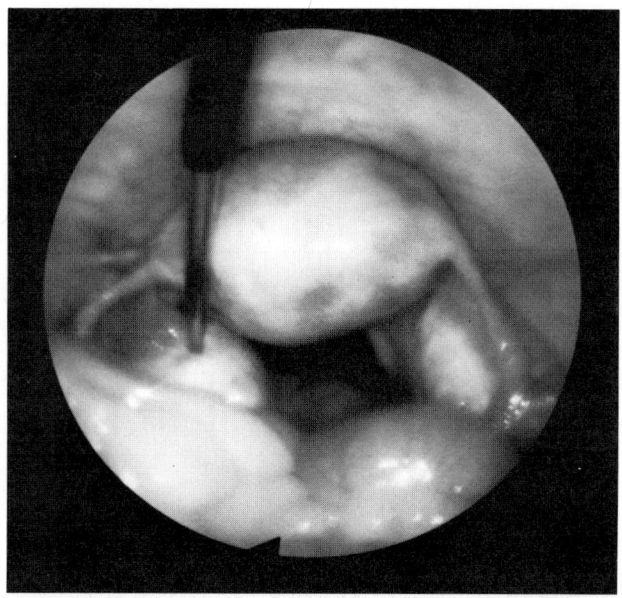

FIGURE 4–11. Laparoscopic view of the pelvis — 80 mm.

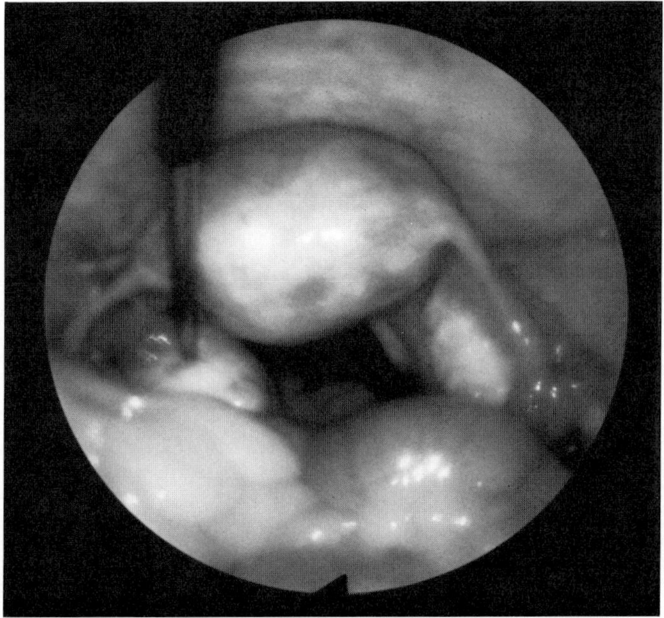

FIGURE 4–12. Laparoscopic view of the pelvis — 90 mm.

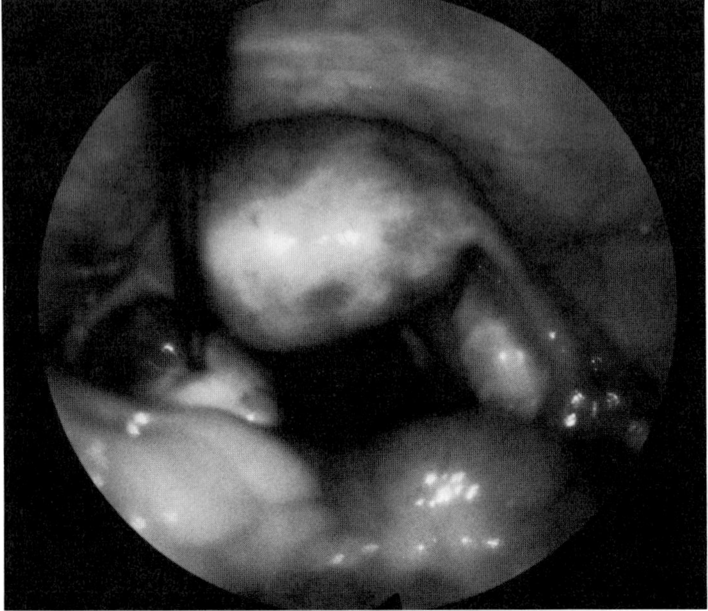

FIGURE 4–13. Laparoscopic view of the pelvis — 100 mm.

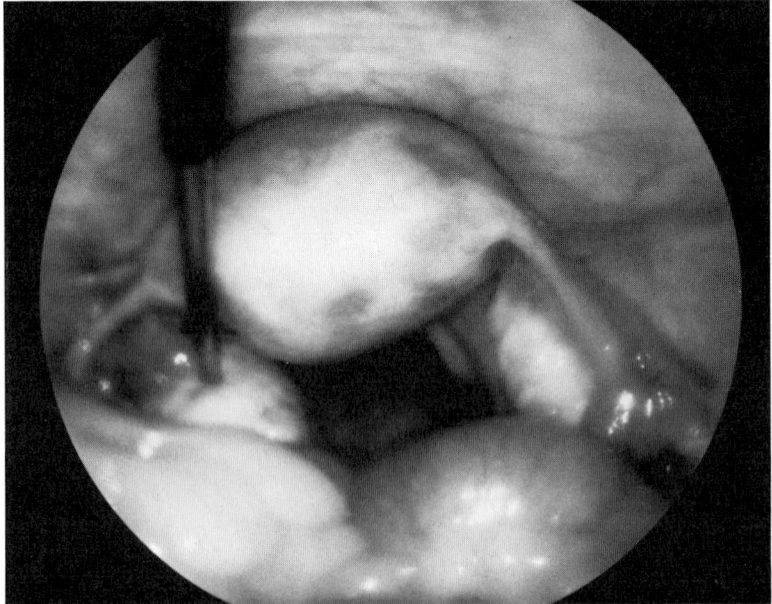

FIGURE 4–14. Laparoscopic view of the pelvis — 110 mm.

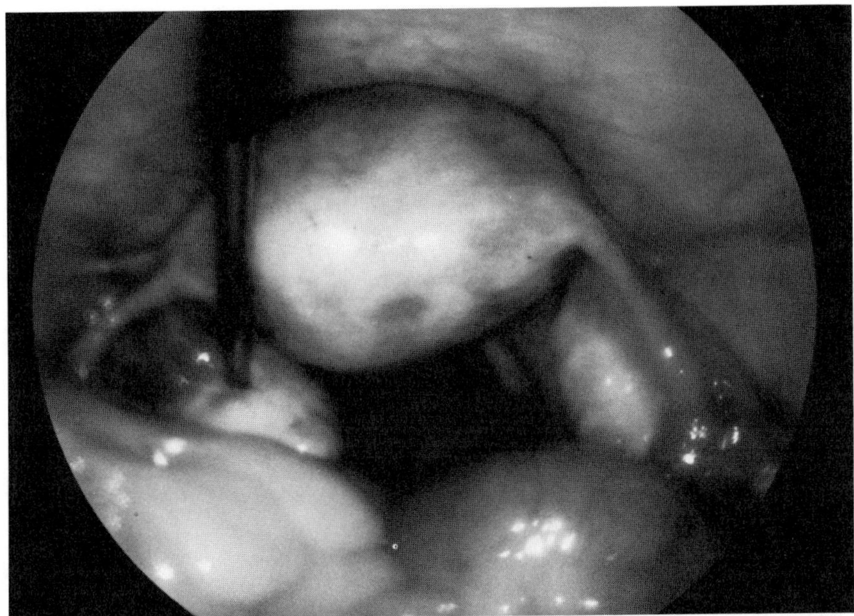

FIGURE 4–15. Laparoscopic view of the pelvis — 120 mm.

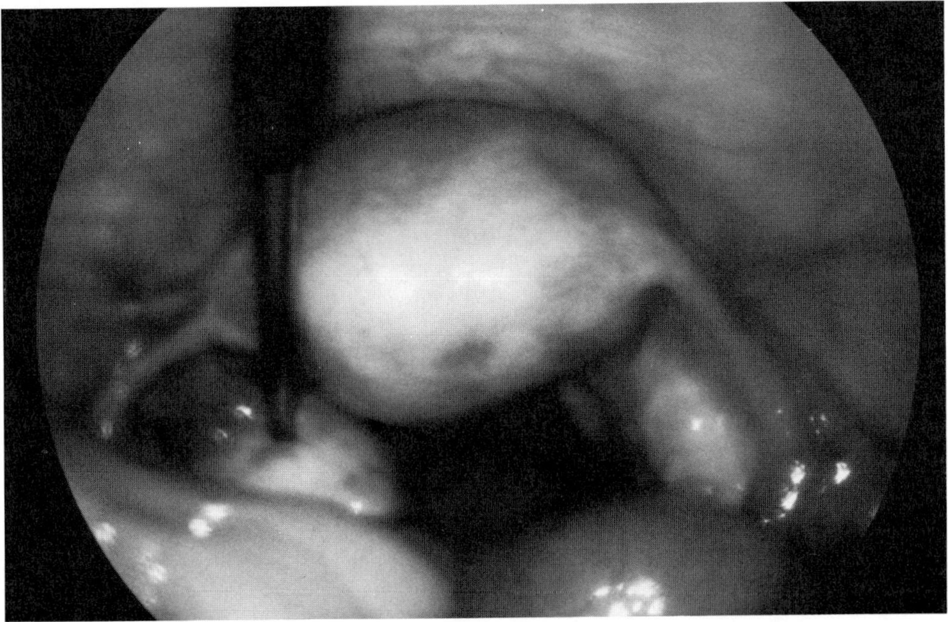

FIGURE 4–16. Laparoscopic view of the pelvis — 130 mm.

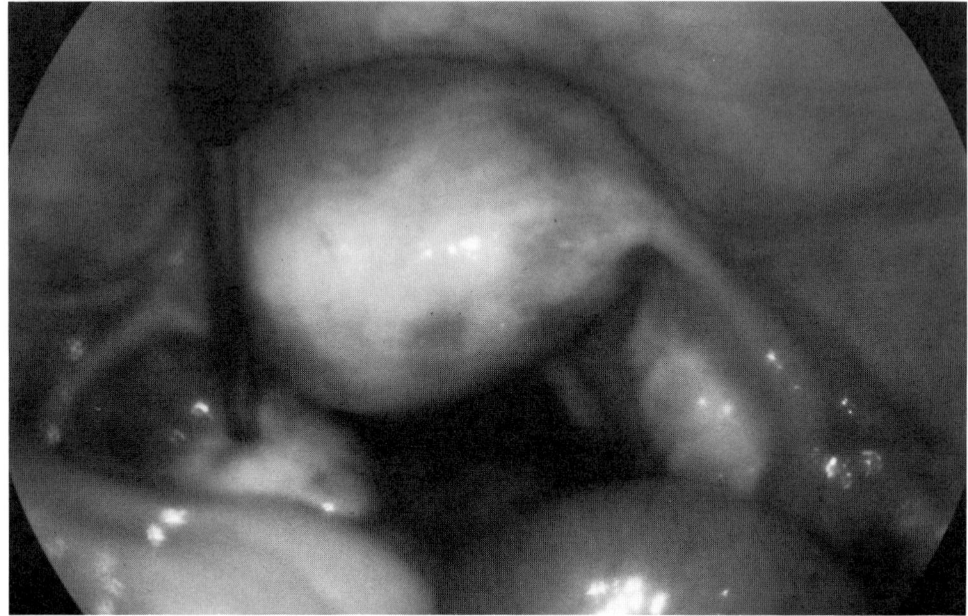

FIGURE 4–17. Laparoscopic view of the pelvis — 140 mm.

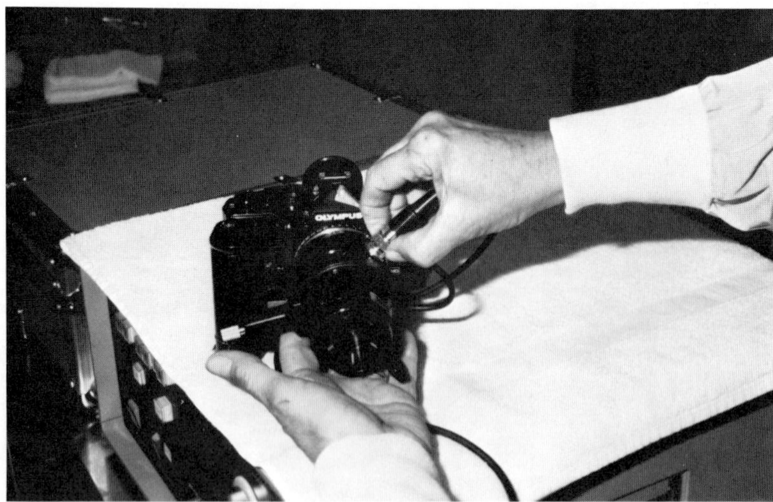

FIGURE 4–18. A photographic assistant assures good contact with the electronic sensing cable.

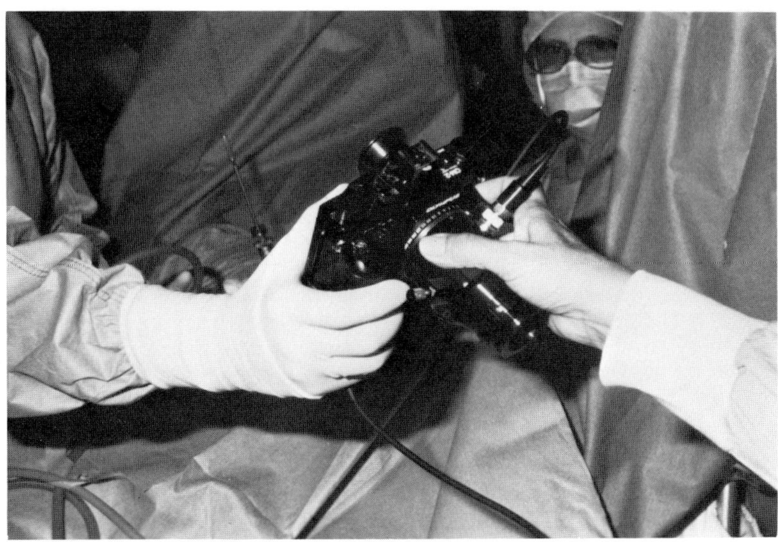

FIGURE 4–19. An assistant hands the camera to the laparoscopic surgeon.

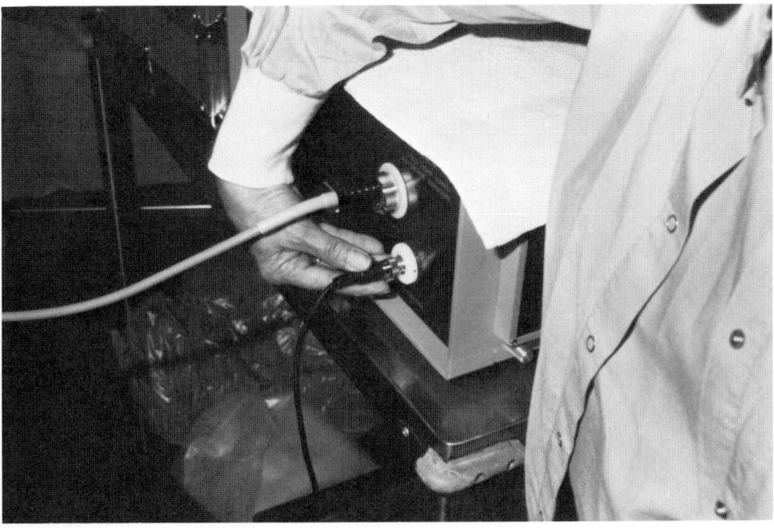

FIGURE 4–20. An assistant inserts the electronic cable into the flash generator.

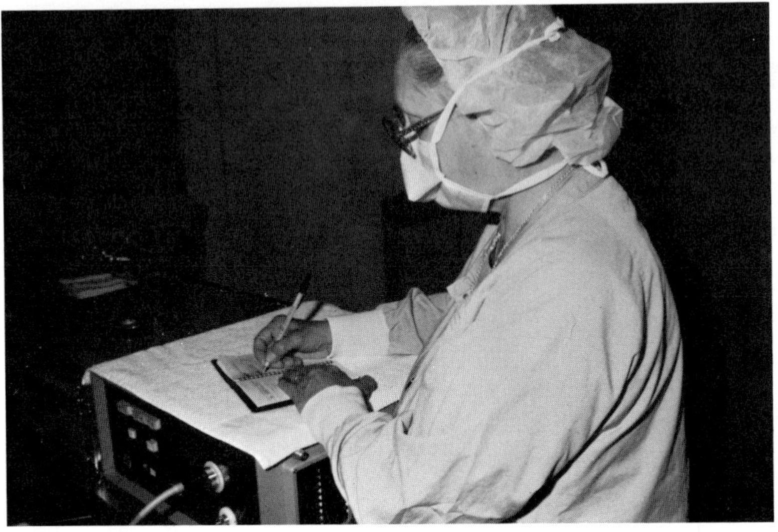

FIGURE 4–21. A photographic assistant records the appropriate settings in pictures for a patient.

Microscope/Colposcope

A beam splitter is required to direct the image to the camera as well as to the operator (Fig. 4–22). The Olympus OM-2N or OM-10 with a C-mount adapter is used in conjunction with a Sanyo remote-control transmitter and receiver (Fig. 4–23) to activate the shutter. Thus, the microscope is not subjected to jarring, which would be magnified through the optics and result in a blurred photographic image.

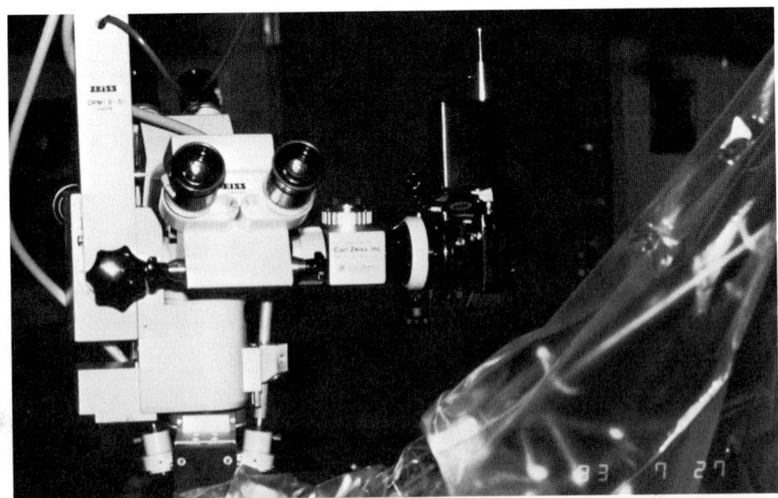

FIGURE 4–22. Olympus camera with a beam splitter and remote control attached to a Zeiss microscope.

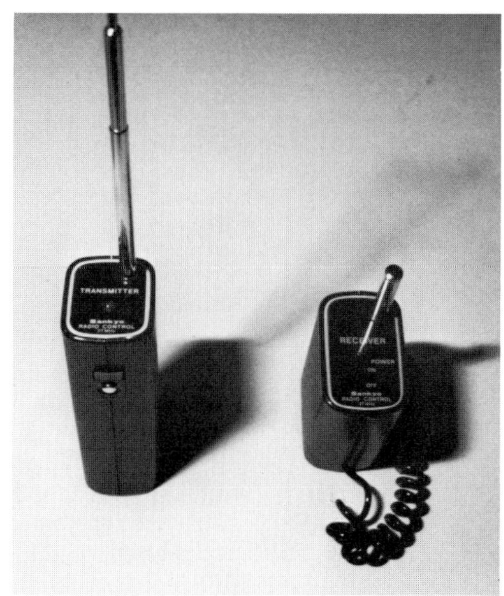

FIGURE 4–23. Sanyo remote-control transmitter and receiver used to activate the shutter for microscopic photography.

Filing

Slides may be developed at home or commercially, sorted on a light table (Fig. 4–24), categorized, and filed (Fig. 4–25). Polaprints may be made for the patient or chart (Fig. 4–26), or black and white prints may be made for publications (Fig. 4–27).

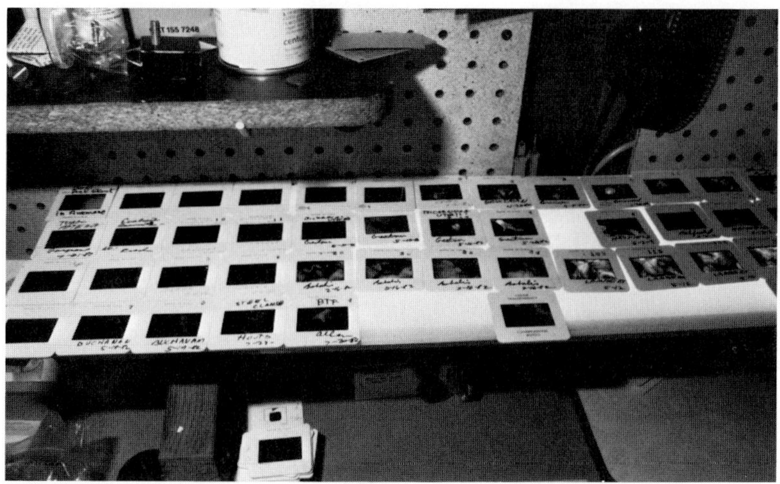

FIGURE 4–24. Slides to be sorted on a horizontal light table.

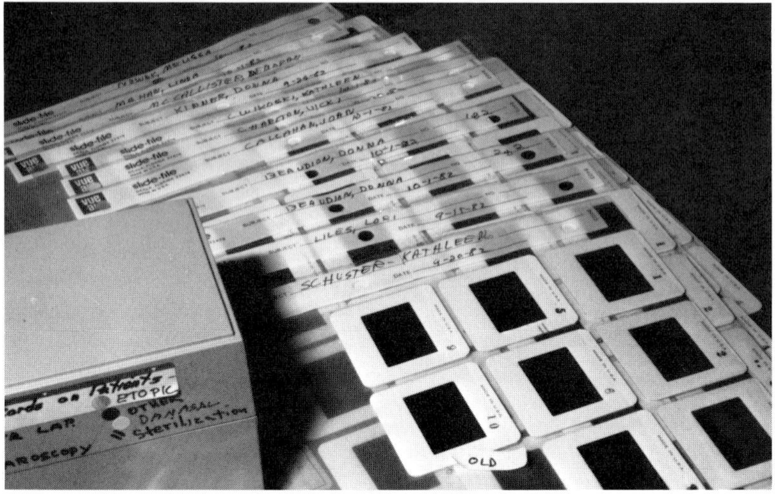

FIGURE 4–25. Slides categorized for filing.

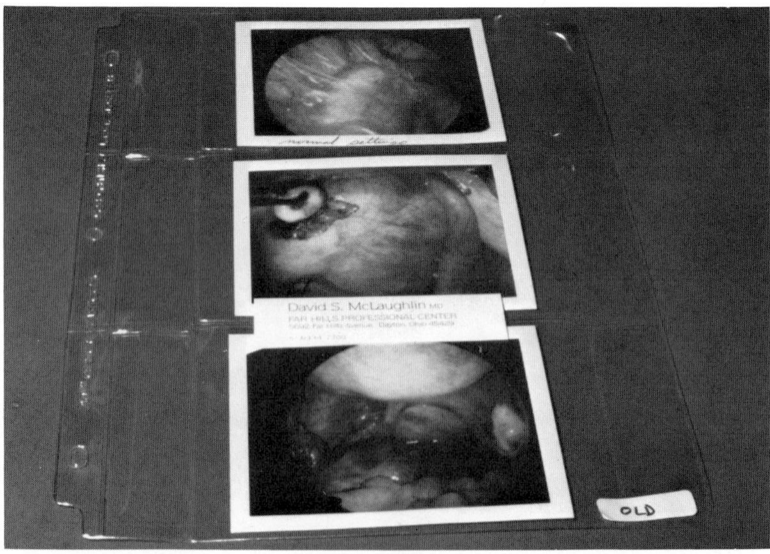

FIGURE 4–26. Polaprints made from slides for patient education.

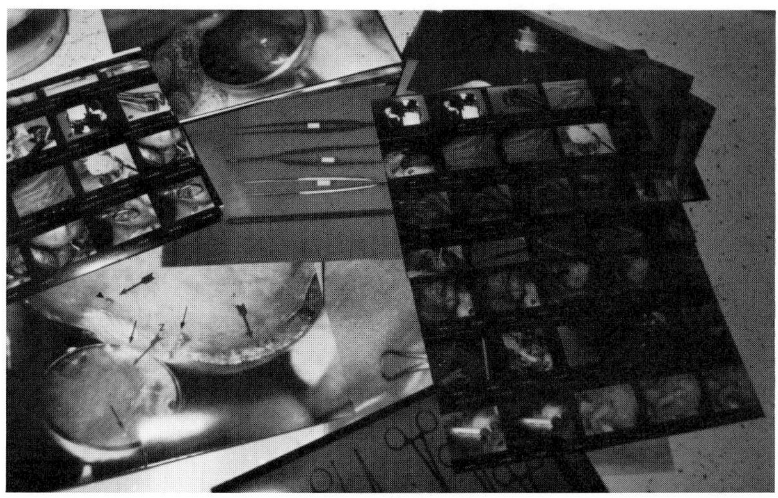

FIGURE 4–27. Black and white prints for publication.

Video

A video camera may be mounted to the microscope by means of a beam splitter (Fig. 4–28); however, the most common use for video in gynecology today is in conjunction with laparoscopy. Small CCD (charge couple device) chip cameras (Figs. 4–29 through 4–31) have revolutionized gynecological endoscopic photography. They may be coupled directly to the endoscope (Fig. 4–32), and a surgeon may perform endoscopic surgery indirectly by viewing the pelvic anatomy on a high-resolution video monitor (Fig. 4–33). Another common use is to couple the camera

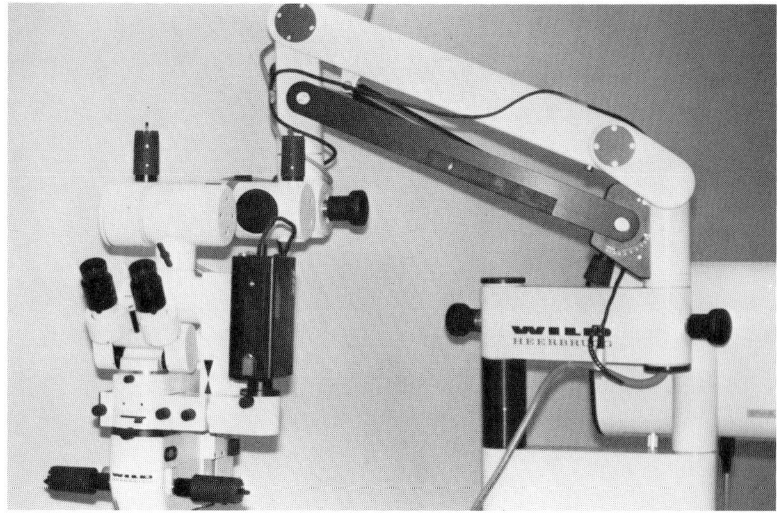

FIGURE 4–28. Microscopic video camera attached to a Wild microscope.

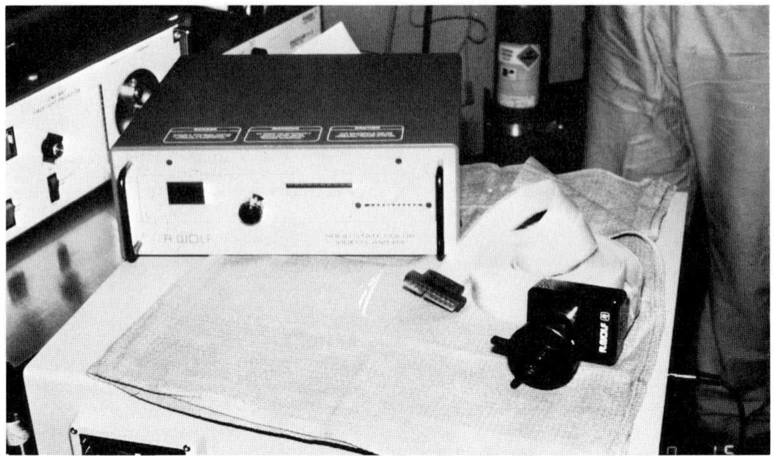

FIGURE 4–29. Wolf chip camera with a direct coupler.

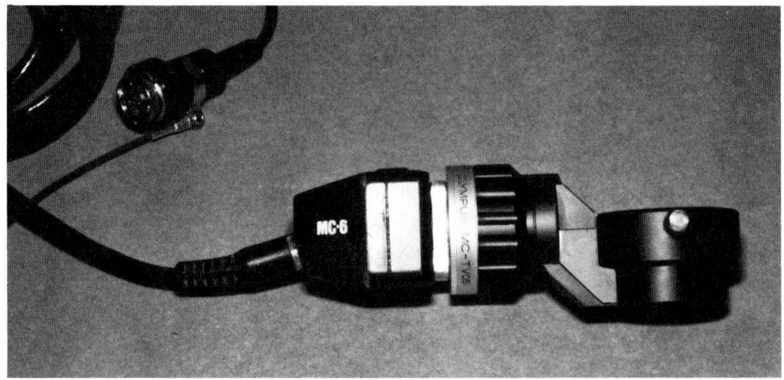

FIGURE 4–30. Olympus video camera with a beam splitter.

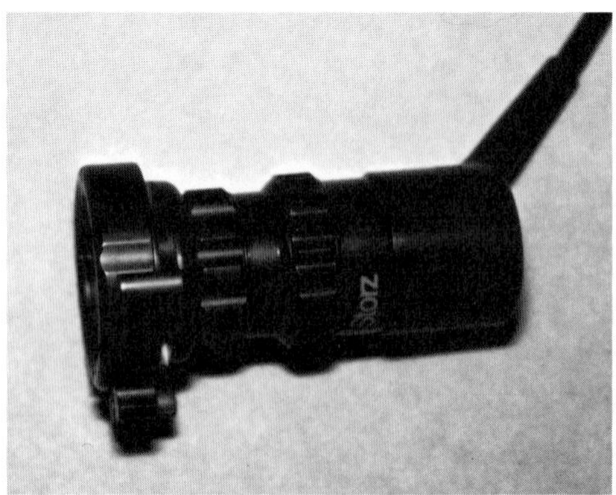

FIGURE 4–31. The most recent Storz chip camera with a direct coupler.

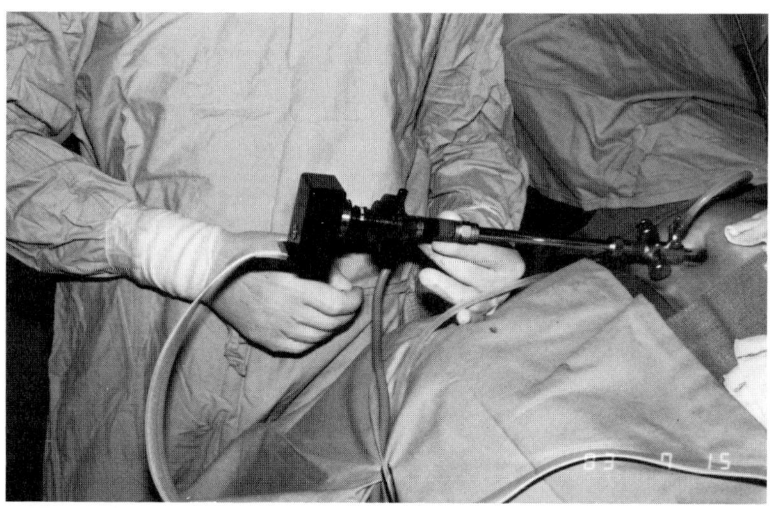

FIGURE 4–32. Wolf chip camera directly coupled to the laparoscope for video monitor viewing.

(Fig. 4–34) to a small beam splitter (Fig. 4–35) and attach it to the laparoscope (Fig. 4–36) for direct pelvic viewing by the surgeon (Fig. 4–37) while the operating room personnel observe the surgery on the video monitor (Fig. 4–38). Freeze-frame video image recording allows instant still photography from the monitor by Polaroid photography (Fig. 4–39) or electronic digitalization (Fig. 4–40).

The ease of video recording while simultaneously performing endoscopic surgery has popularized this method of photographic documentation. Patients are often pleased with the instant documentation of their procedure, which also allows for simultaneous audio narration to enhance patient education.

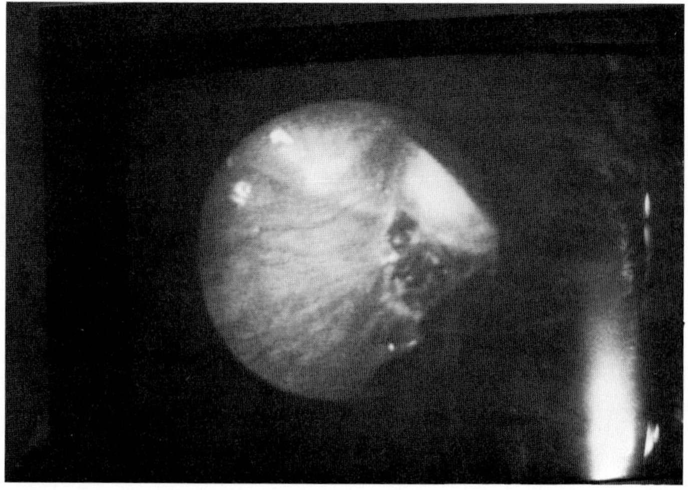

FIGURE 4–33. Video monitor displaying a laparoscopic image from the direct coupler.

(text continued on page 58)

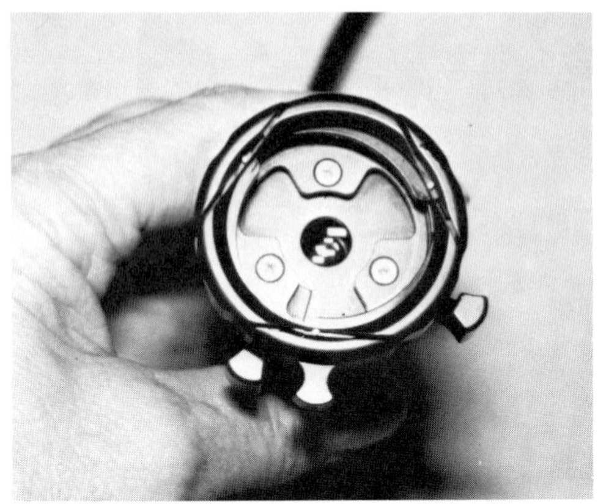

FIGURE 4–34. Storz chip camera that may be attached directly to the laparoscope or to a beam splitter.

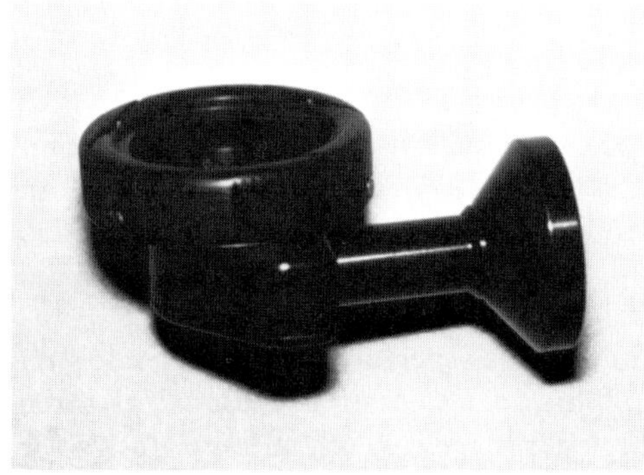

FIGURE 4–35. Storz video beam splitter.

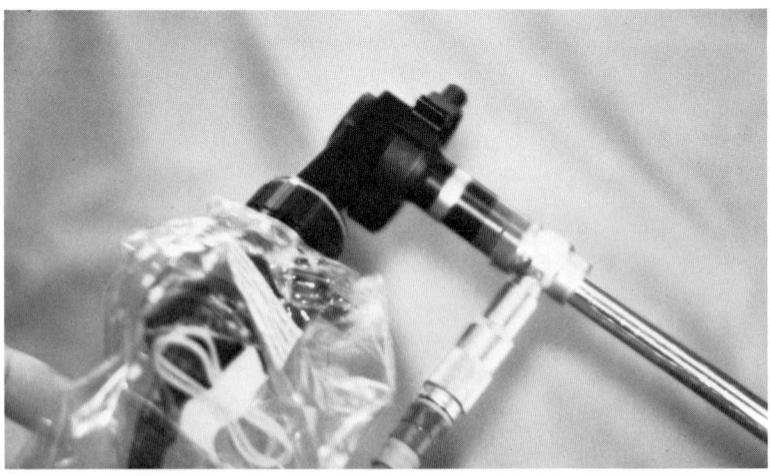

FIGURE 4–36. Olympus camera and beam splitter coupled to a laparoscope.

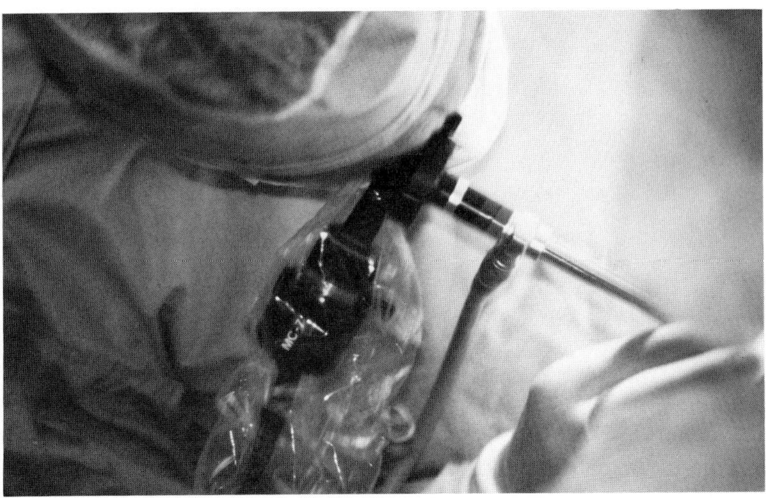

FIGURE 4–37. A surgeon's direct laparoscopic view of the pelvic viscera through the Olympus beam splitter.

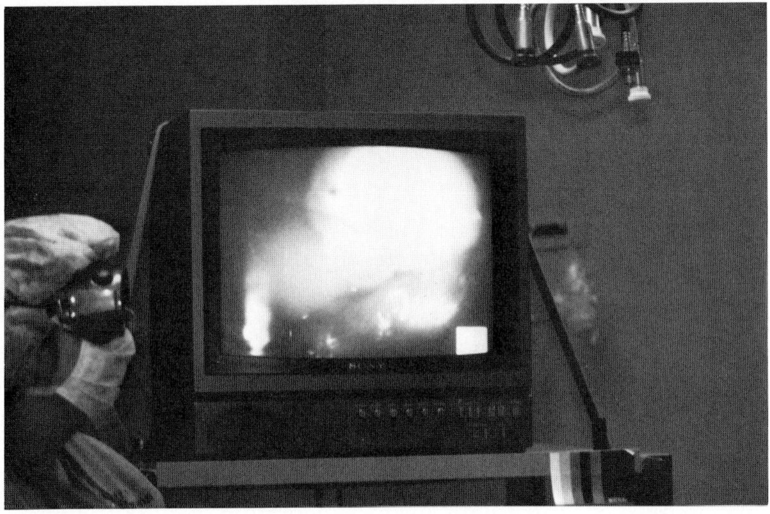

FIGURE 4–38. Operating room personnel observing laser laparoscopic surgery.

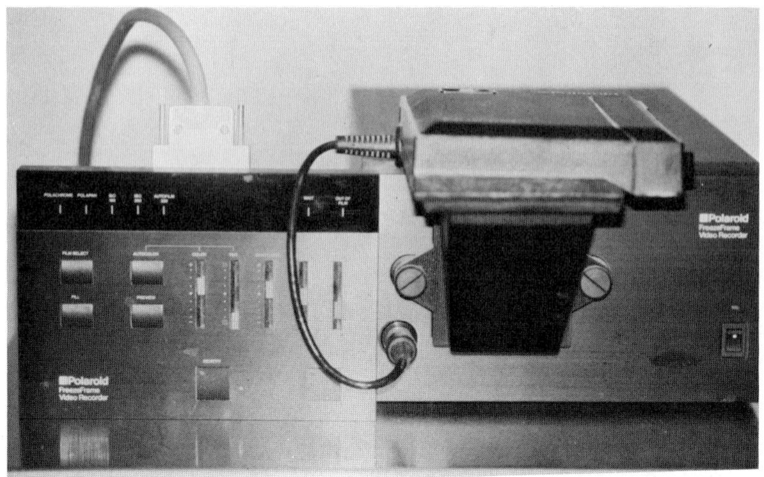

FIGURE 4–39. Polaprinter.

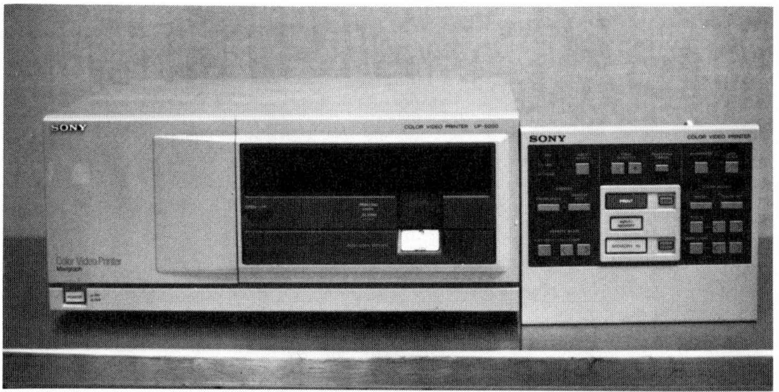

FIGURE 4–40. Sony Mavigraph.

SUMMARY

Gynecological photography adds an interesting dimension to a clinician's surgical armamentarium, whether it be through an endoscope, microscope, or second person (Table 4–4). By means of still or video photography, gynecological surgeons are able to continue to learn new techniques as well as to educate patients and health personnel (Table 4–5). Photographic documentation is becoming vital to survive in today's legal climate. Professor Kurt Semm has stated, "There is no other operative field in medicine in which photography and cinematography play the same essential role to introduce the methods into clinical practice, as has been the case for laparoscopy and pelviscopy."[7] Armed with adequate education, proper equipment, and a desire to succeed, almost any gynecologist should repeatedly be able to produce top-quality slides, prints, and videotapes.

TABLE 4–4
35-mm Photography

	LAPAROSCOPE/ HYSTEROSCOPE	MICROSCOPE/ COLPOSCOPE	SECOND PERSON
Camera	Olympus OM-2N, Auto-winder II, Recordadataback	Same	Same
Viewfinder	1-9 clear focusing screen	Same	T-12 micro/split image focusing screen
Film	ASA 200 or 400, daylight	ASA 160 Tungsten	ASA 200 daylight
Flash	NA	NA	Olympus T-32, Power Grip 2, TTL connector
Light source	CLE-F or CLV-10	NA	NA
Lens(es)	SLE-F or SLR-SN	Beam splitter with 250 and 300-mm lens	28 mm, 50 mm, zooms (30–70 and 80–200)
Cord	EC-24 or EC-30	NA	NA
Light cable	A 3062 with 5 mm condenser lens	NA	NA
Remote control		Sanyo transmitter/ receiver	

NA = not applicable.

TABLE 4–5
Video Recording Devices Used in Gynecology

	LAPAROSCOPE/HYSTEROSCOPE	MICROSCOPE/COLPOSCOPE
Camera	Olympus MC-7	Same
Beam splitter	Olympus AR-7F 2	Zeiss/Wild
Light source	CLV-10	NA
Monitor	Sony 20-inch video monitor	Same
Videocassette recorder	Panasonic no. 8950	Same
Videotape	Fuiji, 30 minute	Fuiji, 2 hour

NA = not applicable.

REFERENCES

1. Cohen MR: What's new in endoscopic still photography. J Reprod Med 29:589, 1984
2. Cos LR, Linke CA, Frank IN et al: Simplified new approach to endoscopic photography. Urology 21:410, 1983
3. Gingell JC, Sweet W, Bowyer N: Low cost endoscopic photography. Br J Urol 56:442, 1984
4. Gow JG: The evolution of modern endoscopic photography. Eur Urol 10:133, 1984
5. Marlowe JL: Endoscopic photography. Clin Obstet Gynecol 26:359, 1983
6. Marlowe JL: Hysteroscopic photography. In Baggish MS, Barbot J, Valle RF (eds): Diagnostic and Operative Hysteroscopy, A Text and Atlas, ed 1. Chicago, Year Book Medical Publishers, 1989
7. Semm K: Operative Manual for Endoscopic Abdominal Surgery, ed 1, p 242. Chicago, Year Book Medical Publishers, 1987

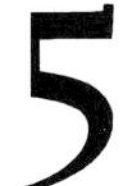

5

Laser Training

William M. Jamieson

The first use of the CO_2 laser was reported in 1967.[10] Since that time, an explosion in surgical uses and technology has taken place. In 1973, Kaplan and colleagues[9] were the first to report using the laser for cervical erosion. Bellina[1] reported its use intra-abdominally in reconstructive pelvic surgery in 1977. Laparoscopic use of the CO_2 laser was subsequently introduced by Bruhat and colleagues,[2] Daniell and associates,[4] and Tadir and co-workers.[15]

Newer lasers for gynecological use have also been developed. Among the more popular lasers in gynecological use today are the argon laser, popularized by Keye and colleagues,[11] and the Nd:YAG laser, pioneered by Goldrath and associates.[7] With new lasers and technical advancements developing so rapidly, it is of utmost importance for today's gynecologists to be well trained in their uses and have a proper understanding of their different roles in the surgical setting.

Laser surgery is a new concept for most gynecologists because it often involves operating with a "no-touch" technique. Cutting without resistance requires developing new skills, which in turn requires new educational training techniques. Because most of these surgical concepts have only been developed within the past 5 to 6 years, teaching these techniques at the residency level is at this time both unpredictable and in most cases inadequate. Surgeons, old and new alike, must seek proper training before they can consider themselves laser surgeons. Proper use of the laser can result in a dry surgical field, reduced blood loss, reduced edema, limited scarring and stenosis, greater precision, reduced postoperative pain (selectively) and shorter hospital stays. Improper use of lasers potentially may result in recurrence of disease, excessive thermal necrosis, scarring, and greater pain for the patient.

With such a fine line between successful laser surgery and disaster, it is therefore imperative that interested surgeons devote the proper amount of time and effort to understanding and mastering this new technology.

BASIC PROGRESSION FOR LASER TRAINING AND SELECTION OF THE FIRST LASER COURSE

Of prime importance in the training of a laser surgeon is an interest in learning a new surgical technique and its appropriate applications to gynecological surgery. Interested gynecologists should begin by learning the language of lasers. This is best accomplished by subscribing to the various laser specialty journals and reading books relating to laser surgery, such as this one. They should have a basic understanding of how lasers differ from the surgical knife and cautery and should appreciate the differences between lasers and their tissue interactions through introductory reading.

Understanding basic physics as applied to light energy is imperative. To use lasers without understanding their physical properties is like performing traditional surgery without knowing anatomy—both may lead to disastrous outcomes.

It should be readily apparent from the literature that the laser is an instrument not a technique, but the proper applications of this instrument require surgical techniques that are alien to most surgeons. With the carbon dioxide (CO_2) laser, cutting tissue without feeling resistance is at first difficult. The proper use of this laser requires the use of high power densities, which in turn requires a speed and eye-hand coordination that is not normally needed for traditional surgery. Even the use of the fiberoptic technology for the argon, KTP, and Nd:YAG lasers, which sometimes touch the tissue, requires that the surgeon let the laser instrument do the work and not apply excessive pressure to the fiber.

It should become readily apparent that the surgical tissue effects are more visual than sensual with any laser. If surgeons try to use these new instruments in the same fashion that they use a knife or cautery, the advantages of the laser will be lost.

Selection of the first laser course is critical because the course should fit a physician's needs as well as meet his or her expectations. For first-time attendees, the course should be from 14 to 16 hours in length. The didactic lecture portion of the course should include basic laser physics and safety precautions. A discussion of laser physiology emphasizing the unique qualities of laser light and its tissue interactions should also be part of a good basic laser course. Finally, the didactic portion of the course should have appropriate clinical lectures on how the laser is used to better treat gynecological diseases. Comparisons of treatments and results should be included. If a physician has no prior experience with lasers, he or she should choose a basic course that emphasizes the use of hand-held lasers in its laboratory session. Basic does not mean short. The selection of any laser course should be based on not only the faculty giving the course but also on the amount of time allowed for hands-on instruction in the laboratory. Any laser course that does not have a laboratory session should be viewed as informational only and not as a credentialing course. A practical guide for a proper hands-on laboratory would be 2.5 hours in the laboratory for every type of laser discussed in the didactic portion of the course. According to the American Society for Lasers in Medicine and Surgery, approximately 50% of the course should be devoted to hands-on laboratory exercises.

The hands-on experience should involve no more than three physicians to a laser, thus assuring the participants adequate time to practice their techniques and understand the principles discussed in the didactic session of the course. There should also be one expert laser monitor for every three attendees during the hands-on laboratory. If these guidelines are not followed, participating physicians will not be able to adequately visualize the principles that are so important in continuing their laser education.

Finally, the broadening of endoscopic laser surgery in gynecology requires physicians to work in small areas, often with multiple instruments. This spacial confinement can be compounded by a limited visual field that is often not viewed in its true form because of colored lenses that are used to protect the operator's eye from the laser backscatter. (Endoscopic laser surgery should only be attempted by those gynecologists who have mastered traditional laparoscopic and hysteroscopic surgical procedures.) For these reasons, endoscopic use of lasers should be the final step in a laser surgeon's progressive education.

Although advanced laser surgery may not be for everybody, training in laser surgery should benefit all surgeons. A good course emphasizes precision, hemostasis, eye–hand coordination, and the delicate handling of tissues. Lasers will never completely replace traditional gynecological surgery, nor will they make a poor surgeon a good one, but re-emphasis of these surgical principles will benefit surgeons even if they find only occasional uses for the laser.

TRAINING WITH THE CO_2 LASER IN LOWER GENITAL DISEASES

The beginning course for gynecologists should be uses of lasers in lower genital disease. A prerequisite for laser use in the lower genital tract should be that the physician also be well trained in colposcopy. The greatest bulk of laser surgery being performed today for lower genital disease is with the CO_2 laser.

Often called the workhorse of lasers, the CO_2 laser is considered a precision surgical tool because of its high degree of soft-tissue absorption and limited peripheral damage. The CO_2 laser produces light in the infrared portion of the electromagnetic spectrum of 10,600 nm. Depending on the power densities used, its capabilities include excising, vaporizing, and coagulating tissue. It may provide hemostasis, but usually only in vessels less than 1 mm in diameter.

The depth of incision using the CO_2 laser is a function of both power density and time of application (speed of stroke). The lateral zone of necrosis with proper use and power densities should be less than 0.5 mm from the incision, compared with 5 to 10 mm with electrocautery. This precision, coupled with the sealing effects of the beam, produces minimal edema, scarring, and necrosis. Learning proper technique is essential for achieving these results.

A surgeon controls three parameters in CO_2 surgery:

1. Size of the beam (spot size).
2. Power (watts).
3. Time of exposure.

In the surgical laboratory of the laser course, physicians should experiment with these parameters and notice the subsequent effect on tissues. The depth of the cut with this laser depends on the wattage, spot size, and speed of the stroke. This feel and control of depth are only developed with practice.

Because some of the first uses of CO_2 lasers in gynecology were for lower genital diseases, it seems appropriate that gynecologists begin their laser training with a course demonstrating uses of the laser in cervical, vaginal, and vulvar diseases. The superiority of the CO_2 laser for cervical intraepithelial neoplasia and vulvar intraepithelial neoplasia[14,16] and condylomata[5] has been well established. The reason to start laser training with use on the lower genital tract is because the lesions are clearly visible and damage to other areas or organs is minimal. The physician has a clear view of the laser effects and can immediately correct any laser-related bleeding problems.

The laboratory portion of the laser course in treating lower genital diseases should include exercises that demonstrate the range and capabilities of the CO_2 laser. By using various inanimate objects and tissues, the exercises should demonstrate laser coagulation, ablation, and excision. Expertise should be gained by using the hand piece connected to the articulating arm of the laser. The goal of the laboratory exercises should be to develop the ability to cut and ablate tissue evenly and in a controlled fashion. As expertise is developed, higher power densities should be used in order to reduce lateral thermal damage and take full advantage of the principles of laser surgery (Figs. 5–1 and 5–2).

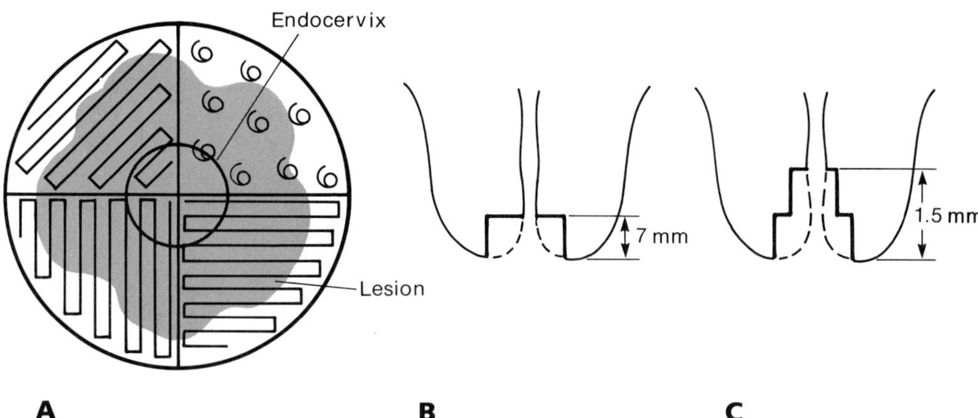

FIGURE 5–1. The technique of CO_2 laser cervical vaporization. (*A*) Vaporization. The CO_2 laser should first be attached to the colposcope through the micromanipulator. Then, using a piece of liver or cow tongue for practice, the trainee should mark a circular area into four quadrants. Next, using a comfortable power density, the trainee should practice smoothly lasering each quadrant using a repeat pulse. There should be no troughs or ridges at the completion of the exercise. Various cross-hatching techniques can be used, but the end result should be even, smooth ablation of the specimen. After control is established, the trainee should use a continuous-pulse mode and increase the power densities. Fine eye-hand coordination and speed are needed to accomplish the same precise surgical ablation with the higher power densities. (*B*) This diagram shows in cross section what the ablation procedure should finally look like. The trainee should strive for an even depth of 7 mm. (*C*) Once all four quadrants are finished using different techniques, attention is turned to the "endocervix." This should be ablated to a total depth of 1.5 cm. The base should be flat and even.

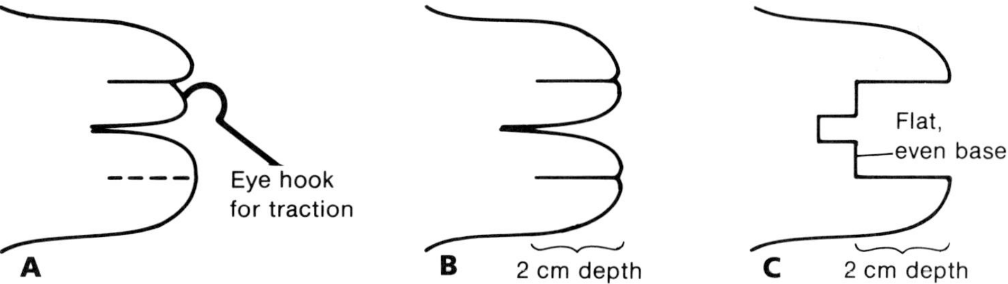

FIGURE 5–2. The technique of CO_2 laser cervical excision. (A) The CO_2 laser should be set at the smallest spot size and the highest power density that the trainee can control. Using the micromanipulator, outline the "lesion" leaving a 2-mm margin of normal tissue. Next, using an eye hook for traction, carry the incision to a depth of 2 cm circumferentially. The incisional planes should be parallel and clean, as seen in Figure 2B. Finally, as seen in Figure 2C, the cylindrical specimen should be excised from its apex using the laser beam perpendicularly. This exercise should then be repeated using the hand piece on the articulating arm of the laser. After removal of the specimen, the beam should be defocused to coagulate the base of the excision.

THE PRINCIPLE OF POWER DENSITY

Surgeons who understand power density understand the laser and are well on their way to becoming successful laser surgeons. We know the following from basic physics:

$$\text{Power density (PD)} = \frac{\text{watts} \times 100}{\pi r^2} = \text{watts/cm}^2$$

Therefore, the surface area of the spot (beam) and the power (watts) of the laser determine the power density of the laser. This is true of all lasers, not just the CO_2 laser. Both the spot size and the wattage are controlled by the surgeon. The wavelength of the light and the lens focal length determine the size of the spot. All other things being equal, the smaller the wavelength, the smaller the size of the spot. But even though an argon or Nd:YAG laser may have smaller spots, lasers should be chosen for their tissue effects rather than for their spot size.

The other determinant of spot size is the focal length of the lens. The smaller the focal length, the smaller the spot size.

Applying these simple principles allows surgeons to understand and equate the power density.

Let's look at an example. Calculate the power densities (PD) when one surgeon uses 30 watts of power and a 1-mm spot size and another surgeon uses the same 30 watts of power but a 2-mm spot size:

$$\text{PD} = \text{watts/cm}^2$$

$$\text{Surgeon 1: PD} = \frac{30 \text{ watts}}{0.1 \text{ cm}^2} = 3000$$

$$\text{Surgeon 2: PD} = \frac{30 \text{ watts}}{0.2 \text{ cm}^2} = 750$$

What is readily apparent is that doubling the spot size but maintaining the same wattage reduces the power density four times. Conversely, to obtain the same power density at one half the spot size means reducing the wattage by a factor of four.

Surgeon 1, although using the same wattage on the laser machine as surgeon 2, is getting a much more precise and effective use of the laser. Surgeon 1's tissue effect will show histologically far less lateral necrosis and edema than will surgeon 2's.

The principle to learn is that cleaner surgical incisions and vaporization are achieved by using higher power densities for shorter duration rather than lower power densities for longer periods. Surgeons should strive for controlling the highest power density that they can. This requires speed and superb eye-hand coordination, which is only achieved through persistent practice.

AFTER THE COURSE—A PRECEPTORSHIP

It is important that physicians begin to apply their knowledge soon after the first laser course. If much time elapses after a laser course, physicians forget the learned principles and techniques. Just because a physician has taken a laser course, it doesn't mean that he or she is qualified to begin using lasers clinically. Experimentation with laser techniques should always take place in the laboratory with inanimate objects. Although the number of precepted cases for credentialing varies from hospital to hospital, most good hospital credentialing committees require the surgeon to have a preceptorship with another physician who has had more laser experience. If no physicians at the hospital perform a particular type of laser surgery, then a recently trained surgeon has to seek out a preceptorship in another locale. As recommended by the American Society for Lasers in Medicine and Surgery, individual physicians should have a minimum of 6 to 8 hours of observation and hands-on involvement with the more experienced operator. After concluding this prescribed preceptorship, a surgeon should apply to the credentialing committee for laser privilege for the particular laser surgeries learned.

This educational triad of didactic material, hands-on laboratory experience, and preceptorship training should be required for all surgical lasers. These criteria should be strictly enforced before any new surgical laser or new procedure is used by a physician in an operating room. This sequence of training and credentialing protects physicians, hospitals, and most importantly patients from incompetent use of this rapidly developing and unique technology.

SECOND LEVEL OF LASER EDUCATION— USING LASERS ENDOSCOPICALLY

Several lasers are now being used in conjunction with the laparoscope and hysteroscope. Laparoscopic use of the CO_2 laser was first reported in 1979 by Bruhat and colleagues,[2] and since that time use of the CO_2 laser laparoscope has become widespread. Numerous investigators in this country have reported it to be safe and effective when using it to treat various gynecological conditions.[3,4,6,13]

Endometriosis continues to be the main disease treated laparoscopically by the CO_2 laser. Gynecologists now have the ability to treat the disease immediately at the time of diagnostic laparoscopy. This offers tremendous advantages to the patients in terms of both cost and disability. Subsequent pregnancy rates and relief of pain have also been shown to be equal or superior to other forms of surgical or hormonal therapies.[6,12]

Although the CO_2 laser laparoscopy system presents several problems and frustrations, it remains the most commonly used laser for laparoscopic surgery. Its continued use and popularity are due to its versatility and reliability. For these reasons, it is suggested that the first laparoscopic laser course chosen by physicians be one that emphasizes use of the CO_2 laser.

Before attending the first course in laser laparoscopy, certain prerequisites should first be met. As previously discussed, physicians should be expected to have some knowledge of lasers from a course in laser treatment of lower genital diseases. Also, they should have gained some practical experience with laser use not only in lower genital disease, but also intra-abdominally by using the hand piece. Finally, laparoscopic laser use should only be attempted by those physicians who have demonstrated abilities with advanced non-laser laparoscopic surgery. Such procedures should include performing operative laparoscopic surgery with multiple puncture sites, using electrocautery, scissors, and forceps. Performing routine sterilization procedures should not be considered advanced laparoscopic surgery.

Selection of the laser laparoscopy course should again be based on the experience of the faculty and the amount of time devoted to a hands-on laboratory experience. This laboratory session should devote most of its time to using the laser in conjunction with a laparoscope by demonstrating its use of both single- and double-puncture laser laparoscopy. Both inanimate objects and animal models should be used to simulate the actual clinical procedures during the laboratory session. Physicians should gain experience using multiple puncture sites while noting the tissue effects of the different power densities and modes of delivery, including superpulse (Fig. 5–3).

THE PRINCIPLE OF SUPERPULSE AND ITS USE IN LASER LAPAROSCOPY

Although the superpulse modality has been available on several CO_2 lasers for years, gynecologists have just recently discovered the advantages of its uses. A thorough understanding of this mode of operation adds an entirely new dimension to the surgical application of the CO_2 laser.

The precision of a CO_2 laser is determined by the degree of thermal spread from the CO_2 laser's point of impact. The greater the heat spread, the greater the destruction and the hemostatic properties of the laser but the less precision. Using low powers for long periods of time causes heat buildup in the form of carbon. Cleaner surgical vaporization with the laser can be achieved by using higher power densities for shorter periods of time. For most surgeons, the problem with using

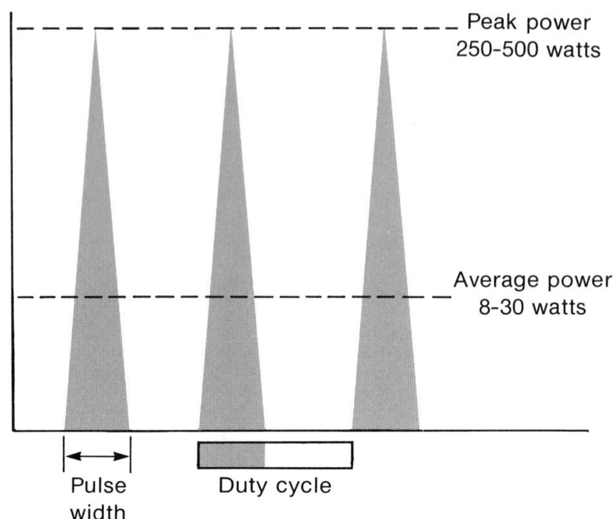

FIGURE 5–3. The superpulse mode. Although the laser beam is emitted the entire time the foot pedal is depressed, the laser energy is actually cycling on and off at a rate of up to 1000 times per second. This high energy output (peak power) with the cooling in between (duty cycle) gives the surgeon the most effective use of the CO_2 laser—high precision, minimal lateral damage, and a predictably controlled beam.

high power densities is control. High power densities when used for longer periods may get out of control and cause direct thermal damage. The answer is, of course, high power densities for short durations that can be controlled by using short pulse times that allow cooling in between "laser bursts." It is this mode of delivering high power densities for short pulses that is called superpulse. It provides surgeons with the greatest precision and least thermal destruction of any of the laser delivery systems.

Although the *peak* power of the superpulse mode is 250 to 500 watts, the *average power* is 8 to 30 watts depending on the specific CO_2 laser being used. Therefore, the superpulse mode results in less thermal destruction and carbonization, which in turn creates less smoke plume. Less thermal destruction and carbonization also lead to a lessened probability of adhesion formation. This advantage is particularly important in infertility surgery. The less smoke produced, the greater the visibility in the surgical field, and thus the more rapidly the procedure progresses. Concomitantly, the lower average power density slows down the speed of making an incision and, therefore, allows cutting to be more controlled by the operator. The result is more precise excision of tissue. For gynecologists performing laser surgery, a thorough understanding of these principles is important.

COMMON PROBLEMS
OF CO$_2$ LASER LAPAROSCOPY
AFTER THE INITIAL TRAINING

After attending a laser course on laser laparoscopy, newly trained physicians are often surprised to discover that they must overcome many minor frustrations before they can become accomplished and confident laser laparoscopic surgeons. The courses for the most part have the same didactic material, and the procedures seem rather straightforward until physicians attempt their first "solo case." Correcting some of these common problems and pitfalls of CO$_2$ laser laparoscopy can make the difference between an accomplished surgeon and a hopelessly frustrated one.

KNOWLEDGE OF EQUIPMENT

The first goal of the beginning laser laparoscopist should be to *know the equipment* that is being used and to know how to troubleshoot if a problem develops in the operating room. Although the technology of lasers and the ancillary equipment may be sophisticated, these devices are built to withstand the rigors of constant daily use. Seldom is the problem strictly within the laser equipment being used. Most often the problems encountered are the result of improper use of the equipment by a physician or nurse.

Laser surgery, more so than with traditional gynecological surgery, requires that the operating room be staffed with well-trained and dedicated personnel. Registered nurses and technicians who work in laser surgery should be hand-picked and extensively trained in courses similar to those attended by physicians. Most hospitals designate a nurse to be the laser coordinator in the operating room. It is this person's responsibility not only to maintain all the laser equipment, but also to troubleshoot if problems arise during laser use.

Even if the hospital has a laser coordinator, it still behooves physicians to be equally knowledgeable about the equipment being used.

The Laser
Regardless of the type of laser being used, physicians should know the basics of the laser machine. With regard to the CO$_2$ laser, physicians should know how to start the machine, the maximum wattage of the machine, and how to set the machine for the desired wattage and mode of delivery. In addition, physicians should be able to correctly focus the helium–neon beam as it exits the articulating arm.

The Laser Laparoscope
Single-puncture laser laparoscopes all are approximately 10-mm operating laparoscopes with smaller operating channels (5 to 7.5 mm). (The equipment made by various manufacturers is rarely interchangeable, with sizes varying up to 1 mm in diameter.) The operating channel is used for either the delivery of instruments, such as forceps, or for the delivery of the beam from the CO$_2$ laser. When surgeons use the laser, they simply attach the articulating arm of the CO$_2$ laser to the operating

laparoscope, which has been fitted with a special coupler that contains a mirror and a focusing lens. Using the CO_2 laser through the operating channel of the laparoscope allows a surgeon to aim the CO_2 laser with its helium–neon aiming beam directly on the targeted tissue in the abdomen. A suprapubic probe is also placed in the abdomen to vent off the accumulated plume and irrigate the vaporized tissue.

The advantages of single-puncture laser laparoscopy are its ease of use and the avoidance of multiple probes in the abdomen. For beginning laser laparoscopists, this is the easiest way to start and is effective in most gynecological cases. However, more advanced laser laparoscopy often requires the use of second-puncture probes, which have shorter focal lengths, smaller spot sizes, and thus are capable of higher power densities. Because these instruments have a larger internal diameter (6 to 8 mm), it is easier to maintain a proper beam alignment. By using these second-puncture probes, surgeons are able to cut more precisely and excise tissue, as is often needed in more advanced cases.

Incorrect abdominal placement of the second-puncture laser probe is a pitfall that should be avoided. Placement too low in the abdomen renders the laser unable to reach the cul-de-sac and deep pelvic structures. Placement too high causes the infamous "clashing of swords" as the operating laparoscope and the second-puncture laser probe constantly run into each other. The optimum placement is approximately one third the distance from the pubic symphysis to the umbilicus and about 2 cm off the midline (Fig. 5–4).

Insufflation Machine with Electrocautery

During laser surgery, it is not uncommon to use 30 L or more of CO_2 to maintain an adequate pneumoperitoneum. This is the result of the frequent evacuation of the smoke plume that is created with tissue vaporization. To decrease the length of the overall procedure, a *high-flow* insufflator should be used. These machines should deliver a minimum of 3 L of CO_2 per minute. Newer electronic automatic high-flow insufflators have recently been developed; they are able to deliver up to 6 L of CO_2 per minute and maintain constant intra-abdominal pressure automatically. Newer developments such as these should not only decrease the time for most CO_2 laser laparoscopy procedures, but should make them safer as well.

It is important to remember to attach the tubing from the high flow CO_2 insufflator to the *outer channel* of the operative laparoscope as opposed to attaching it to the trocar channel sleeve. This constant high flow infusion of CO_2 prevents the laser plume from condensing on the laser laparoscope coupling lens, which could obscure the helium–neon aiming beam and thus render the laser useless.

Electrocautery should be available before initiating any laser laparoscopy procedure. As surgeons gain experience and confidence, they will attempt more difficult cases, and the risks of bleeding will likely increase. The availability of cautery for hemostasis is important, due to the relatively poor coagulation properties of the CO_2 laser.

Finally, laparoscopic surgery should not be started without proper consent, including the possibility of open laparotomy. If bleeding is not able to be controlled with electrocautery or if injury to bowel or bladder is suspected, then a surgeon must immediately perform open laparotomy. Discussing the special risks of laser

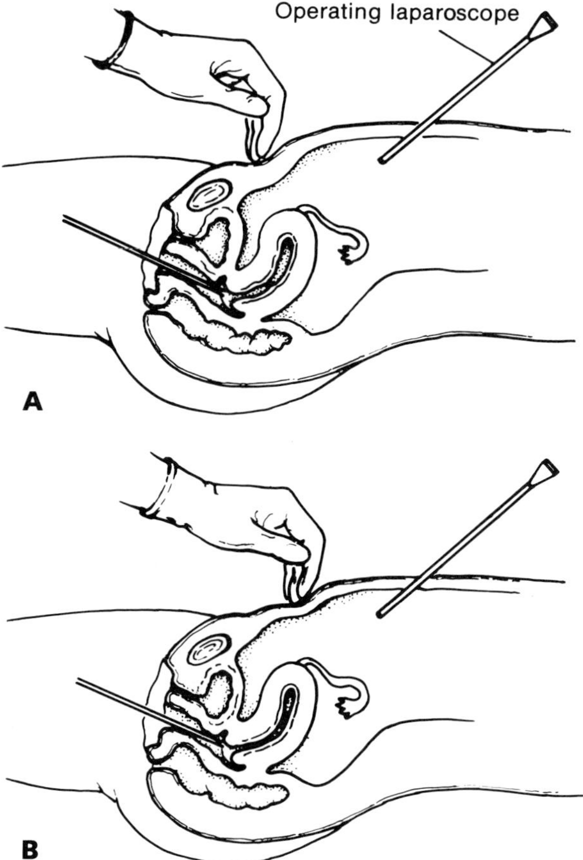

FIGURE 5–4. Abdominal placement of multiple probes when using the CO_2 laser. Advanced cases using the CO_2 laser require a minimum of three abdominal punctures. Proper placement of these instruments is crucial for success with this surgery. (*A*) The proper position of the suprapubic suction-irrigation probe: midline 2 inches above the symphysis pubis. (*B*) The proper position of the second puncture laser: one-third the distance between the symphysis and the umbilicus and 2 cm off the midline.

surgery and obtaining proper consent for the possibility of laparotomy is imperative before the surgery is scheduled.

LOSS OF THE HELIUM-NEON BEAM

Probably two of the most frustrating aspects of CO_2 laser laparoscopy are the loss of the helium–neon beam and the collection of laser plume (smoke) in the abdominal cavity. These two problems are often related because the plume not only decreases a surgeon's visibility, but its condensation causes the inadvertent loss of the helium-neon beam during the procedure. Understanding these potential problems and knowing how to remedy them will decrease frustration as well as operating time. *The CO_2 laser should never be fired without clear visualization of the helium-neon beam.*

Before any CO_2 laser laparoscopy is begun, the nurse should check the beam alignment not only as it exits the laser articulating arm, but also through the laser laparoscope itself. Movement of CO_2 lasers from operating room to operating room often results in mirror misalignment in the articulating arm, which would require realignment by a laser technician. Once the helium–neon beam is focused and the joystick of the coupler is locked in place, readjustment is seldom needed. Loss of the helium–neon aiming beam after initial alignment is most often due to condensation, as previously mentioned. Attaching the CO_2 tubing to the outer channel of the laparoscope keeps the laser plume from rising out of the abdomen and entering the lens system of the coupling device. This technical error is the most common problem relating to loss of the helium–neon beam intraoperatively.

By reducing the laser plume in the abdomen, surgeons not only increase visibility but also reduce the likelihood of losing the helium–neon beam. In order to clear the plume as rapidly as possible, the suction–irrigation probe, which is introduced suprapubically, should be as close to the site of laser impact as possible. This keeps the plume from widely dispersing in the abdomen. Avoiding the direct lasering of irrigation fluid in the pelvis as well as the use of superpulse also reduce the production of laser plume and hence increase the operator's visibility and efficiency.

Loss of the beam is occasionally not due to fogging of the lens system. Once all the lenses have been checked for condensation and have been found to be clean, then realignment of the beam is in order. Manually realigning the knuckles of the articulating arm is often all that is needed to bring the beam back into focus. This can sometimes be accomplished easily by raising or lowering the column on the laser machine. If this fails to correct the problem, the laparoscope should be removed from the abdomen and the beam rechecked on a wet tongue blade. Failure to obtain a proper beam at this point requires unlocking the joystick and refocusing the beam.

TRAINING WITH THE USE OF FIBEROPTIC LASER SYSTEMS LAPAROSCOPICALLY: ARGON, KTP/532, AND Nd : YAG

Because of the mechanical problems sometimes associated with CO_2 laser laparoscopy, other lasers that can be delivered fiberoptically have been developed for use through the laparoscope. Fiberoptic delivery systems have many advantages over the CO_2 system. The use of a flexible fiber to deliver the laser energy eliminates much of the bulky, cumbersome equipment that is required for the CO_2 system. These laser fibers can often be more precisely and easily delivered to a lesion deep in the pelvis. Because less of the laser's energy is absorbed in water, less smoke is created; thus, the laser laparoscopic procedure can be accomplished more rapidly. Finally, because there are no mirrors in an articulating arm, there is no need to focus and realign the beam as has to be done with the CO_2 laser.

The fiberoptic lasers in use for gynecology today (argon, KTP/532, and Nd : YAG) all differ from the CO_2 laser regarding their tissue effects. Because of these lasers' unique properties, surgeons should undergo the same training process for these lasers as for the CO_2 laser. Special training courses are offered for these lasers, which should include adequate hands-on experience in the laboratory (at least 2½ hours per laser). The same educational triad of lecture, hands-on laboratory, and preceptorship should be followed.

Sapphire contact tips have been developed for use with the fiberoptic Nd : YAG laser. By attaching the contact tip to the Nd : YAG laser, the laser energy is focused more precisely and the backscatter (which may be 40% when using the bare fiber) is reduced to approximately 5%.[8] This allows safer use of the Nd : YAG laser when working through the laparoscope. Whereas other noncontact laser systems often must be positioned at awkward angles to impact the tissue at a 90-degree angle in order to achieve the desired tissue effect, this laser system actually touches the tissue at various angles. Power density is predictable, with a uniform tissue effect. If a bare quartz fiber contacts blood or tissue, the tip melts. It then becomes necessary to recleave and polish the fiber end. The new contact technique allows laser surgeons a tactile sense that is lacking with other laser systems. With these sculptured sapphire tips, the Nd : YAG laser is transformed into a multipurpose surgical laser that is able to cut as cleanly and precisely as the CO_2 laser yet retain the coagulative properties of the noncontact YAG laser.

TRAINING WITH THE CONTACT TIP Nd : YAG LASER

Only a few laser courses that teach gynecologists the use of the Nd : YAG laser delivered through contact tips are now offered. The course should emphasize the physical properties of this laser and demonstrate the tissue effects in the laboratory. The laboratory sessions should begin with the use of this laser through a hand piece and progress to its fiberoptic use laparoscopically and hysteroscopically. The laboratory exercises should demonstrate that the contact tips must be placed in direct contact with the tissue *before* the power is turned on and, most importantly, the power should be *kept on momentarily* while disengaging the tip from the tissue. The likelihood of the tissue sticking to the probe and causing inadvertent tearing or bleeding from the contact point is thus reduced. These unique properties and techniques must be practiced diligently in the laboratory before surgeons attempt their first case in the operating room.

These contact tips require either gas or water cooling and must be used only in direct contact with tissue, in order to avoid damage to the tips. This principle is exactly opposite to the recommended use of the other fiberoptic delivery systems, in which the operator should avoid touching the tissue.

The contact tips range in diameter from 0.2 to 1.2 mm. The geometric configuration of the sapphire tip and its diameter determine its power density and tissue effect. Depending on the tip used, cutting, coagulation, vaporization, and interstitial irradiation all can be accomplished with this laser. The training course should allow adequate time for physicians to use all the probes and observe the tissue effects of each. Even though powers less than 25 watts are recommended, one should realize that recommended power settings are of less importance than the actual observed tissue effect (Fig. 5–5).

Cutting. When using the contact probe for cutting, physicians may use the scalpel, conical, or chisel probe, taking care to understand that each has different spot sizes and energy distribution patterns. The technique of cutting with these probes is different from traditional surgery. While holding the tissue taut, a surgeon should lightly draw the sapphire tip across the surface of the tissue. If too much pressure is used, as when using a knife, there is a tendency to separate or tear the tissue—again losing the unique and beneficial effects of the laser. It is the laser energy, not the physical pressure of the sapphire tip, that creates the incision. Although incising with the contact tips may appear slow at first, the fact that small vessels are simultaneously being coagulated rapidly makes up for lost time. With this technique, damage to adjacent healthy tissue is reduced by up to 75%, along with tissue edema and postoperative pain.[8]

Coagulation. To demonstrate the coagulative properties of the contact laser probes, the participant physician should use the flat or frosted probes. These tips seal vessels up to 3 mm in diameter using powers less than 15 watts. To demonstrate the coagulative effects of these probes, live animal tissue must be used in the laboratory. The vessel should not merely be coagulated in one spot. The most effective method involves forming a rosette around the periphery of the bleeding vessel to first initiate edema (Fig. 5–6). Then the vessel is mechanically cut and coagulated using short pulses of energy.

Vaporization. When vaporization of tissue is required, as would be needed for endometriosis, higher power densities are used. The most effective

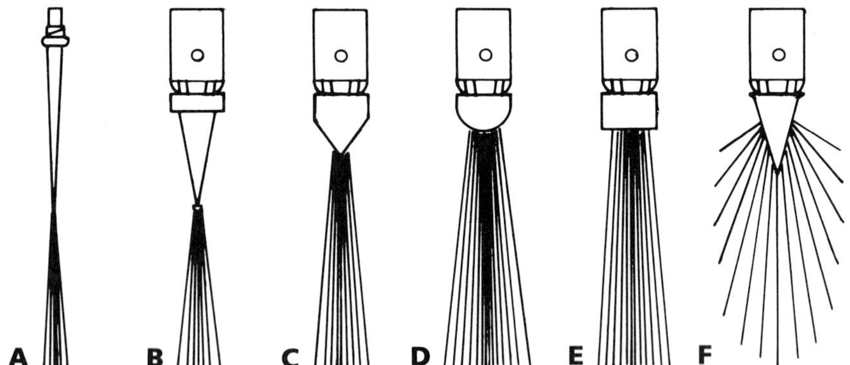

FIGURE 5–5. The various geometric configurations of the Nd : YAG contact sapphire tips produce different tissue reactions and can be interchanged for different gynecological conditions: A, Scalpel tip, for fine incisions. B, Cone tip, for excisional cone biopsies and lysis of intra-abdominal adhesions. C, Chisel tip, a multifaceted probe useful for incision, excision, and vaporization—an excellent tip for laparoscopic treatment of endometriosis. D, Round tip, for vaporization of vulvar condylomata and endometriosis. E, Flat tip, best for coagulation of vessels. F, Frosted tip, for coagulation and interstitial irradiation.

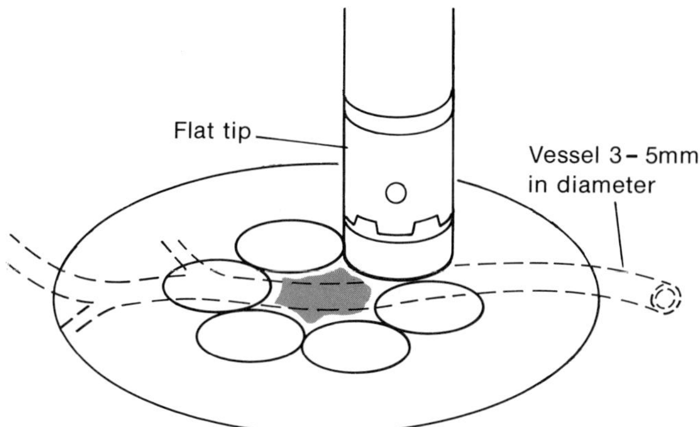

FIGURE 5–6. The best method for achieving hemostasis in large vessels when using contact sapphire tips is illustrated here. The flat or frosted tip delivers its energy in a rosette fashion, creating edema and partial coagulation before actually cutting the vessel.

probe for this is the rounded probe, which evenly disperses the Nd:YAG laser's energy and allows for rapid removal of tissue. The chisel or wedge probe may also be used for vaporizing when cutting is also desired.

Interstitial Irradiation. At the present time, the frosted probe is used for deep coagulation, but its major future applications may become the preferred delivery system for administering local hyperthermia and photodynamic therapy.

HYSTEROSCOPIC LASER TRAINING

For years, gynecologists were taught that the hysteroscope was an instrument waiting for an indication. With improved optics and illumination along with the advent of lasers, the waiting is over. Hysteroscopy has become popularized and has emerged as a widely used diagnostic and operative procedure in gynecology. No longer is it prudent to perform a "blind" dilatation and curettage. Additionally, several conditions that at one time required correction with laparotomy may now be safely and effectively treated by hysteroscopic surgery.

Common sense dictates that interested physicians first be skilled in using the diagnostic and operative hysteroscope before endeavoring to use lasers through the hysteroscope. Experience should be gained after attending a diagnostic and operative hysteroscopy course before seeking a laser hysteroscopy course.

Although any fiberoptic laser may be used hysteroscopically, thus far, only the Nd:YAG laser has been consistently and effectively used to treat several gynecological conditions. Goldrath and colleagues first described the effective use of the Nd:YAG laser by photoablating the endometrial cavity for intractable menorrhagia.[7] This procedure is rapidly becoming a viable alternative to hysterectomy in selected cases for women who wish relief from intractable menorrhagia. As the procedure becomes more widespread, it could potentially replace 30% to 40% of hysterectomies currently being performed. In addition to the ablation procedure, uterine septa and submucosal fibroids may easily and bloodlessly be resected through the hysteroscope.

Gynecologists who are interested in learning hysteroscopic laser surgery should seek a course that consists of a minimum of 8 to 10 hours with at least 50% of the time devoted to laboratory hands-on training. The laboratory session should allow participant physicians enough time to visualize the tissue effects unique to the Nd:YAG laser. The beam's backscatter effect must be emphasized and thoroughly understood by every participant. Proper eyepieces must be attached to the hysteroscope used in the laboratory exercises to protect against retinal damage from the backscatter effect of the YAG laser. The course should also provide each participant with an extirpated cow uterus in order to simulate an endometrial ablation procedure. After completion of the course, physicians should be precepted by a more experienced surgeon for a series of cases before credentialing by the appropriate hospital committees.

OVERCOMING COMMON PROBLEMS WITH Nd:YAG HYSTEROSCOPIC LASER SURGERY

After the initial training course and before physicians actually begin to perform the Nd:YAG laser photoablation procedure, they should understand some of the common problems and pitfalls that may be encountered with this unique type of surgery.

Anesthesia. Obviously, one of the most important aspects of any surgical procedure is anesthesia. In the ablation procedure, it is important, first of all, to keep the patient "dry" and not preload her with intravenous fluids. This is done to help reduce the risk of fluid overload, which is the most common complication of the procedure. Several anesthesiologists have observed that a narcotic anesthesia technique results in less fluid overload than does an inhalation anesthesia technique, which tends to produce uterine relaxation and vasodilation. The anesthesiologist should also be reminded to auscultate the patient's lungs periodically for possible fluid overload throughout the course of the procedure. The first sign of pulmonary edema often is decreased oxygen saturation noticed by the anesthesiologist. Nd:YAG endometrial photoablation has been performed under spinal or epidural anesthesia for those patients who are not candidates for general anesthesia, but again, caution should be exercised.

Positioning of the Patient. Patients should be placed in the dorsal lithotomy position with approximately 5% to 10% Trendelenburg. Their buttocks should extend over the edge of the table in order to facilitate the hysteroscopic maneuvering required to treat the entire endometrium. The table should be at a comfortable height so that the operator does not have to bend over for prolonged periods of time. Also, in order to facilitate movements during the procedure, a stool with rollers is used.

Draping the Patient. Because fluid overload and pulmonary edema can be complications of this procedure, it is important that all the infused fluid be accurately accounted for. This endeavor can be facilitated by appropriately draping the patient for meticulous fluid collection. The following draping technique has been found to be not only extremely efficient, but also very easy to perform for each surgery. Using standard urologic drapes, the following procedure is carried out: The first urologic drape is placed across the patient's sacrum and secured at the patient's hips. A standard dilatation and curettage preparation is then performed before continuing with the rest of the draping. The second urologic drape is next used to cover the patient's perineum close to the anus. The adhesive part of the drape is initially applied to the middle of the perineum and then laterally to the buttocks to avoid any open channels between the drape, which might allow fluid to escape onto the floor. Tincture of benzoin is often used over the perineum to secure a fluid-tight seal. Standard dilatation and curettage drapes are then used to cover the patient. The bottom of the drape is cut off, and finally the third urologic drape is placed—again first at the perineum—this time closer to the introitus and then secured laterally over the standard dilatation and curettage drape. If draping is properly carried out, all the fluid used to distend the uterus during the procedure will be suctioned into the collection bottles and will be readily accounted for at all times.

Transfusion Pump. In order to obtain proper distention of the uterus during the ablation procedure, lactated Ringer's solution, normal saline, or dextran is delivered through the hysteroscope under constant pressure by using a rapid transfusion pump. A 3000-ml bag of fluid is placed in the pump, and by stepping on the foot bulb, a constant flow of fluid is delivered at up to 150 mm Hg pressure. The operator is thus afforded excellent visibility as well as enough pressure to wash away any blood or debris that is created during the procedure. To avoid "down time" during the procedure, two of these pumps are used and are connected with a standard Y tubing. When this setup is used, the procedure never has to be interrupted in order to change fluid bags. This is important because when the procedure is stopped and the fluid is not running into the uterus, one loses the tamponade effect of the fluid that maintains visibility and avoids clots from forming in the uterine fundus. If the clots have to be removed through the hysteroscope, valuable time is lost during the procedure. It is not uncommon to use as much as 12,000 ml of fluid during the course of a single procedure. *Under no circumstances should operative hysteroscopic laser surgery be performed using coaxial CO_2 gas (to cool the fiber tip) because fatal air embolism can occur rapidly.*

The Surgical Laser. A Nd:YAG laser capable of producing 100 watts is recommended for this procedure. Although the procedure is normally performed using a power setting of 60 watts, the ability to deliver higher powers is often useful. A liquid-cooled, 600-micron silica-silica fiber 3 meters long delivers the laser energy. This silica cladding is much harder than standard silicone cladding and, therefore, reduces damage to the fiber as it is dragged across the endometrium. This feature is important because the less the fiber is damaged, the more predictable is the power output from the laser. The result is that the fiber has to be removed from the hysteroscope less frequently to be changed, so the procedure is accomplished more rapidly. The length of time the procedure takes is directly proportional to the amount of fluid absorbed by the patient. Therefore, anything that can be done to increase the speed of the operation without compromising technique reduces the patient's risk of pulmonary edema.

The Hysteroscope. The hysteroscope that is used is a dual-channel 7-mm hysteroscope. It allows the distending fluid to flow to and from the uterus through separate channels. Before the procedure is begun, the hysteroscope is measured 4 cm from the tip and marked with sterile tape. This safety measure informs the assistant when the operator is to the internal endocervical canal and that the endometrial ablative procedure is complete. At the tip, it may also have a flexible bridge that can be used to direct the fiber into difficult areas of the uterus.

Cervical dilatation is usually performed using progressive Hegar dilators to no. 9. The dilatation must be carefully performed to avoid uterine perforation and excessive bleeding from the endocervical canal. If perforation occurs, the procedure must be terminated. If cervical stenosis is discovered, laminaria tents may be used to slowly dilate the cervix to the proper diameter.

The operating room personnel are instructed to put protective eye wear on themselves and the patient. The surgeon then places a filtered eyepiece on the hysteroscope. The irrigation system and light source are then connected to the hysteroscope, and the uterine cavity is explored. The laser fiber is then threaded through the operating channel of the hysteroscope.

THE ABLATION PROCEDURE

Two basic types of surgical techniques can be used when performing the ablation procedure. The difference in the techniques is whether the laser is fired when the fiber is a few millimeters away from the tissue (noncontact technique) or touching it directly (contact technique). The contact technique appears to produce better results in terms of amenorrhea and is actually easier and faster to perform. The difference between treated and untreated endometrium is readily apparent.

A combination of the two techniques is usually used, depending on the area of the uterus being ablated. In medically compromised patients (*i.e.,* renal or heart disease), the noncontact technique certainly seems to be the more appropriate in order to minimize the risk of fluid overload and pulmonary edema.

The procedure should begin by identifying both tubal ostia and obliterating them. The fiber is subsequently repetitively withdrawn using either the noncontact or contact technique. *The laser should only be fired while the laser fiber is either stationary or being withdrawn from the uterine cavity and the helium-neon beam is clearly visible.* The possibilities of uterine perforation and inadvertent bowel or bladder damage are thus reduced.

Care must be taken when the ablation is being performed on the lateral side walls of the lower uterine segment and upper endocervical canal, where the cervical branch of the uterine artery is located. If too vigorous ablative technique is performed there, the resulting necrosis may cause either immediate or delayed hemorrhage. If heavy bleeding should occur, tamponading the endometrial cavity with an inflated 30-ml Foley balloon usually stops it.

The average fluid absorption is usually between 500 and 800 ml. The procedure should probably be terminated if greater than 2000 ml is absorbed or if rales are heard in the patient's lungs. In healthy patients, 40 mg of furosemide (Lasix) usually causes immediate diuresis.

CONCLUSION

It has been said that laser is to light what music is to noise. Gynecologists who wish to be successful in the applications of this new technology will train diligently and learn to orchestrate these subtle interactions of light and tissue. In so doing, they will create a successful harmony between their traditional surgical training and tomorrow's technology.

Physicians who follow a diligent basic program to learn laser surgery will find this new field not only challenging but also satisfying, in that they are able to offer their patients safe and effective state-of-the-art medicine.

REFERENCES

1. Bellina JH: Carbon dioxide laser in gynecology. Obstet Gynecol Ann 6:371, 1977
2. Bruhat MA, Mage G, Mahner M: Use of the CO_2 laser via laparoscope. In Kaplan I (ed): Proceedings of the Third International Congress for Laser Surgery, pp 271–273. Tel Aviv, 1979
3. Daniell JF, Brown DH: Carbon dioxide laser laparoscopic surgery; initial experience in experimental animals and humans. Obstet Gynecol 159:761, 1982
4. Daniell JF, Pittaway DE: Use of the CO_2 laser in laparoscopic surgery: Initial experience with the second puncture technique. Infertility 5:15, 1982
5. Ferenczy A: Treating genital condylomata during pregnancy with the carbon dioxide laser. Am J Obstet Gynecol 148(1):9–12, 1984
6. Feste JR: Laser laparoscopy: A new modality. Fertil Steril 41:745, 1984
7. Goldrath MH, Fuller TA, Segal S: Laser photovaporization of endometrium for the treatment of menorrhagia. Am J Obstet Gynecol 104:14, 1981
8. Joffee SN: Contact Nd : YAG laser surgery in gastroenterology: A preliminary report. Lasers Surg Med 6:155–157, 1986
9. Kaplan I, Goldman JM, Ger R: The treatment of erosions of the uterine cervix by means of the CO_2 laser. Obstet Gynecol 41:795, 1973
10. Ketcham AS, Hoye RC, Riggle GC: A surgeon's appraisal of the laser. Surg Clin North Am 47:1249, 1967
11. Keye WR Jr, Matson GA, Dixon J: The use of the argon laser in the treatment of experimental endometriosis. Fertil Steril 39:26, 1983
12. Martin DC: CO_2 laser laparoscopy for the treatment of endometriosis associated with infertility. J Reprod Med 30:409, 1985
13. Nezhat D, Trowgey SR, Garrison CP: Surgical treatment of endometriosis via laser laparoscopy. Proceedings of the Annual Meeting of the American Fertility Society, Chicago, 1985
14. Reid R: Superficial laser vulvectomy. Am J Obstet Gynecol 151(8):1047–1052, 1989
15. Tadir Y, Kaplan I, Zukerman Z et al: New instrumentation and technique for laparoscopic carbon dioxide laser operations: A preliminary report. Obstet Gynecol 63:582, 1984
16. Wright VC: CO_2 laser surgery for CIN. Lasers Surg Med 4:145–152, 1984

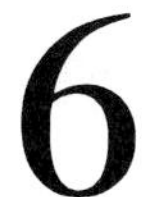

6

Credentialing of the Gynecologic Laser Surgeon

James H. Dorsey

Credentialing is the process by which a hospital grants permission to physicians or to appropriate health care professionals to perform surgery or administer specialized procedures involved in patient care. As health care providers, hospitals have a corporate responsibility to consumers (patients) to ensure that reasonable care has been exercised in the selection of physicians and other professionals who are practicing within its jurisdiction. In the specialty of obstetrics and gynecology, there are many procedures that vary in complexity, in frequency of use, and in the length of time required for physicians to achieve reasonable surgical skill and competency. For these reasons, hospital credentialing committees require staff physicians to review a list of accepted surgical procedures in their particular specialty and to supply justification of competency to perform those operations for which privileges are requested. This specific listing of surgical and other special procedures that physicians or health care professionals are allowed to perform in the hospital is referred to as the "delineation of privileges." The ultimate responsibility for credentialing rests with the governing board of the institution. Because this board is usually not composed of physicians, the responsibility is relegated to a committee of the medical staff, which then makes a recommendation to the board. Thus, the final credentialing decisions are actually made by a peer group of physicians.

RATIONAL APPROACH TO CREDENTIALING

It is necessary for the credentialing committee to develop objective criteria for credentialing and delineation of privileges. Objective criteria help minimize liability and provide a rational aid for departmental chairpersons and the credential board for decision making. The criteria also supply objective benchmarks to physicians who desire staff privileges. Certainly the burden of proof to demonstrate competency to perform special procedures rests with the applicant; however, the objective criteria must be applied consistently or the committee may be accused of unfair prejudices.

CREDENTIALING FOR SPECIALIZED SKILLS

Physicians and surgeons usually become expert in the performance of specialty procedures during the course of a formal residency training program. There are, however, some specialty procedures that are not learned in the usual residency program. For example, in obstetrics and gynecology, radical cancer surgery requires training above and beyond that which is received in the usual residency program. Surgeons acquire skills in radical cancer surgery through additional training in gynecologic oncology. Hospitals certainly may legitimately assume that graduates of an approved residency program in obstetrics and gynecology have the ability to perform a procedure such as a routine hysterectomy. On the other hand, physicians who wish to be credentialed for radical surgery must supply additional proof that training in this subspecialty area was sufficient to justify granting the request. In addition to these subspecialty operations, there are other new procedures that are constantly being developed and that have not been taught or incorporated into residency training programs. If physicians wish to be credentialed for those procedures, new skills must be acquired and objective goals met as proof of the acquisition. Physicians then must present evidence of the newly acquired skills to the credentialing body in order to support specific credentialing requests.

DEVELOPMENT OF OBJECTIVE CRITERIA FOR CREDENTIALING FOR GYNECOLOGIC LASER SURGERY

Surgeons are usually trained by a combination of both formal and informal teaching sessions, laboratory experience, assisting at surgical procedures, and finally through the actual practice of surgery on patients. With this sequence in mind, a logical set of credentialing requirements for gynecologic laser surgery can be developed.[1-3] Obviously, laser surgeons must be well trained in conventional surgical technique and understand current medical opinion regarding the diseases to be treated. An example of rational and objective credentialing criteria is given in Table 6–1. Lasers of different wavelengths do not produce the same tissue reactions; therefore, requests for credentialing should specify the types of lasers that a gynecological surgeon wishes to use.

LASER SURGERY COURSES

Courses in laser surgery do not credential physicians but do provide a part of the justification for credentialing requests. These courses should supply the necessary didactics and afford some hands-on laboratory experience for beginning laser sur-

TABLE 6–1
**Credentialing Criteria for Gynecologic
Laser Surgery**

1. Thorough knowledge of the disease or abnormality to be treated by laser
2. Thorough knowledge of the conventional methods of treating
3. Participation in a formal laser course that presents physics, safety techniques, and theory of gynecological laser surgery
4. Hands-on laboratory experience with surgical laser systems
5. Hands-on training with patients
6. Maintenance of skills by continued practice

geons. Because of the complexity of laser endoscopes, many laser courses now deal solely with this topic. Although laser tissue reaction is more easily observed in the lower reproductive tract, it does not appear necessary for laser endoscopists, who do no lower reproductive tract surgery, to spend time learning lower tract technique. On the other hand, endoscopic courses must include all of the necessary laser course elements if they are to legitimately supply justification for credentialing requests. Table 6–2 outlines the necessary ingredients of a satisfactory general introductory laser course.

LASER LABORATORY

During the introductory laser course, it is usually impossible for physicians to gain enough laboratory time to become proficient in laser surgical technique or to fully develop eye-hand coordination. This is particularly true for laser endoscopy, in which surgical procedures are complex and often involve the use of many different instruments. It seems wise for hospitals in which advanced laser surgery is performed to have available laboratories or practice areas where surgeons may develop

TABLE 6–2
Introductory Laser Course Topics

Laser physics
Laser energy and tissue reaction
Laser safety/laser energy delivery systems
Laser surgical theory and technique
Surgical technique with specific wavelengths
Laser laboratory

skills outside the actual operating room. A manual of laboratory exercises should be located in this area so that laboratory time is meaningfully spent. The number of laboratory hours required for credentialing justification is arbitrary of course, but it seems logical to suggest that the more complicated endoscopic procedures should require more practice time.

LASER SURGICAL PRECEPTORSHIPS AND WORKSHOPS

Although the laboratory offers a necessary and highly desirable step in laser surgical training, there is no substitute for actual surgery on patients. A number of qualified surgeons are now able to offer workshops or preceptorships in hospitals where this type of experience may be gained. Workshops usually include advanced laboratory training and participation in the operating room for a limited number of physicians. Preceptorships involve a much smaller number of participants and afford hands-on experience with patients under the direction of a highly qualified laser surgeon. This type of program should be available only to those physicians who have completed a formal course and who have spent time in the laboratory.

TABLE 6–3
Delineation of Laser Surgical Privileges

Wavelengths to be used	**Procedures**
CO$_2$	**Lower reproductive tract laser surgery**
Argon	Cervix
KTP	Vagina
Nd : YAG	Vulva
Other (specify)	**Laparotomy**
Delivery system	Use in all open abdominal procedures
Micromanipulator	**Laparoscopy**
Laser hand piece	Lysis of adhesions
Laparoscope	Vaporization endometriosis
Hysteroscope	Ovarian cystectomy
Other (specify)	Salpingostomy of fimbrioplasty
	Ectopic pregnancy
Types of surgery	Vaporization uterosacral ligament
Lower reproductive tract	Myomectomy
Laparotomy	**Hysteroscopy**
Endoscopy	Incision uterine septa
	Lysis intrauterine adhesions
	Endometrial ablation
	Resection of submucous myoma
	Other (specify)

There are always medicolegal considerations when hospitals offer this type of training program. In our institution, the preceptee is treated as resident physician or fellow and assists or performs laser surgery in that capacity. Because state laws and hospital requirements vary, preceptorship programs also vary tremendously in structure.

DELINEATION OF PRIVILEGES

The laser is a surgical tool; it should be used only when a surgeon perceives an advantage for laser surgery in specific situations. The laser is often used in combination with conventional techniques. For example, an accomplished laser laparoscopist uses laser energy to vaporize or excise pathologic pelvic lesions but may also use sutures or ties to achieve hemostasis.

Because of the diversity and complexity of the gynecologic operations performed by laser surgeons, the list of procedures relating to laser use has grown tremendously during the past decade. This spectrum should be reflected in the Delineation of privileges form that each hospital develops for the specific credentialing process. An example of such a form is shown in Table 6–3.

SUMMARY

Credentialing is a logical safeguard for patients, physicians, and hospitals. Laser courses and preceptorships do not credential physicians, but they give them logical support for their credentialing requests to hospital boards. Not all surgeons are competent to perform laser surgery even after several courses and preceptorships. It is the duty of the credentialing authority to determine which physicians are able to perform this new type of surgery satisfactorily. It is the credentialing authority's duty to objectively and fairly decide which of the delineated privileges requested should be granted to a laser surgeon based on the available data submitted for analysis.

REFERENCES

1. Dorsey J, Baggish M: Initiating a CO_2 laser program. In Baggish M (ed): Basic and Advanced Laser Surgery in Gynecology. Norwalk, Appleton Century Crofts, 373–381, 1985
2. Dorsey J, Baker C: Credentialing of the gynecologic laser surgeon. Colpo Gyn Laser Surg 1:79, 1984
3. Dorsey J: The education of the gynecologic laser surgeon and a board of laser surgery. Colpo Gyn Laser Surg 1:83, 1984

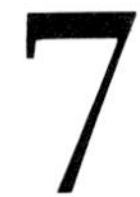

Developing a Laser Program: Humana Women's Hospital— Indianapolis as a Model

John Harryman and Jay Williams

Two decades ago, only a handful of lasers were in use throughout the United States. Today there is a rapid diffusion of laser technology in outpatient medical centers and in hospitals throughout the United States.

This rapid growth in the use of laser technology has created both problems and promises for hospitals, physicians, nurses, and medical personnel. Laser technology is complex; it requires considerable training for the entire medical team. Laser equipment must interface; installation, maintenance, and safety are of primary consideration. However, this technology has many advantages. The clinical "no-touch" technique that the laser offers enhances surgical precision and reduces blood loss. This modality can be less invasive (when coupled with additional equipment) and can thereby minimize surgery time. Consequently, laser use has allowed some operations to be performed on an outpatient or same-day basis.

It is not surprising that more and more hospitals are considering incorporating laser technology. What is somewhat surprising is the dearth of literature available on implementing a laser program. Ball[1] briefly outlines how to develop a laser program, and Bauman[3] details a four-pronged approach to implementing such a program. Cerne[4] probes whether or not lasers can cut hospital costs, and Ball[2] discusses the legal aspects of laser surgery.

With fewer than six articles describing the administrative considerations for a modality that is growing in tremendous proportion, it is believed that those implementing laser programs should be encouraged to share their insights with others in the field.

Because Humana Women's Hospital–Indianapolis has successfully incorporated laser technology into its services, it was thought the hospital could briefly outline the protocol it developed and the problem solving it faced during implementation.

The assumption at Humana Women's Hospital was that this hospital could effectively develop a laser program because it shared the Humana corporate mission of "providing state-of-the-art technology and equipment as well as qualified personnel that allow physicians to provide the highest standard of care for their patients." The laser program was also viewed as a catalyst for the hospital's long-standing infertility program. In essence, (1) executive management was interested in the practical and economic advantages offered by lasers, (2) administration viewed laser technology as an enhancement to marketing, and (3) management was encouraged by a group of physicians who wanted to remain current and competitive to pursue the development of a laser program.

Humana Women's Hospital could have chosen the dedicated operatory/single laser route, but the hospital viewed this option as ineffective because it limits growth.

Some hospitals may purchase a single laser to accommodate a sole surgeon with expertise in this technique. If the physician's skill is well known, the laser may be used. If not, the laser may be significantly underused. The hospital may not recoup its investment or may do so only after a protracted period of time.

At Humana Women's Hospital, carbon dioxide (CO_2) lasers were initially purchased, followed by the addition of the argon laser for use by all qualified members of the medical staff.

Perhaps the most critical component of a successful laser program is education. It should dispel myths and may create enthusiasm for the new laser technology. Seminar participation by surgeons, nurses, and other hospital personnel should be encouraged. Laser manufacturers and distributors are usually more than willing to bring equipment onsite to conduct hands-on workshops. Although each workshop at Humana generally was field specific, taken as a whole, they significantly enhanced cooperation and understanding. Attendance in off-site, 2-day workshops should also be encouraged.

The hospital's position is that in order to obtain laser privileges, an individual physician must seek appropriate training backed by written certification and must also demonstrate competency in laser surgery. According to the Medical Staff Rules and Regulations, "Any surgeon requesting privileges for laser surgery must be precepted for the first two cases. The surgeon will be provided with a listing of those Medical Staff Members who are credentialed for laser privileges. It is the requesting surgeon's responsibility to find his preceptor."

The Surgery Proctoring Report provides an internal quality check for the hospital (Fig. 7–1). It must be completed after the procedure and then sent to the Medical Staff Office for evaluation. The goal is to maintain an overall high-quality laser program; continuing education is necessary in order for that goal to be realized.

Because setup and equipment safety checks are the responsibility of the operating room nurses, it is essential that laser nurses be skilled in handling the equipment. Initial and subsequent training updates are often included as part of the initial contract that the hospital signs with the laser manufacturer.

OBSERVER: Please complete the information required below immediately after the procedure and send to D. Mingus, Medical Staff Office.

NAME OF PROCEDURE: _________________   MEDICAL RECORD NO. _______________

SURGEON: ____________________________   PROCTOR: ___________________________

DIAGNOSIS: ____

TYPE OF LASER: CO_2 Argon   YAG   KTP

APPLICATION: Intra-abdominal   External

OTHER PROCREDURE: ____

COMMENTS ON:

   Preoperative workup ____

   Preoperative preparations ____

   Operative judgment ____

   Surgical technique ____

   Results of procedure ____

   Postoperative care ____

RECOMMENDATIONS OF PROCTOR:

   Qualified for this procedure? ____

   Needs further observation? ____

   Not qualified for this procedure? ____

COMMENTS:

____   ___________________

Signature of Preceptor   Date

FIGURE 7–1. Surgery proctoring report.

Administration at Humana Women's Hospital held sessions with specialty physicians to determine needs and then evaluated equipment that could satisfy those needs. Quality, durability, maintenance, and cost were factored into the purchase price. During the past 5 years, the hospital spent $814,000 on lasers and related equipment. Annual budgeting is based on needs identified by physicians and staff. Appropriate budgeting took place each year as physicians identified equipment that would be beneficial to their practices at the hospital.

In our experience, it quickly became apparent that annual service contracts are essential for proper preventive maintenance and timely repairs of laser equipment. Contract expenses are more than recovered, and a line of accountability for timely service is established with the vendor.

Humana Women's Hospital currently has five operating rooms equipped with two Sharplan lasers (1100 and 743, at 100 and 60 watts, respectively), a 60-watt CooperVision laser, one HgM model E-20 argon laser, two operating room Wild microscopes, and four video monitors (two of which are portable). The hospital has always intended to move toward fully equipped operating rooms containing at least one CO_2 laser as well as a fixed video system. The capital cost and the fact that there was a learning curve for laser technology necessitated approaching this goal gradually.

One of the main concerns of a laser program is safety. The protocol followed at Humana Women's Hospital is based largely on issues identified and resolved in other existing laser programs. The hospital established standards of practice for using the laser that were in compliance with regulations set forth by the Food and Drug Administration; it reviewed equipment design and function with safety in mind; and it assessed established standards and criteria as well as the safety records of the laser surgeons on a regular basis. Although the hospital has developed a detailed protocol for all laser usage, the policies and procedures regarding the CO_2 laser are represented in Table 7–1 and may provide greater insight into the process.

The marketing of the laser program at Humana Women's Hospital is integrated into the overall strategic marketing plan. The 150-bed hospital provides for acute inpatient and outpatient services for women, children, and adolescents. The hospital acknowledges the practice patterns of referring physicians and the strengths of its staff. The marketing campaigns emphasize these points in general; the laser program is part of the service afforded patients.

SUMMARY

Some preliminary evaluations based on what has been observed may be noted.

First, the hospital laser program has proved to be cost-effective. The original cost-benefit analysis weighed the costs of equipment, training, and safety against the

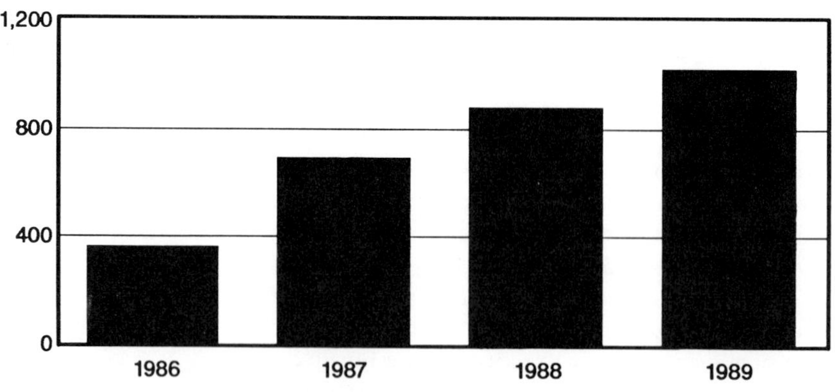

FIGURE 7–2. CO_2 laser utilization in Humana Women's Hospital in Indianapolis.

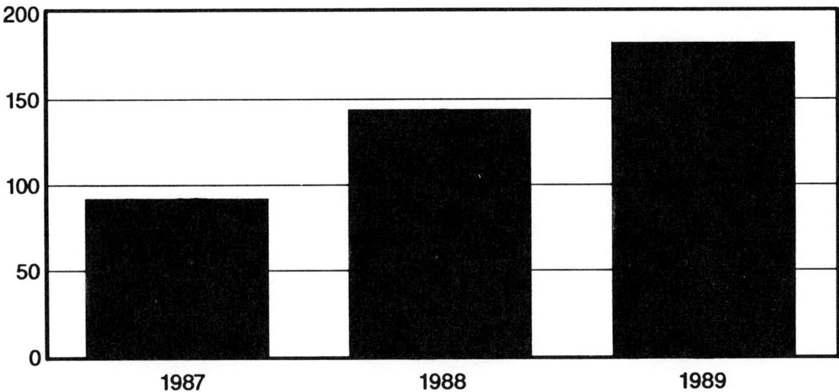

FIGURE 7–3. Percentage of growth in fiscal year 1986 of CO_2 laser utlization at Humana Women's Hospital in Indianapolis.

benefits of offering this modality. The hospital has experienced an increase in laser surgery (Figs. 7–2 and 7–3) but has also witnessed an increase in laser treatment being done as a result of laser surgery. For example, many infertility patients who have had laser surgery return to Humana Women's Hospital for obstetric and subsequent gynecological procedures as well. Additionally, the hospital has seen a tremendous link between laser surgeries and alternative reproductive therapies such as *in vitro* fertilization, tubal ovum transfer, and gamete intrafallopian transfer.

The laser program has enhanced the image of the hospital within the community and has broadened the service market to out-of-state patients as well. In turn, the hospital's ability to serve as a referral base for other complicated procedures has been enhanced.

The final judgment is still out on the long-range benefits of the laser program, but the initial overview is favorable.

REFERENCES

1. Ball K: How to develop a laser center. Indiana Med 81:332, 1988
2. Ball K: Legal aspects of laser surgery. Today's OR Nurse 9:23, 1987
3. Bauman N: A recipe for a laser program—commitment, equipment, education and money. Lasers Med Surg News 5:10, 1985
4. Cerne F: Can lasers cut hospital costs? Hospitals 62:63, 1988

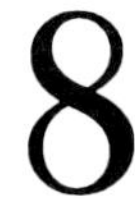

8

The Perioperative Role of the Clinical Nurse During Laser Laparoscopy

Carolyn J. Mackety

The explosion of medical care technology has begun to have noticeable effects on our daily practice and with the concurrent compression of the clinical experience in nursing education, has created an increased need for continuing education.

Patients undergoing laparoscopy benefit from current advances that allow safe use of equipment for minimally invasive procedures. Telescopelike instruments (*i.e.,* cystoscopes, bronchoscopes, hysteroscopes, and laparoscopes) make direct visualization possible for therapeutic or diagnostic procedures.[1]

We expect nurses who work in a surgical environment to have perioperative responsibilities for care of patients. The perioperative role has since 1975 been described by the Association of Operating Room Nurses.[2] Operating room nurses perform their duties during their practice according to these philosophical guidelines. The perioperative role has three phases:

The *preoperative* phase is an opportunity to assess patients' understanding of the risks, expectations, and outcomes of their surgical intervention. This is done before surgery, in various environments: the patients' unit, at the time of preadmission testing, in the preoperative phone call, in the holding room, and just before the surgical procedure.

The *intraoperative* objectives are to provide competent care for patients during surgical intervention, using a plan of care that has been defined for the procedure by the physician, and an evaluation of the patient assessment process.

The *postoperative* phase provides surgical nurses with the opportunity to evaluate a patient's progress toward wellness and to document his or her satisfaction with care provided while in the operating room.

Providing care for patients undergoing surgical intervention requires understanding of scientific nursing theory and application of skills learned during the basic nursing education process. Complex interventional procedures such as laparoscopy require knowledge of procedure principles, perioperative routines, and the risks and outcomes. Nurses must be able to recognize postoperative complications, must be cognizant of their treatments, and must have the knowledge to individualize patient education.

Endoscopy developed about 1863, but it was not until 1969 that instrumentation evolved sufficiently to perform endoscopic procedures in the pelvis safely. By 1981, laparoscopic techniques were a requirement for all obstetrics and gynecology residency programs and were taught to operating room nurses as part of the orientation experience.

Before performing nursing assessments of patients presenting for laparoscopic procedures, nurses should have a basic understanding of the following indications for laparoscopy:

1. To provide a method of visualization of the internal pelvic anatomy for diagnosis during physical examination.
2. To provide the physician an opportunity to perform minimally invasive therapeutic procedures.
3. For sterilization procedures, which currently are the most frequent indication.

Laparoscopy does not replace laparotomy but is considered an alternative in certain circumstances. Recuperation seems to be faster, and the period of hospitalization is decreased. Patients have less discomfort and return more quickly to activities of daily living, including sexual activity.

Laparoscopy may be contraindicated in certain patients:

1. Patients with cardiopulmonary disease, who may be compromised because of the Trendelenburg position.
2. Patients who have severe pathological obesity.
3. Any patient who may be compromised by having increased intra-abdominal pressure caused by the pneumoperitonieum, such as patients known to have a diaphragmatic hernia.

The pathophysiology and surgical indications for laparoscopic procedures will be presented in subsequent chapters in this book. The nursing preoperative informational objectives are met, and nurses acquire a basic understanding of the pathophysiology and the psychosocial influences on health and illness based on the surgical indications. Then, using the nursing process, an intraoperative plan of care is developed for patients requiring endoscopic procedures.

The operating room nurse collaborates postoperatively with the health care givers to provide continuity of care and positive patient outcomes for the period of convalescence. This rationale is based on understanding the physical, psychosocial, cultural, and ethnic responses to illness and health. The principles of nursing science are used to assist the patient and family in adapting to the activities of daily living until the patient has recuperated.

As the operating room nurse undertakes the development and maintenance of perioperative care for patients requiring endoscopic procedures, the following information will be required:

I. Preoperative
    A. Physical preparation
        1. Laboratory studies and x-rays
        2. Evacuating the contents of the bowel, as ordered
        3. Shower with bactericidal soap
        4. Preoperative medication
    B. Psychosocial
        1. Answer questions or refer them to the physician
        2. Explain the risks and expected outcomes of the procedure
        3. Tell the family where to wait and that the physician will see them postoperatively

II. Intraoperatively
    A. Physical preparation
        1. Anesthesia is usually general, but epidural or local may be used
        2. The patient is in the dorsal lithotomy and then a Trendelenberg position
        3. The abdomen, perineum, and vagina are prepared with a antimicrobial solution
        4. The bladder must be emptied
    B. Instruments that may be required (not all-inclusive)
        1. Dilatation and curettage set
        2. Laparoscopy set with multipuncture trocars
        3. Variable high-flow insufflator
        4. Light source
        5. Video equipment or teaching scope, as needed
        7. Electrocautery
        8. Laser of specific wavelength, as scheduled

III. Postoperative care of the laparoscopic equipment
    A. A hospital policy and procedure must be developed and approved for cleaning, disinfecting, and sterilizing the equipment
        1. Supplies needed
            a. Long brush
            b. Cidex
            c. Soak pans
            d. Rinse pans
            e. 60-ml syringe
            f. 3000 ml water

       g. Hibiclens (or other bactericidal solution)

       h. Alcohol

       i. Soft cloth and lens paper

B. Cleaning techniques

  1. Clean all debris and body fluids from the scope and accessories

  2. Fill 60-ml syringe with warm water and Hibiclens solution and flush the lumen of the scope vigorously

    a. Use a brush to clean debris

  3. Rinse well

  4. Dip a cotton swab in alcohol, squeeze it to dampness, and clean the ocular lens. Dry it with lens paper or a soft cloth

C. Cleaning the adaptors

  1. Disassemble

  2. Clean with an antimicrobial solution

  3. Rinse well and apply silicone lubricant sparingly

  4. Check the seals and replace them as needed

D. Between-case disinfectant procedure

  1. Follow the above cleaning procedure

  2. Soak the scope in Cidex for 10 minutes using the soak pan

  3. Do not immerse the optical head unless it is recommended by the manufacturer

  4. Rinse well, usually twice

  5. Flush the lumen of scope with clear water

Note: Cidex can be toxic to mucous membranes and to the skin

E. Sterilization

  1. Clean the scopes following the above procedures

  2. Prepare them for terminal sterilization using ethylene oxide

Note: Sterilization of the equipment after each use is recommended, but economic reality may prevent the facility from compliance. In that case, the institution must develop strict policies and procedures regarding the cleaning, maintenance, and sterilization of consumer equipment.

F. Care and maintenance of laser equipment

  1. Carbon dioxide

    a. The body of the laser and the articulated arm are wiped each day with a bactericidal solution, at the beginning of each day.

    b. The articulated arm is usually draped during the operative procedure, not to include the endoscope

  2. Nd:YAG laser

    a. Wipe off the body of the laser daily with bactericidal solution

    b. Check YAG fibers for integrity; replace them as needed

      c. Noncontact fibers must be checked for a polished surface and polished if necessary

      d. All noncontact fibers can be wiped with warm soapy water, dried, and sterilized

      e. Contact YAG fibers must be checked for fiber transmission before each use

   3. Visible wavelength lasers

      a. Lasers are wiped with a bactericidal solution before each use

      b. Hand pieces and fibers are cared for according to manufacturers' recommendations

IV. Postoperative care

  A. Immediate

    1. On emergence from anesthesia, patients may complain of

      a. Abdominal discomfort

      b. Discomfort in the neck and shoulder area from positioning and free upward flow of absorbed CO_2

    2. Mild analgesics will be sufficient for local discomfort

    3. Patients having general anesthesia require special consideration

      a. They may complain of throat discomfort

      b. They need to be observed for airway obstruction

    4. Patients who are having local or epidural anesthesia and who are awake during a procedure must have adequate preoperative information and individualized education about their procedure

  B. Discharge instructions

    1. Depending on the reason for the laparoscopic procedure, the following information may need to be discussed with patient:

      a. Refrain from lifting for 2 weeks

      b. Refrain from sexual intercourse for 1 week to prevent possible infection

      c. Patients may need specific medication information if infertility drugs are necessary

There are very few potential complications from having a laparoscopic procedure. If complications do occur, they can be attributed to four factors:

1. A physician's inexperience

2. Equipment defects or mishandling

3. Anesthesia problems, depending on other medical conditions of the patient

4. The type of procedure performed

  a. Perforation of abdominal organs

  b. Primary puncture and insufflation of CO_2 gas during pneumoperitenium may cause subcutaneous emphysema, insufflation of the bowel or stomach, or injury to the bladder

The nursing responsibilities are to recognize the signs and symptoms of these complications and notify the physician immediately:

1. Bowel injury causes fever and the sudden occurrence of abdominal pain.
2. Cardiac dysrhythmias may occur because of the extended pressure in the thorax. These respond well to decreased pressure and improved ventilation.

Laparoscopic procedures are generally performed on healthy young women. A positive nursing interaction contributes to a patient's satisfaction with health care delivery. Maturity, motivation, and the adjustment of the individual or couple seeking medical or surgical intervention play a key role in wellness and satisfaction with health care delivery. Nurses spend even more time with patients than do physicians, and they can positively influence patients' acceptance and impression of health care and caregivers. Nurses must therefore be well informed about all aspects of medicine and surgery and must establish collaborative practice techniques with physicians and other health team members, to provide sophisticated consumers with meaningful information so they can make informed decisions about their health care. It is difficult in today's technological environment to maintain expertise in all fields of nursing, and nurses are entering into subspecialties within the operating room. We are encountering more opportunities to influence our daily practice, to give quality patient care, and to become those recognized specialists.

REFERENCES

1. Daniell J: Laser laparoscopy. In Baggish M (ed): Basic and Advanced Laser Surgery in Gynecology, pp. 343–346. East Norwalk, Appleton-Century-Crofts, 1985
2. Davis D, Kneedler J, Manuel B: Surgical experience; a model for profession practice in the OR. AORN J 1978

Part Two

EXTERNAL LASER THERAPY

9

Carbon Dioxide Laser Surgery for the Cervix: Indications, Operative Methods, Complications, and Results

V. Cecil Wright
Mary Ann Riopelle

Carbon dioxide (CO_2) laser surgery allows precise and complete tissue eradication; however, the success of laser surgery depends on removing all obviously diseased and potentially involved tissue. A growing number of gynecologists have adopted laser surgery and incorporated it into routine practice in offices and operating rooms. Laser surgery has, in fact, become the primary method of treatment for many gynecologic diseases, especially for preinvasive cervical neoplasia.

The wavelength (or its inverse, the frequency) determines the particular effect a laser beam will have on biologic tissues. CO_2 laser energy, which is absorbed on the surface of tissues with a high water content, vaporizes the tissue, producing steam and scattered carbonized particles. Tissue necrosis, caused by thermal denaturing of proteins, occurs within 50 to 100 μm of the crater with limited exposure time (Fig. 9–1). The inherent hemostatic effect is the result of heat sealing smaller blood vessels in the zone of thermal necrosis. A wider zone of injury, caused by elevated temperature, surrounds the zone of necrosis, but the tissue will recover.

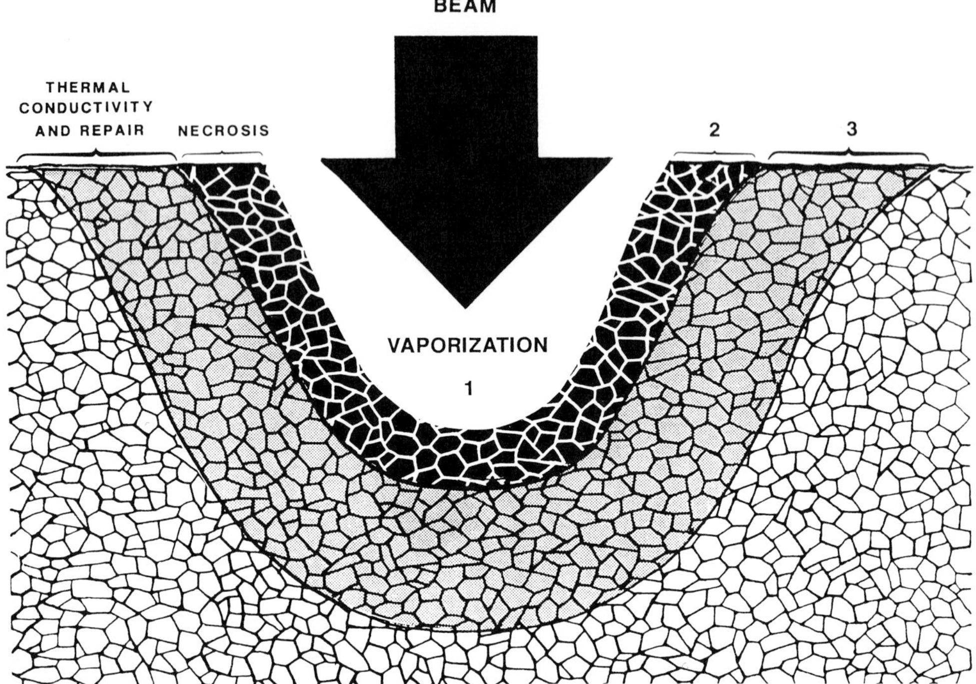

FIGURE 9–1. Zones of injury. The shape of the actual tissue defect, resulting from laser vaporization of tissue, reflects the spacial intensity of the laser beam and is deepest in the center where the intensity is greatest. The heat effect in zone two accounts for the sealing of blood vessels. (With permission from Wright VC, Riopelle MA: Gynecologic Laser Surgery: A Practical Handbook. Houston, Biomedical Communications, 1982)

SURGICAL APPROACH BASED ON DISEASE SOLID GEOMETRY

The CO_2 laser permits surgeons to destroy tissue in place or excise it, creating surgical craters, defects, or specimens of virtually any size or shape. A surgeon can limit vaporization or excision to only the diseased tissue, sparing surrounding normal tissue. In the cervix, four geometric patterns account for the distribution of cervical intraepithelial neoplasia (CIN). The laser surgical procedures based on disease patterns include the following:

1. Vaporization of a shallow domed cylinder for ectocervical CIN, when the disease has a radial linear length of 8 mm or less.
2. Vaporization of a central domed cylinder with peripheral vaporization of a lesser depth when ectocervical CIN has a radial linear length of more than 8 mm.
3. Excision of a tall cylindrical specimen for canal disease.
4. Excision of a moderately tall cylinder surrounded by vaporization of a doughnut or innertube configuration for disease occupying the

endocervical canal and extending beyond a radius of 8 mm onto the portio.

Surgery based on these four geometric configurations will eradicate CIN because of the following well-established concepts:

1. Tissue susceptible to developing squamous cell intraepithelial neoplasia lies between the original squamocolumnar junction and the histologic internal os. This area of susceptibility, which includes but is not limited to the transformation zone, can be as much as 2.0 to 2.5 cm in radial linear length (Fig. 9–2).

2. CIN can extend into the underlying cervical crypts (Fig. 9–3). Higher-grade lesions (severe dysplasia and carcinoma *in situ*) extend into cervical crypts up to 5.2 mm,[1,2] but in most cases crypt depth varies between 1.24 and 1.6 mm.[1,8] In CIN III lesions (severe dysplasia and carcinoma *in situ*), 85% to 95% will have some crypt extension.[3] However, 96% of these cases have depth of disease extension less than 2.9 mm (Table 9–1 and Fig. 9–3).[13] It has been hypothesized that destruction of lesions to a depth of 3.8 mm will eradicate all involved crypts in 99.7% of patients.[1]

3. The radial linear length of CIN can vary between 2 and 22 mm (Figs. 9–4 and 9–5),[8,9] but the usual linear length varies between 6 and 8 mm.[8,9]

4. CIN lesions do not extend more than 22 mm up the endocervical canal when measured from the lowermost border of the lesions.[8]

5. The transformation zone recedes into and up the endocervical canal with age[5] (Fig. 9–6). In women of reproductive age, CIN lesions do not extend above the level of the anatomical internal os.

6. Invasive cancer occurs on the canal side—that is, the worst pathology is located centrally.[2,4]

(text continued on page 106)

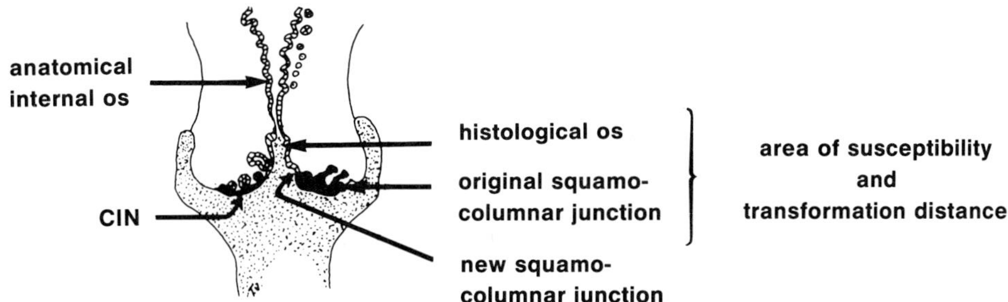

FIGURE 9–2. Cervical topography. The area of susceptibility (transformation distance) to develop CIN lies between the original squamocolumnar junction and the histologic os. CIN usually occupies only the caudal part of this area. (With permission from Wright VC: Laser surgery for cervical intraepithelial neoplasia—Principles and results. In Wright VC, Lickrish GM: Basic and Advanced Colposcopy: A Practical Handbook for Diagnosis and Treatment. Houston, Biomedical Communications, pp 161–172, 1989)

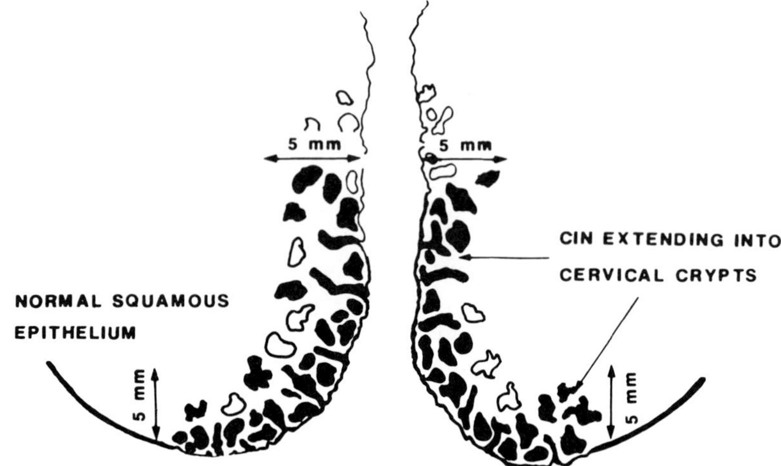

FIGURE 9–3. Involvement of cervical crypts with CIN. CIN III (severe dysplasia and carcinoma *in situ*) can extend into the underlying cervical crypts as much as 5 mm, regardless whether they occupy the ectocervix or line the endocervical canal. However, 96% of these high-grade lesions extend only 2.9 mm or less into the underlying crypts. (With permission from Wright VC, Riopelle MA: Gynecologic Laser Surgery: A Practical Handbook, 2nd ed. Houston, Biomedical Communications, 1990)

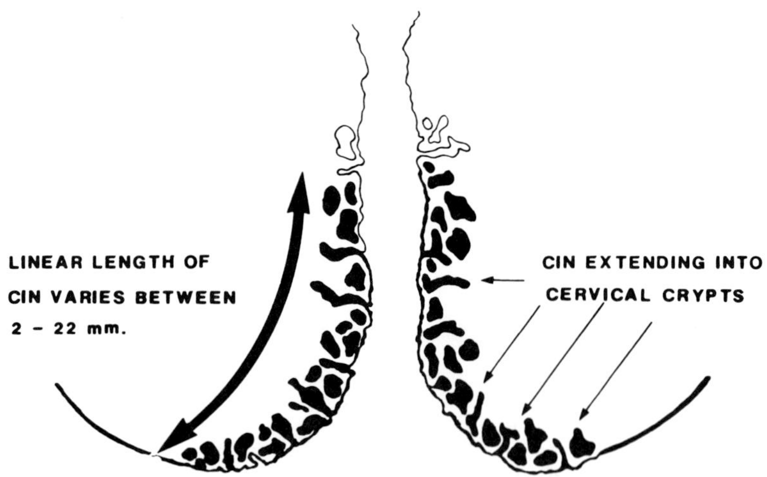

FIGURE 9–4. The linear extent of CIN. The linear extent of CIN (from the lowermost to the uppermost edges of the obvious lesion) measures 2 to 22 mm regardless of its location. The radial linear extent of the usual lesion measures 6 to 8 mm.

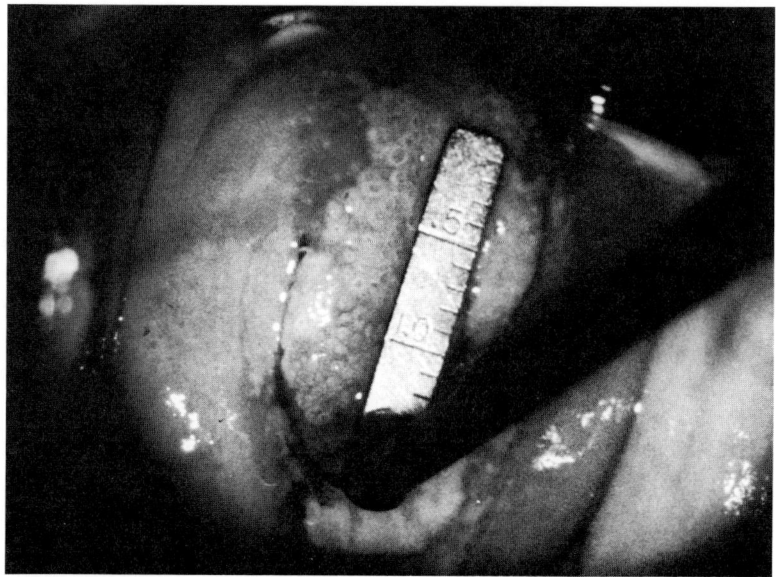

FIGURE 9–5. This photograph demonstrates measurement of the radial linear length of a CIN III lesion, which is 12 mm. (With permission from Wright VC, Riopelle MA: Gynecologic Laser Surgery, 2nd ed. Houston, Biomedical Communications, 1990)

TABLE 9–1
Cervical Crypt Involvement with CIN III

CRYPT EXTENSION	NO.	%	%	%
0 mm	26	11.8		
0.1–0.9 mm	140	63.6	86.8	95.9
1–1.9 mm	25	11.4		
2–2.9 mm	20	9.1		
3–3.9 mm	5	2.3		
4–4.9 mm	2	0.9		
5–5.9 mm	2	0.9		
All cases	220	100.0		

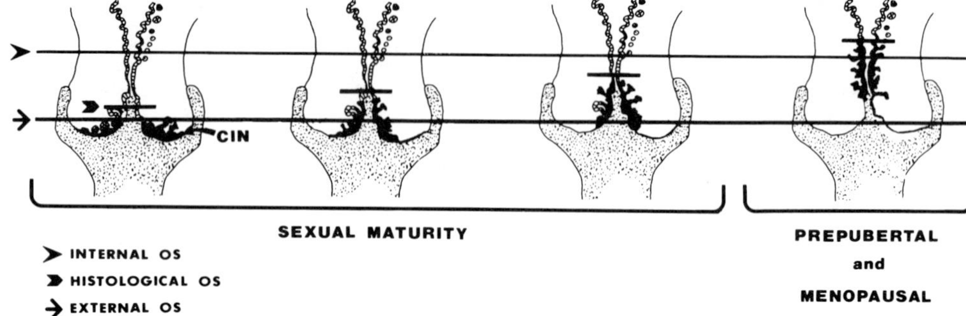

FIGURE 9–6. Cellular distribution on the cervix as a function of age. The proportion of columnar epithelium on the ectocervix or in the canal is a function of age. (With permission from Wright VC: Laser surgery for cervical intraepithelial neoplasia—Principles and results. In Wright VC, Lickrish GM: Basic and Advanced Colposcopy: A Practical Handbook for Diagnosis and Treatment. Houston, Biomedical Communications, pp 161–172, 1989)

INDICATIONS FOR THE LASER VAPORIZATION PROCEDURES FOR ECTOCERVICAL CIN

The criteria to be fulfilled for laser destruction are the following:

1. Cytology, colposcopy, and pathology must be correlated to establish an accurate cervical tissue diagnosis.
2. The entire atypical transformation zone must be colposcopically defined.
3. The colposcopist must be certain from the qualitative assessment of the transformation zone that no invasive cancer is present.
4. The CIN must occupy the ectocervix at or below the level of the external os with no extension into the endocervical canal.

OPERATIVE TECHNIQUE FOR ECTOCERVICAL LESIONS WITH A LINEAR LENGTH OF 8 mm OR LESS

To create a vaporized cylindrical defect (Fig. 9–7), a surgeon couples the CO_2 laser to an operating microscope or colposcope. A working distance of 300 mm is standard and is achieved by having a 300-mm main objective lens in the operating microscope. The total magnification of the operating microscope should be in the range of 3.5 to 7 times. This gives an adequate diameter of view ranging from approximately 28 to 57 mm (Fig. 9–8). Higher magnification permits more colposcopic detail, but these lower magnifications allow an operator to see the entire operative field during surgery. An effective laser beam diameter of 2 mm is used,

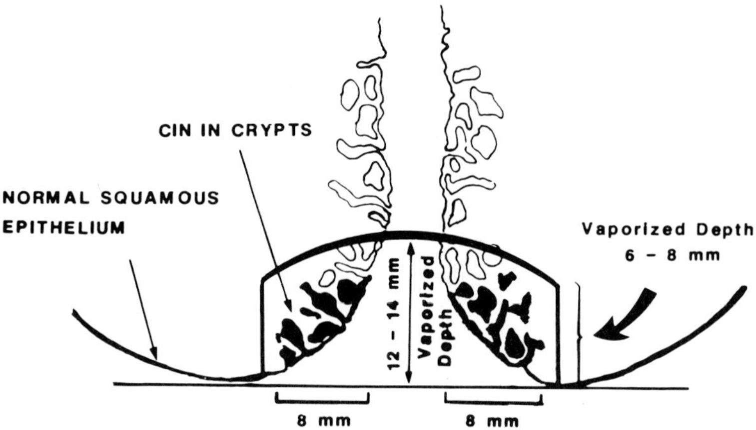

FIGURE 9–7. Laser vaporization. Schematics of ectocervical CIN with a linear radial length of 8 mm or less. When CIN occupies the ectocervix and has a radial linear length of 8 mm or less, a central cylindrical dome-shaped defect measuring 12 to 14 mm centrally at the dome and 6 to 8 mm at the sides is vaporized. (With permission from Wright VC: Laser surgery for cervical intraepithelial neoplasia—Principles and results. In Wright VC, Lickrish GM: Basic and Advanced Colposcopy: A Practical Handbook for Diagnosis and Treatment. Houston, Biomedical Communications, pp 161–172, 1989)

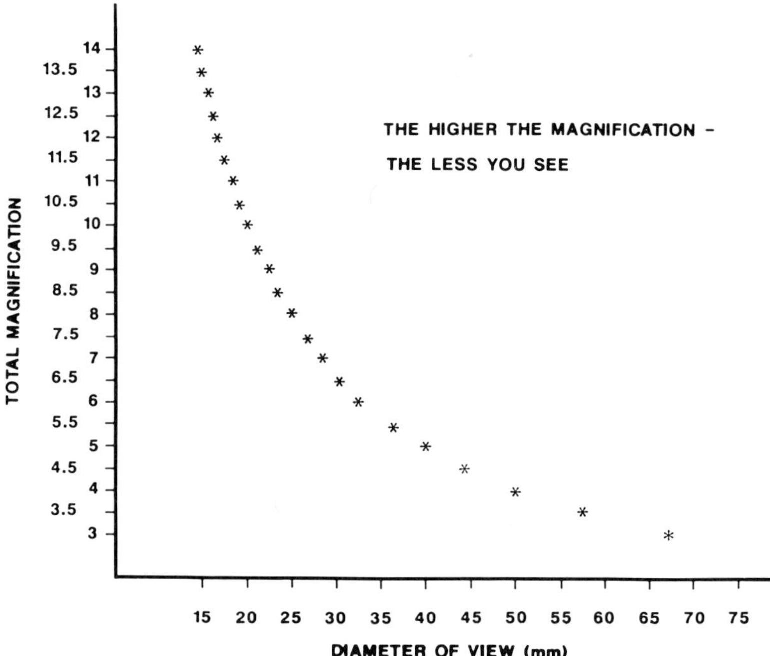

FIGURE 9–8. Diameter of view as a function of total magnification of the scope. The higher the magnification, the less is the diameter of view. (With permission from Wright VC: Understanding the operating microscope. In Wright VC, Riopelle MA: Surgical CO_2 Laser Fundamentals. Houston, Biomedical Communications, pp 45–66, 1988)

and a power density ranging from 650 to 1200 watts/cm^2 is recommended. The surgeon operates through a speculum with the plume evacuated by a suction device attached to the upper blade. In order to eradicate the disease completely, the laser beam first encircles the lesion, including normal tissue 2 to 3 mm beyond the diseased area. The entire transformation zone, including the area of pathology, is then vaporized to a minimum depth of 6 to 8 mm, with the surgeon beginning at the 6-o'clock position and never leaving an area until proper depth is achieved. Centrally a further vaporization of 4 to 8 mm is recommended (see Fig. 9–7), creating the dome shape. The latter step takes into account the topographical anatomy of the cervix and removes part of the remaining area of susceptibility in order to prevent new disease from developing in the future. This procedure usually takes 1 to 5 minutes to perform in an office or clinic setting. Approximately 10% to 20% of patients require local injection of anesthesia into the cervix. The detailed operative techniques for this procedure have been previously published.[9]

OPERATIVE TECHNIQUE FOR ECTOCERVICAL LESIONS HAVING A LINEAR LENGTH GREATER THAN 8 mm

There is a limit to the amount of central loss of cervical tissue that will regenerate. The authors have found that when lesions have a radial linear length exceeding

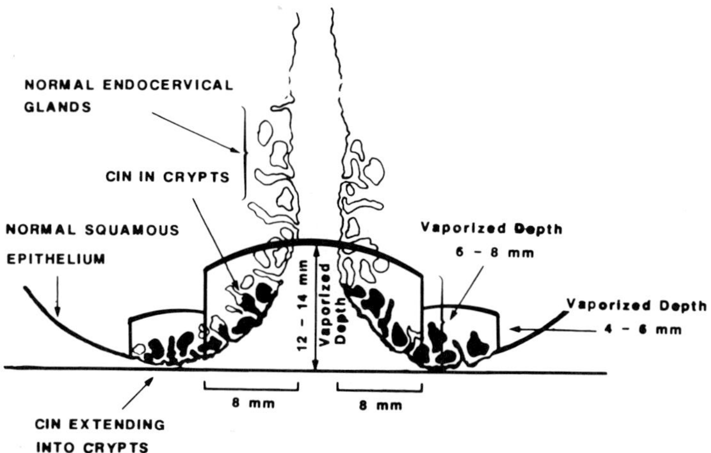

FIGURE 9–9. Laser vaporization. Schematics of ectocervical CIN extending beyond a radial linear length of 8 mm. When CIN occupies the ectocervix and has a radial linear length exceeding 8 mm, a central cylindrical dome-shaped defect measuring 12 to 14 mm centrally at the dome and 6 to 8 mm at the sides is vaporized. CIN peripheral to the 8-mm radial length is vaporized to a depth of 4 to 6 mm. (With permission from Wright VC: Laser surgery for cervical intraepithelial neoplasia—Principles and results. In Wright VC, Lickrish GM: Basic and Advanced Colposcopy: A Practical Handbook for Diagnosis and Treatment. Houston, Biomedical Communications, pp 161–172, 1989)

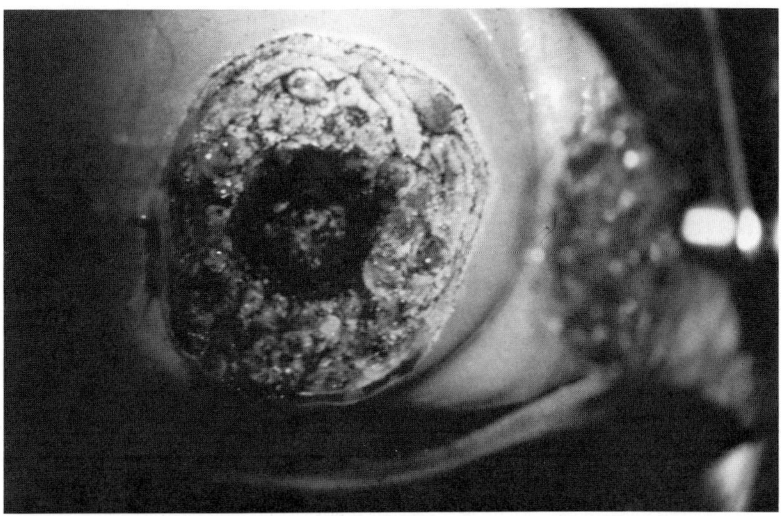

FIGURE 9–10. Combination vaporization. Colpophotograph of the completed procedure showing two different depths of vaporization in an extensive lesion.

8 mm, vaporizing the typical dome-shaped cylindrical defect as previously described should be done first, leaving some disease on the cervix. The CIN peripheral to the defect should then be vaporized to a depth of 4 to 6 mm (Fig. 9–9), producing a "cowboy hat" configuration (Fig. 9–10).[9] Should the CIN extend farther onto the vagina, laser vaporization will be continued to incorporate all disease but at a depth not exceeding 1.5 mm.

INDICATIONS FOR LASER CYLINDRICAL EXCISION FOR ENDOCERVICAL LESIONS

Laser cylindrical excision for endocervical lesions is indicated in the following instances:

1. When discrepancies exist between cytology, colposcopy and histology.
2. When lesions are located in the endocervical canal and require tissue for histologic evaluation.
3. When either cytology or colposcopy suggests invasive carcinoma that has not been proved by colposcopically directed biopsy.

Figure 9–11 illustrates the geometry of endocervical disease (shown in two dimensions). In this case, the disease extends to a maximum depth of 5 mm into the underlying cervical crypts (indicated by horizontal arrows) and involves the endocervical canal to a maximum height of 1.5 cm (indicated by vertical arrows). By removing a cylinder rather than a cone, a surgeon excises half as much tissue as

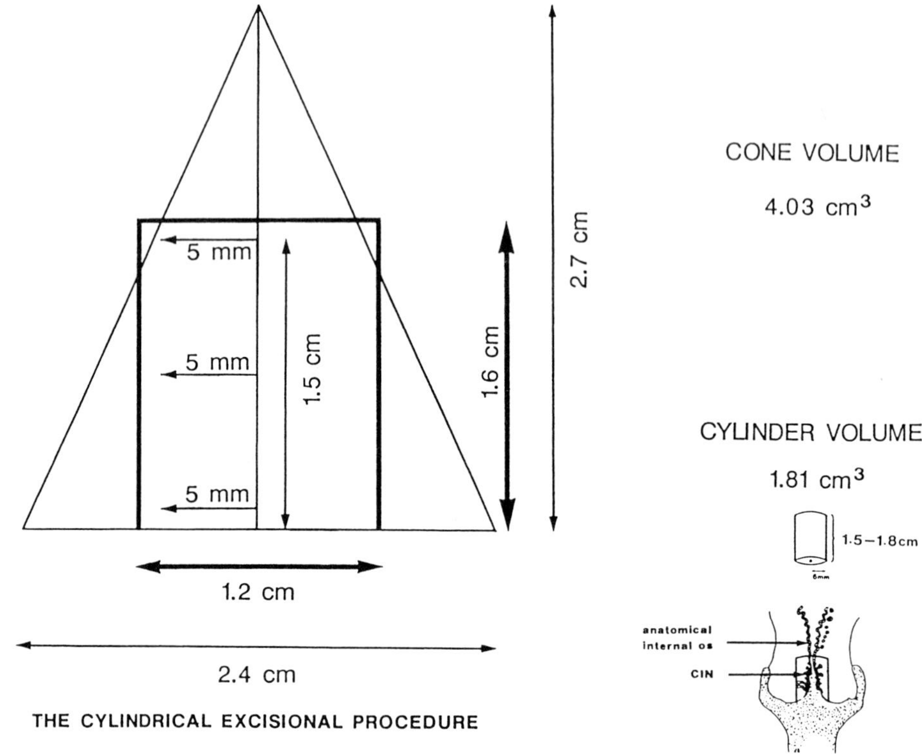

FIGURE 9–11. The geometry of CIN for endocervical disease. To incorporate a lesion 1.5 cm in height and to account for maximal crypt involvement, a cylinder (volume 1.81 cm³) removes considerably less volume than a cone defect (volume 4.03 cm³) when cure is anticipated and all diseased tissue is contained in the specimen. (With permission from Wright VC: Laser surgery for cervical intraepithelial neoplasia—Principles and results. In Wright VC, Lickrish GM: Basic and Advanced Colposcopy: A Practical Handbook for Diagnosis and Treatment. Houston, Biomedical Communications, pp 161–172, 1989)

required to incorporate all disease when cure, not just diagnosis, is the goal. This procedure is performed as outpatient surgery in a hospital or surgery center with a patient under general or local anesthesia.

OPERATIVE TECHNIQUE FOR CYLINDRICAL EXCISION

The CO_2 laser should be attached to an operating microscope with a working distance of 300 mm. Thus, the focal length of the objective lens of the operating microscope equals the 300-mm laser lens, yielding an effective laser beam setting diameter of 0.5 to 0.6 mm. Power density greater than 1500 watts/cm² (usually between 1,500 and 18,000 watts/cm²) is appropriate, providing that the operating surgeon feels comfortable using that power setting. To ensure a bloodless operating field, hemostatic sutures are placed at the 3-o'clock and 9-o'clock positions, and a vasopressin (Pitressin) solution (10 units/30 ml, not exceeding 1 pressor unit) is injected into the cervical stroma. A cylindrical, not a cone-shaped, specimen is removed for histologic interpretation (Figs. 9–12 and 9–13). The specimen usually has a height varying between 1.5 and 1.8 cm (depending on the location of the lowermost edge of the disease) in a woman of reproductive age. Cylinders with a height of 2 cm may be necessary in the menopausal age-group (Fig. 9–6). After the circular incision is made, the upper pole of the specimen is cut transversely with a scalpel or tonsil snare (Figs. 9–13 through 9–16), followed by "flashing" the apex with a 2-mm laser beam diameter to seal the blood vessels and enhance hemostasis (Fig. 9–13). The only thermally damaged tissue is located at the outer margin (less than 100 μm).[9,10] This procedure usually takes less than 8 minutes to complete. The operative details for general anesthesia and scalpel upper cut have been previously described.[9,10] Use of the tonsil snare can enable the proper operation with local anesthesia and a standard speculum. This latter approach is used for patients only under local anesthesia and has allowed some excisions to be done in the clinic or office. Using the laser to "cone-in" the upper margin to sever the specimen is not a good idea, even if the defect is then vaporized further to create the final cylindrical shape. It destroys the most important tissue that contains the most severe histology and, in younger women, possibly the anatomical internal os necessary for cervical competence.

(*text continued on page 114*)

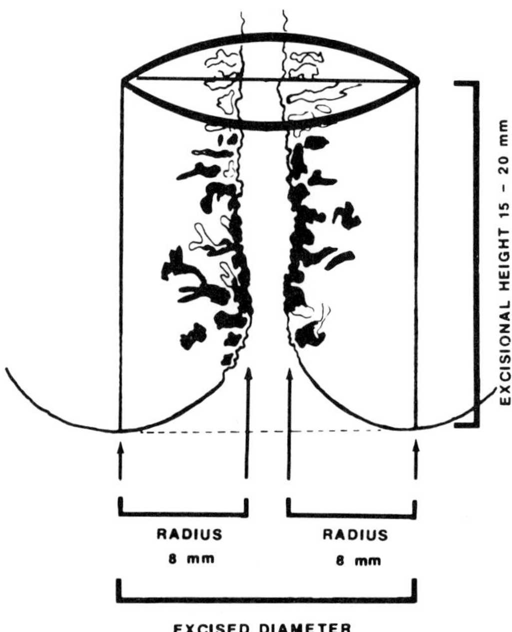

FIGURE 9–12. Laser cylindrical excision. Schematics of the laser cylindrical excisional procedure. (With permission from Wright VC, Riopelle MA: Gynecologic Laser Surgery: A Practical Handbook, 2nd ed. Houston, Biomedical Communications, 1990)

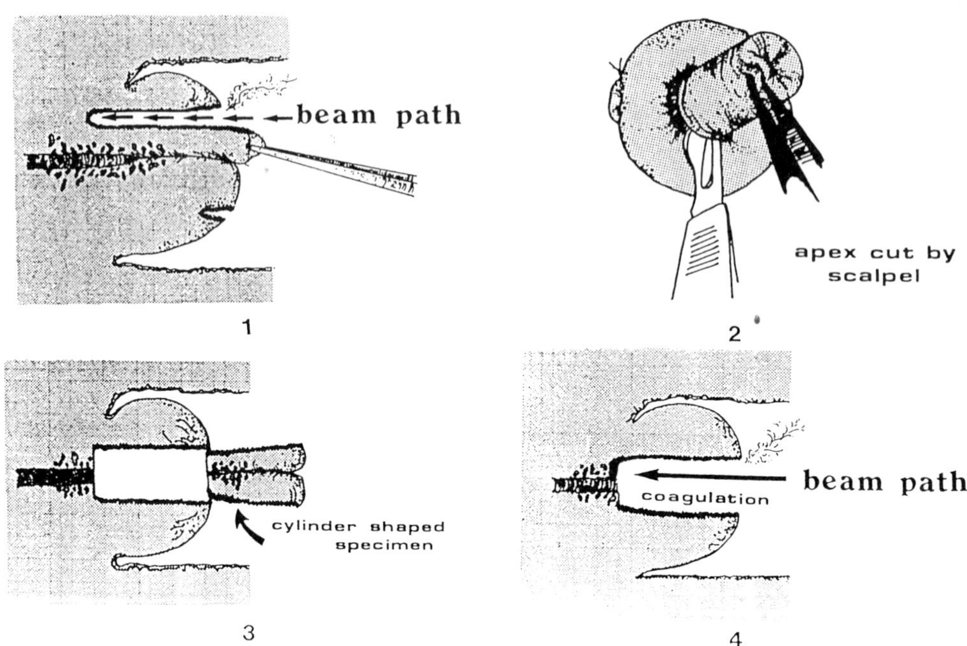

FIGURE 9–13. Steps in the laser cylindrical excisional procedure: 1) A circular incision enclosing a specimen with a radius not exceeding 8 mm is made around the external cervical os. The line of excision is parallel to the endocervical canal. 2) The apex of the specimen is cut with a scalpel. 3) The cylindrical specimen is removed. 4) The blood vessels in the defect's base are sealed by a lower-intensity laser beam. (With permission from Wright VC, Riopelle MA: Gynecologic Laser Surgery: A Practical Handbook. Houston, Biomedical Communications, 1982)

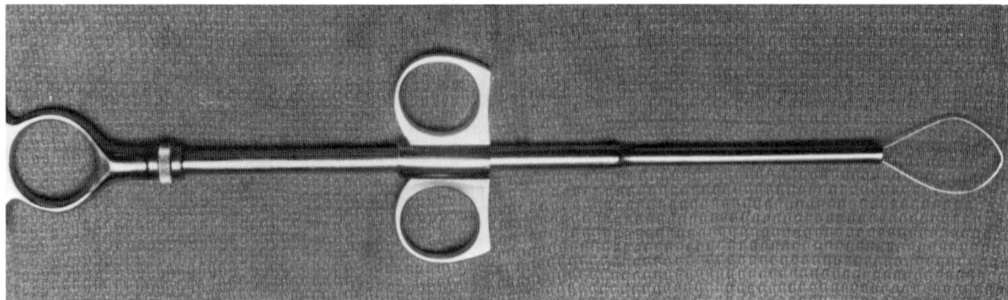

FIGURE 9–14. A standard tonsil snare. This instrument can be used to sever the specimen when working through a bivalved speculum. (With permission from Wright VC, Riopelle MA. Gynecologic Laser Surgery: A Practical Handbook, 2nd ed. Houston, Biomedical Communications, 1990)

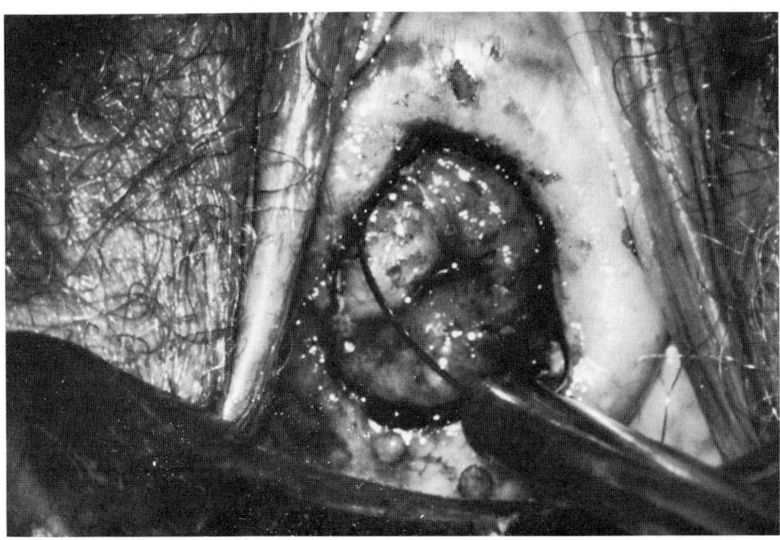

FIGURE 9–15. Insertion of the snare. The wire surrounds the specimen. (With permission from Wright VC, Riopelle MA: Gynecologic Laser Surgery: A Practical Handbook, 2nd ed. Houston, Biomedical Communications, 1990)

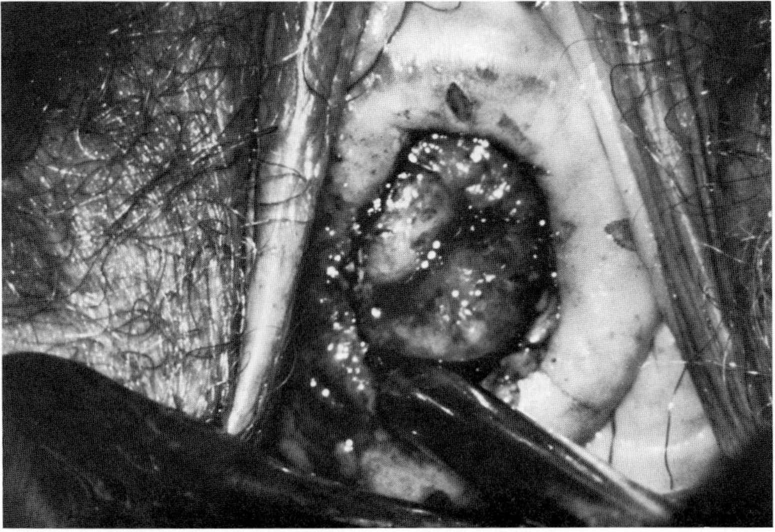

FIGURE 9–16. Severing the base. The snare placed at the incision base is used to sever the cylindrical specimen.

INDICATIONS AND OPERATIVE TECHNIQUE FOR LASER EXCISION AND VAPORIZATION (THE COMBINATION PROCEDURE)

In approximately 18% of CIN cases, extensive disease occupies the transformation zone on the ectocervix but also extends beyond colposcopic vision into the lower endocervical canal. Although cytology and colposcopy indicate only CIN disease, histologic examination of the endocervical tissue is necessary to evaluate this area completely. A suitable defect incorporating the ectocervix and the lower endocervical canal can effectively eliminate this distribution of disease (Fig. 9–17). The combination procedure is used when the ectocervical component has a linear radius greater than 8 mm.

With the patient under local or general anesthesia, the central cylinder is removed first for histologic evaluation. Specimen heights usually range from 1.0 to 1.5 cm (Fig. 9–18). This part of the operation is surgically similar to the laser cylindrical excision. Then, using a 2-mm CO_2 laser beam, the remaining outer disease and transformation zone are vaporized to a depth of 6 to 8 mm. This results in a cowboy hat configuration similar to the vaporized one (Fig. 9–19). By removing a central cylinder with peripheral vaporization, a surgeon removes one half as much tissue as would be required to remove all the disease with a cone-shaped configuration (see Fig. 9–19). The entire procedure takes less than 10 minutes when properly performed. The operative details have been previously described.[8–11]

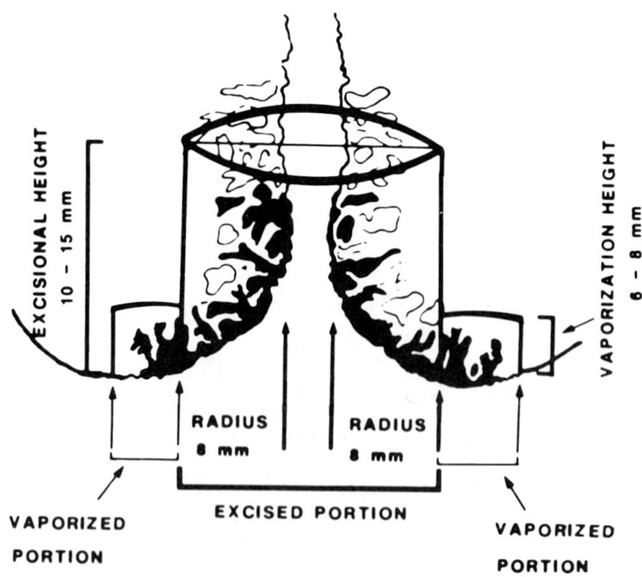

FIGURE 9–17. The schematics of the combination procedure, demonstrating the measurements for the ideal defect achieved by central excision and peripheral vaporization.

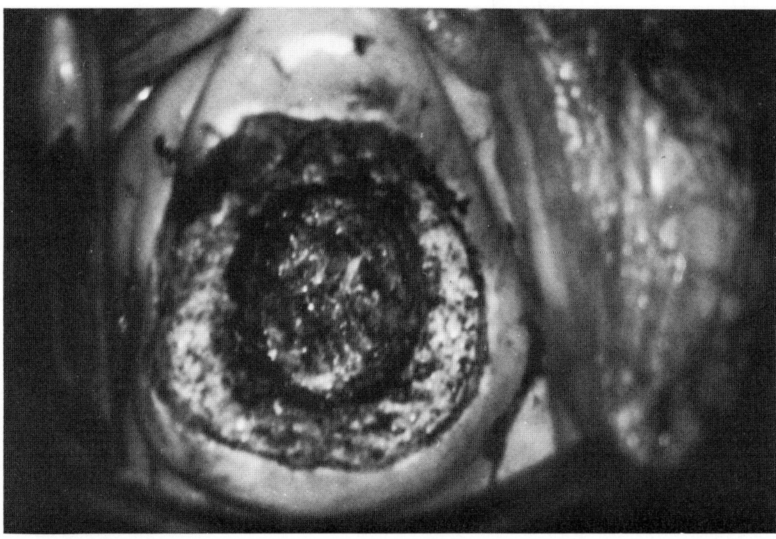

FIGURE 9–18. This photograph demonstrates the "cowboy hat" configuration of a completed combination procedure.

BLEEDING FROM THE LASERED CERVIX

During laser cervical vaporization, bleeding is unusual when a 2-mm laser beam diameter is used. Should bleeding occur, because blood absorbs the laser energy, it will be necessary to remove the blood from the field. The most effective method is to disconnect the plastic suction tube from the speculum and attach it to a long, non-flammable plastic suction tip, and use it to suction the blood away. This method requires a fluid trap in the plume evacuator's suction line. The dry field should then be lasered during the continued suctioning. The aspirated blood goes into the trap and the plume, onward to the suction filtering equipment. This method is efficient, and very little time is lost. The beam's heat effect should seal the vessels. Should this fail, a focal tip cautery may be employed to cauterize the bleeding site. In the authors' experience, using these methods during laser ablation procedures, suturing the cervix for uncontrolled bleeding has been unnecessary.

During the laser excisional procedures, troublesome bleeding is unusual. This is due to the placement of hemostatic sutures at the 3- and 9-o'clock positions, which decreases blood flow to the operative site, as well as the use of vasopressin, which constricts the vessels' lumina to allow the thermal effect of the laser to seal them. Should bleeding occur, the blood is aspirated from the field as previously discussed. When this fails, appropriate hemostatic sutures are placed and tied externally to the excised area. Never chase a bleeder with the CO_2 laser, because the laser beam may vaporize a hole into an undesirable area, with potentially serious damage.

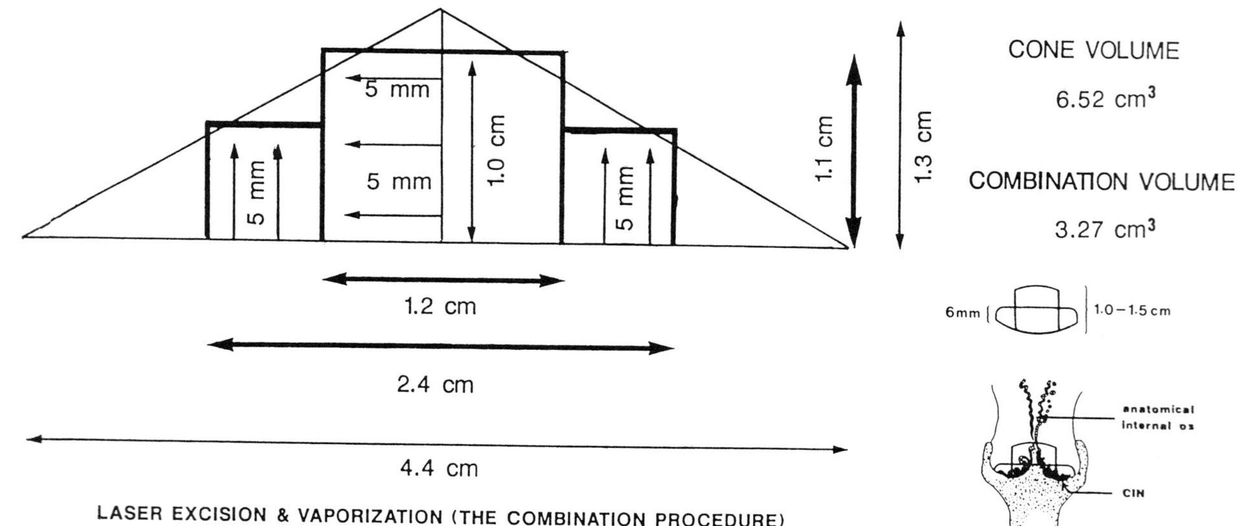

LASER EXCISION & VAPORIZATION (THE COMBINATION PROCEDURE)

FIGURE 9–19. The geometry of endocervical plus ectocervical CIN disease. A combination of a moderately tall cylinder surrounded by a shallower innertube shape incorporates disease in cases of ectocervical lesions extending into the endocervical canal. The cylindrical approach removes one half the volume of tissue that would be required of a cone shape to include all the diseased areas. (With permission from Wright VC: Laser surgery for cervical intraepithelial neoplasia—Principles and results. In Wright VC, Lickrish GM: Basic and Advanced Colposcopy: A Practical Handbook for Diagnosis and Treatment. Houston, Biomedical Communications, pp 161–172, 1989)

CERVICAL HEALING
AFTER LASER SURGERY

The four procedures discussed in this chapter, using excision and vaporization individually or in combination, are designed to treat CIN with any anatomical distribution over the cervix. Healing patterns are well documented.[6] Some sloughing of necrotic tissue and carbon residue occurs during the first 2 days, and cytology reveals the presence of acute inflammatory cells. By day 3, squamous epithelium begins to proliferate in the defect. Specks of carbonized debris from the crater surface can be observed. During days 4 to 7, the cavity is being filled in by squamous epithelium, and the inflammatory reaction subsides. At 20 days, a fragile but histologically normal epithelium is formed. Any trauma at this time will easily detach the epithelial cells in a single sheet from the underlying stroma. Re-epithelialization occurs during 10 to 21 days later.

The original or almost original tissue mass is restored by day 21, with normal topography. At that time, mature epithelium with normal tensile strength has been documented cytologically, histologically, and by scanning electron microscopy (Figs. 9–20 and 9–21).[6]

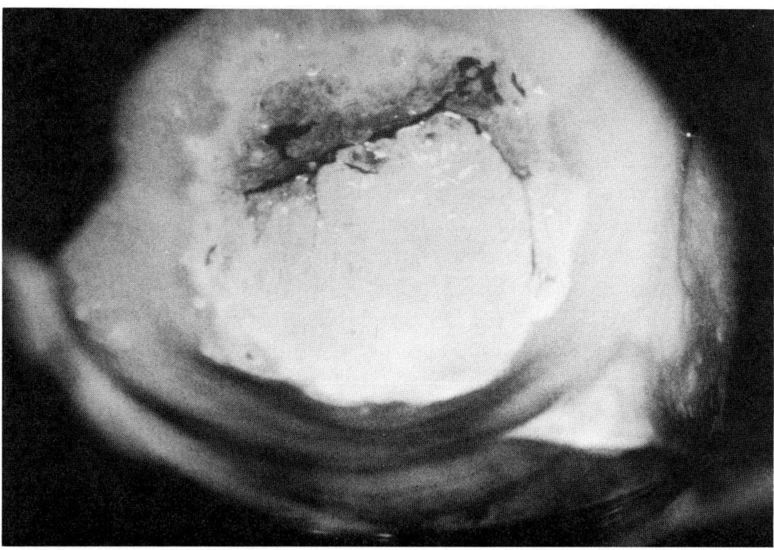

FIGURE 9–20. An ectocervical CIN lesion. This colpophotograph shows a typical lesion suitable for vaporization.

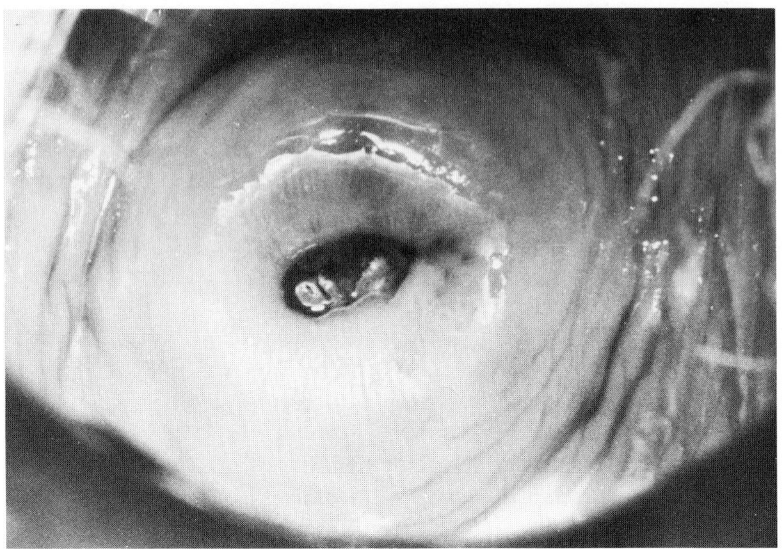

FIGURE 9–21. The healed cervix. This colpophotograph of the case illustrated in Figure 9–21, after complete healing, shows regeneration of organ mass seen at the first postoperative evaluation. Note the ideal location of the squamocolumnar junction at the level of the external os.

RESULTS OF LASER SURGERY FOR CIN USING THE CYLINDRICAL APPROACHES

In a prospective study in the Abnormal Pap Smear Clinic at St. Joseph's Hospital, London, Ontario, 2327 patients with CIN were treated by one of the four methods described in 1978–1986. No other method of treatment was offered as a first intervention. The location of the disease determined which laser procedure was performed. Only 1.1% of patients did not return for at least one postoperative visit, and most of these patients have had long-term follow-up.

Table 9–2 shows the results after one laser surgery. One vaporization procedure cured 93.4% of CIN I, 95.6% of CIN II, and 96.9% of CIN III cases. One

TABLE 9–2
Cure Rates After One Laser Surgery

	VAPORIZATION			CYLINDER AND COMBINATION		
DISEASE	Treated	Cured	% Cured	Treated	Cured	% Cured
CIN I	469	438	93.4	175	162	92.6
CIN II	504	482	95.6	195	183	93.8
CIN III	481	466	96.9	503	483	96.0
TOTAL	1454	1386	95.3	873	828	94.8

TABLE 9–3
**Results of One Laser Surgery
(Vaporization, Excision, and Combination)**

DIAGNOSIS	CASES	FAILURES	% CURED
CIN I	644	44	93.2
CIN II	699	34	95.1
CIN III	984	35	96.4
TOTAL	2327	113	95.1

excision or combination procedure cured 92.6% of CIN I, 93.8% of CIN II, and 96.0% of CIN III cases. Table 9–3 summarizes the success rates after one laser surgery with all procedures combined. Tables 9–4 and 9–5 illustrate the incidence and histology of persistent disease after first laser vaporization (Table 9–4) and laser excision (Table 9–5). In only 11 (of 113) cases of persistent disease was histology more severe than the original diagnosis, and no microinvasive or frankly invasive disease was noted. In all procedures, condyloma accounted for increased failures in the lower-grade lesions. This is probably because laser surgery has activated latent virus. In higher-grade lesions, it is believed that the virus is integrated in cells within diseased areas, and because of this, most virus is removed by the surgery. Table 9–6 illustrates the management of persistent disease after the first laser surgery. Thirteen hysterectomies were performed, 11.5% of primary treatment failures. One truly stubborn CIN III case required three laser vaporizations.

The first follow-up examination was done at the 3-month anniversary. The examination included colposcopy and cytology, with biopsy if appropriate, and was very accurate in identifying persistent disease. Greater than 90% of treatment failures were identified at the first follow-up, with all but one of the remaining failures detected at the second visit 3 months later. The rare case that appeared colposcopically and cytologically normal at two follow-up visits was identified at the third visit

TABLE 9–4
**Percent and Histologic Diagnosis of Persistent Disease Following Primary
Laser Vaporization**

INITIAL DIAGNOSIS	TOTAL CASES		PERSISTENT DISEASE		HISTOLOGIC DIAGNOSIS OF PERSISTENT DISEASE			
	No.	%	No.	%	CIN I	CIN II	CIN III	Condyloma
CIN I	469	32.2	31	6.6	22	3	1	5
CIN II	504	34.7	22	4.4	12	4	2	4
CIN III	481	33.1	15	3.1	4	3	6	2
TOTAL	1454	100.0	68	4.7	38	10	9	11

TABLE 9–5
Percent and Histologic Diagnosis of Persistent Disease Following Primary Laser Excision

INITIAL DIAGNOSIS	TOTAL CASES		PERSISTENT DISEASE		HISTOLOGIC DIAGNOSIS OF PERSISTENT DISEASE			
	No.	%	No.	%	CIN I	CIN II	CIN III	Condyloma
CIN I	175	20.1	13	7.4	4	2	1	6
CIN II	195	22.3	12	6.2	3	5	2	2
CIN III	503	57.6	20	4.0	2	7	11	0
TOTAL	873	100.0	45	5.2	9	14	14	8

(9 months). During follow-up, 20 hysterectomies were eventually performed in women for benign indications. No CIN, microinvasive, or invasive disease was found in the extirpated specimen.

Ninety percent of cases healed with a new squamocolumnar junction located at the external os, and in all cases the cervix appeared to regenerate to its original or almost original tissue mass (Figs. 9–21 and 9–22). No case of cervical stenosis occurred in a menstruating woman. In this series of 2327 patients, 7% experienced bleeding that required attention. Only 1.4% of patients undergoing laser vaporization and only 2.2% of patients having excision or combination procedures required admission to hospital. Five of these required suturing, and only one required a transfusion. No patient required a hysterectomy to control bleeding, either during the procedure or postoperatively.

Table 9–7 illustrates the pregnancy outcome in 95 patients (142 vaporizations and 53 laser excisions). There was no increase above expected in the rates of premature delivery or cesarean section.

SUMMARY

These four procedures—vaporization of a dome-shaped cylinder or domed cylinder plus wide peripheral vaporization, excision of a cylindrical specimen of endocervix, and a combination of excision plus peripheral vaporization, are effective and efficient in eliminating CIN regardless of histologic grade, lesion size, or disease location.[11] It is remarkable that only 13 (0.56%) of all cases required hysterectomy to effect a cure, and therefore it can be concluded that laser surgery is at least as effective as hysterectomy for this disease. This is probably because the surgical approaches are designed to remove appropriate tissue volumes based on the solid (*i.e.,* three-dimensional) geometry of CIN. The defects created always leave a base and an adequate rim to promote healing. The geometry of disease and the surgical defects are cylindrical and differ substantially from the traditional cone in theory, practice, and results. These data further demonstrate that creating the described surgical defects based on the geometry of CIN using proper surgical techniques does not

TABLE 9–6
Management of Persistent Disease After One Laser Surgery

| INITIAL DIAGNOSIS | Cases | PRIMARY TREATMENT | | SECONDARY TREATMENT MODALITY | | | | | |
| | | Failures | | Second Laser | | Focal Cautery | | Hysterectomy | |
		No.	%	No.	%	No.	%	No.	%
CIN I	644	44	6.8	40	90.9	2	4.5	2	4.5
CIN II	699	34	4.9	31	91.2	1	2.9	2	5.9
CIN III	984	35	3.5	25	71.4	1	2.8	9	25.7
TOTAL	2327	113	4.8	96	84.9	4	3.5	13*	(11.5)

* *All extirpated specimens contained CIN III histologically.*

TABLE 9–7
Pregnancy After Laser Surgery

	VAPORIZATION		LASER EXCISION		TOTAL	
	No.	%	No.	%	No.	%
Total pregnancies	142		53		195	
Term deliveries (37+ weeks)	116	93.5	42	89.4	158	92.4
Premature deliveries (20–36 weeks)	8	6.5	5	10.6	13	7.6
Spontaneous abortion	12	8.4	1	1.8	13	6.7
Therapeutic abortion	3	2.1	3	5.6	6	3.1
Extrauterine pregnancy	3	2.1	2	3.7	5	2.7
Vaginal deliveries	106	85.5	44	93.6	150	87.7
Total cesarean sections	18	14.5	3	6.4	21	2.3
Fetal death 23 weeks	1	0.8	0	0.0	1	0.6

increase the rate of premature delivery or produce an incompetent cervix.[11] This outcome is likely related to the fact that the defects are designed to include all disease but not encroach on the anatomical internal os in women of reproductive age.[7,11]

Restoration of almost normal organ mass and an optimal location of the new squamocolumnar junction at the level of the external os enable effective follow-up assessments by colposcopy and cytology.[9] Therefore, any persistent disease is easily diagnosed, usually identified early, and easily retreated, often by further laser vaporization or excision.

REFERENCES

1. Anderson MC, Hartley RB: Cervical crypt involvement by intra-epithelial neoplasia. Am J Obstet Gynecol 55:546–549, 1980
2. Carson RP, Gall EA: Preinvasive carcinoma and precancer metaplasia of the cervix. Am J Pathol 30:15–19, 1954
3. Fluhmann GF: Involvement of clefts and tunnels in carcinoma in situ of the cervix uteri. Am J Obstet Gynecol 83:1410–1419, 1962
4. Gusberg SB, Moore DB: The clinical pattern of intraepithelial carcinoma of the cervix and its pathologic background. Obstet Gynecol 2:1–14, 1953
5. Hamperl H, Kaufmann C: The cervix uteri at various ages. Obstet Gynecol 14:621–625, 1959
6. Holmquist ND, Bellina JH, Danos ML: Vaginal and cervical cytologic changes following laser treatment. Acta Cytol 20:290–294, 1976
   Larsson G: Conization for preinvasive and invasive carcinoma of the uterine cervic. Acta Obstet Gynecol Scand (Suppl) 114:19–40, 1983
9. Kora LA, Plutowa A: Histological topography of carcinoma in situ of the cervix uteri. Cancer 273, 1959
10. Reagan JW: Diagnostic cervical biopsy technique for the study of early cancer: Value of the conization procedure. JAMA 160:343–348, 1956
   Davies E, Riopelle MA: Laser surgery for cervical intraepithelial neoplasia: Principles Obstet Gynecol 145:181–185, 1983

11. Wright VC, Davies E, Riopelle MA: Laser cylindrical excision to replace conization. Am J Obstet Gynecol 150:704–709, 1984

12. Wright VC, Riopelle MA: The geometry of cervical intra-epithelial neoplasia as a guide to its eradication. The Cervix 4:21–38, 1986

13. Wright VC: Carbon dioxide laser surgery for the cervix and vagina: Indications, complications, and results. Compr Ther 14:54–64, 1988

10

Laser Therapy for
the Vulva and Vagina

Richard Reid
Mitchell D. Greenberg

Within just one decade, the carbon dioxide (CO_2) laser has become the modality of choice for treating various anogenital epithelial disorders associated with human papillomavirus (HPV) infection. However, it should be emphasized that the great majority of these disorders can and should be managed by simpler therapies. Although sexually transmitted HPV infections are remarkably common, disease expression appears to be the exception rather than the rule.[17] When disease expression does occur, differences in host susceptibility produce enormous variability in clinical outcome.[10] Lesions may be unicentric or multicentric, and severity ranges from minute to massive. Clinical course varies from trivial and self-limiting to extensive and refractory. Even with high-risk types, the lifetime risk of progression from benign infection to cancer is probably no more than 1%.[8] Hence, the use of the CO_2 laser for vaginal and vulvar disease must be approached with restraint.[14]

THERAPEUTIC PRINCIPLES FOR VULVAR AND VAGINAL DISEASES

Benign Condylomata

Treatment of vulvar and vaginal condylomas should take account of the four phases in the natural history of papillomavirus infection.[11]

1. *An incubation phase* (6 weeks to 8 months before lesions appear). Incubation begins with inoculation at sites of microtrauma, leading

to HPV invasion of the basal layer cells underlying the sites of entry.[7] Thereafter, the virus spreads horizontally within susceptible tissues, eventually establishing a steady-state latent infection of the entire anogenital epithelium.[18]

2. *An active expression phase* (3 to 6 months from the time of the first lesion). After a period of latent expression, focal areas of maturing keratinocytes switch over to active viral expression, inducing both epithelial and capillary proliferation. If vascular overgrowth is prominent, these lesions will manifest as focal, clinically apparent papillomas. Alternatively, when epithelial effects exceed the degree of capillary proliferation, a diffuse field of subclinical acetowhitening results.

3. *A containment phase* (6 to 9 months from lesion occurrence). As a result of a B- and T-cell response,[23] about 20% of patients will undergo spontaneous regressions and another 60% will respond to simple office therapies. However, the 15 to 20% of women with extensive, refractory, or dysplastic lesions constitute a therapeutic problem for which laser surgery is indicated.[14]

4. *A late stage* (beyond 9 months). After about 9 months, patients can be divided into two groups: those who remain in sustained clinical remission and those who relapse into continued active disease expression. Even though women in the first group no longer present with new condylomata, it is important to understand that latent HPV infection persists within the anogenital epithelium. Some "cured" patients may even remain contagious to other sex partners. In contrast, the second group of patients (who either remain in active disease expression or who have a recurrence after a lesion-free interval) represent the subset most likely to undergo neoplastic progression.[22]

Aggressiveness of treatment must be counterbalanced against the degree of disease expression in an individual patient. Obviously, simple problems should have simple solutions. Benign, asymptomatic, subclinical lesions of the vulva or vagina do not require any treatment. Among patients who do present with overt condylomata, the great majority can be managed by scissor excision, caustic agent application, or focal physical destruction. However, extensive, refractory, and dysplastic lesions respond poorly to office methods.

Vulvar Intraepithelial Neoplasia

During the past decade, there has been a dramatic increase in the prevalence of vulvar intraepithelial neoplasia (VIN) in young women, particularly of the multifocal Bowenoid variety. Treatment of VIN is controversial, with recommendations ranging from wide excision to skinning vulvectomy. Although the treatment originally proposed for carcinoma *in situ* of the vulva was wide local excision, fears that the disease was preinvasive led to the widespread use of simple vulvectomy.[4] However, most documented instances of invasion have occurred in immunosuppressed or elderly women.[1] In young patients, the risk of malignant progression is insufficient to justify such mutilating surgery. Moreover, despite the mutilation, simple vulvectomy is an ineffective treatment for multifocal VIN (Fig. 10–1). Wide excision of small foci produces excellent results, but multifocal or extensive lesions are difficult to treat by this method. Hence, in the past, the only reasonable alternative was skinning vulvectomy with grafting. Although this technique is a definite improvement over conventional vulvectomy, cosmetic and functional results are unpredictable. Fortunately, the CO_2 laser offers an escape from this dilemma by providing an effective but nonmutilating treatment.

Vaginal Intraepithelial Neoplasia

Vaginal intraepithelial neoplasia (VAIN) has also been seen with increasing frequency during the past decade. In contrast to premalignant changes of the vulva, VAIN has a well-defined potential for malignant progression. Indeed, about one third of the invasive cancers following therapy for cervical neoplasia have occurred in the original squamous epithelium of the vaginal vault.[9] Because HPV-associated neoplasia within the lower genital tract does not affect tissues proximal to the upper limit of squamous metaplasia, removal of the normal endometrium adds nothing to prophylaxis. In other words, not only does hysterectomy provide incomplete protection against subsequent cancer, but the operation complicates matters by burying islands of HPV-infected squamous epithelium beneath the scar.[13]

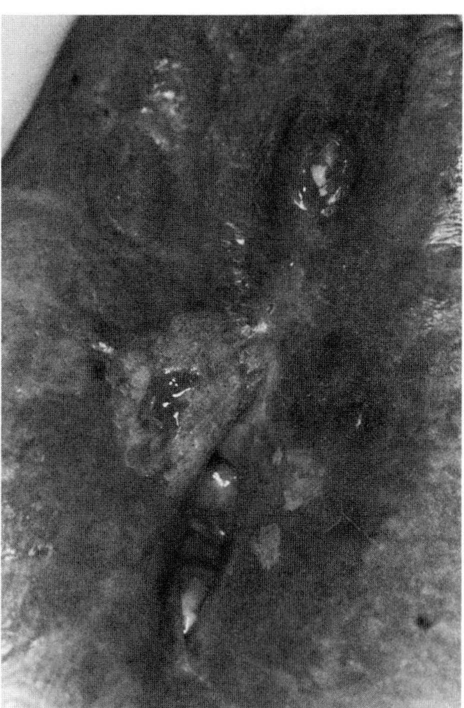

FIGURE 10–1. Recurrence of extensive VIN 3 with focal superficial invasion at the margins of a previous simple vulvectomy for Bowen's disease.

Although the CO_2 laser is ideal for treating vaginal lesions when the uterus remains *in situ*,[2] VAIN following hysterectomy often requires excision of the vault scar. In a series of 23 British women managed by laser vaporization of recurrent VAIN, Woodman and colleagues[25] reported that only six patients remained free of disease at 30 months after treatment. Of the 21 women in whom VAIN involved the vault scar, three developed invasive cancer in islands of buried vaginal epithelium. Hence, ablation should be reserved for foci of VAIN that can be seen in their entirety.[6]

Idiopathic Vulvodynia

An illness characterized by itching or burning of the vulva, plus intense tenderness around the vaginal opening, was recognized by gynecologists during the last two decades of the nineteenth century.[24] For mysterious reasons, this disease then disappeared from our society for the next 70 years. However, since 1975 there has been a dramatic increase in the numbers of women who present with complaints of idiopathic vulvodynia.[5]

Physical examination shows that this syndrome has three components:[21]

1. An irritative acetowhite reaction of the vulvar epithelium, apparently attributable to chronic HPV infection (Fig. 10–2*A*). This irritative acetowhitening always involves the mucosa of the vestibule but extends to the minimally keratinized, hairless skin of the interlabial grooves, clitoris, and perineum in about 50% of women, and to the hair-bearing skin of the labia majora and perianal region in about 25% of patients.
2. Ectasia of small vessels within the mucosal surface of the vulvar vestibule. Strangely, these hyperemic vessels contribute to the diffuse burning symptomatology, and are often tender to touch. Disruption of epithelial maturation and vascular growth appear to represent the immediate consequences of an irritant factor (probably low grade HPV infection) upon the surface mucosae of susceptible hosts. In contrast, deep inflammation surrounding vestibular glandular elements (component 3) constitutes a later, more severe stage in the evolution of this syndrome.
3. Painful inflammation within the connective tissue surrounding the minor vestibular glands (embryologic remnants of the endothelial portion of the cloaca, which persists as shallow clefts that are located in the hymenal sulcus [Fig. 10–2*B*]). In severe cases, this inflammation also involves the other structures derived from cloacal endothelium: namely, Skene's complex (shallow glands adjacent to the external urethral meatus) and the ducts of Bartholin's gland (two 1-mm orifices located just proximal to the mucocutaneous junction, on the posteromedial surface of the labia minora).

These three components are often associated, the irritative acetowhitening perhaps representing an earlier and milder manifestation of the syndrome, and the painful vestibular erythema denoting a more severe form.

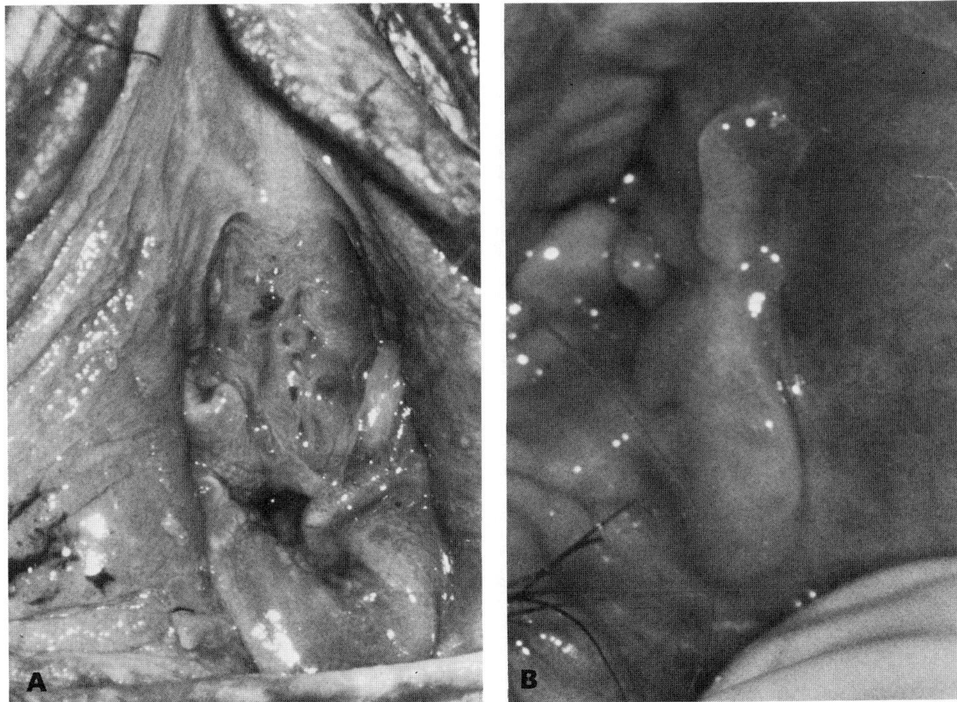

FIGURE 10–2. (A) The irritative acetowhite component of vulvodynia. **(B)** Painful red gland openings, at the hymenal margin. (Reproduced with permission from Reid R, Greenberg M, Daoud Y et al: Colposcopic findings in women with vulvar pain syndromes. A preliminary report. J Reprod Med 33:523–532, 1988)

Although the surface papillomavirus infection often responds to topical 5-fluorouracil cream, the inflammation surrounding the minor vestibular glands is resistant to anti-inflammatory medication, including topical or injected steroids. The standard therapy has been an operation described by Woodruff,[26] in which the posterior three quarters of the hymenal ring (including the minor vestibular glands) are excised, and the defect closed by downward advancement of the posterior vaginal wall. Woodruff's procedure is unsatisfactory for three reasons[21]:

First, excision of the minor vestibular glands cannot cure chronic burning discomfort that is caused by lateral extension of the HPV infection to involve the interlabial grooves or labia majora.

Second, even when hymenal resection is successful, the cosmetic results are somewhat dismaying (Fig. 10–3). Although it is accepted that a cosmetic deformity may be preferable to a functional inability to have coitus, it is also clear that hymenal resection should be a treatment of last resort (rather than an initial surgical approach).

Third, the success rate for hymenal resection is only about 50%. Moreover, trying to approximate the vaginal mucosa to the perineal skin often causes scar formation. Such scarring can exacerbate any incipient inflammation in the stroma surrounding Skene's and Bartholin's glands, sometimes resulting in a marked wors-

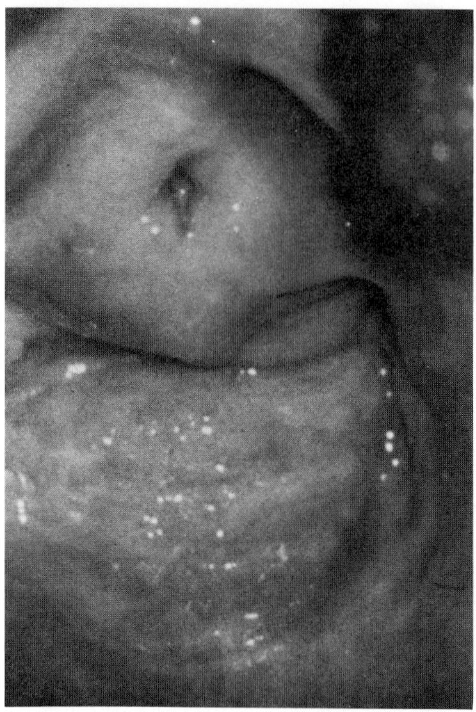

FIGURE 10–3. End result showing removal of hymenal ring and approximation of the vaginal mucosa to the perineal skin. Cosmetic appearances of this operation are poor, and efficacy is low. (Reproduced with permission from Reid R, Greenberg M, Daoud Y et al: Colposcopic findings in women with vulvar pain syndromes. A preliminary report. J Reprod Med 33:523–532, 1988)

ening of symptoms (Fig. 10–4*A*). Areas of painful erythema that occur following previous surgery have usually proved to be very difficult to treat.

When faced with patients who had suffered a postoperative recurrence of Skene's and Bartholin's gland inflammation, the only surgical option was re-excision of the original scar and an *en bloc* dissection of the periurethral tissue, Bartholin's ducts, and Bartholin's glands.[21] Although generally successful, such surgery is technically difficult and produces even more vulvovaginal deformity. Moreover, excising all of the inflamed mucosa sacrifices a very large proportion of the vestibular epithelium.

Based on this experience, we are presently investigating the use of lasers to achieve the same surgical objectives while avoiding the unnecessary disfigurement of a radical excision of the inflamed vestibular glands. Preliminary results with superficial CO_2 laser photovaporization of the irritative acetowhite epithelium and deep CO_2 laser photovaporization of inflamed vestibular glands have been encouraging. However, the problem of ectopic erythema due to telangiectatic overgrowth of stromal blood vessels is not controllable by CO_2 laser destruction. Some of these complications have been controlled by argon laser photocoagulation of these hyperemic vessels (Fig. 10–4*B*).[21] However, attempting to treat such highly vascularized areas with the argon laser carries a risk of severe burning. Hence, our protocol also employs a flash pumped dye laser to produce selective photothermolysis of these target blood vessels.

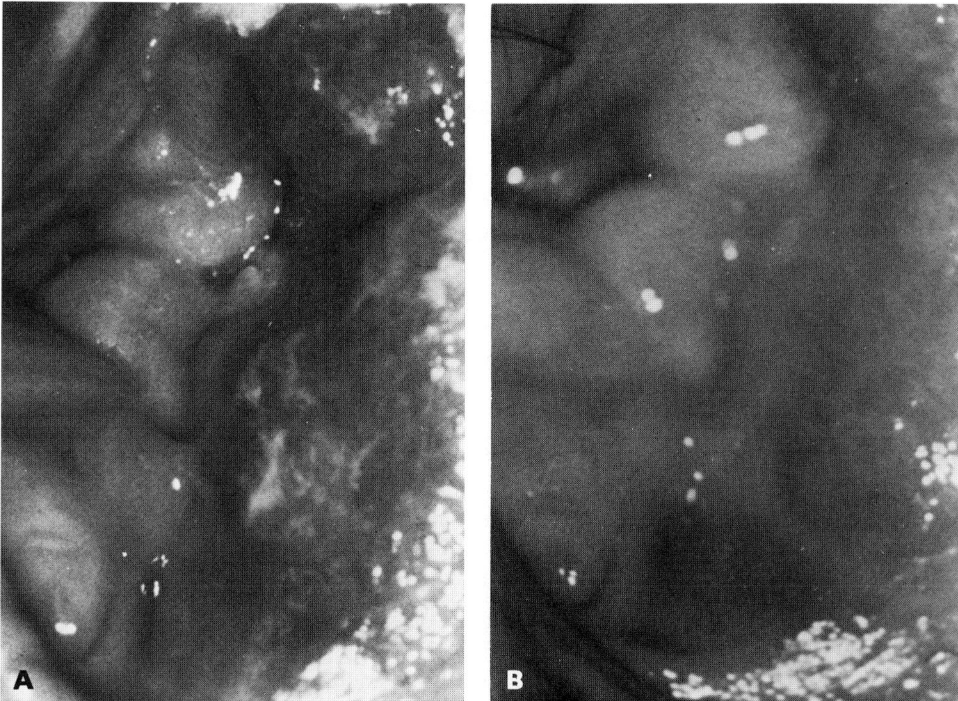

FIGURE 10–4. **(A)** An intensely painful focus of vestibular erythema arising adjacent to the hymenal scar. **(B)** Appearance 2 months after argon photocoagulation, showing almost complete resolution. The symptoms resolved completely during the next 4 months of colchicine therapy. (Reproduced with permission from Reid R, Greenberg M, Daoud Y et al: Colposcopic findings in women with vulvar pain syndromes. A preliminary report. J Reprod Med 33:523–532, 1988)

WHAT ADVANTAGES DOES THE CO$_2$ LASER OFFER?

Laser use has expanded enormously during the past decade, particularly in the male and female genital tracts. Results are generally reported in glowing terms, and there is widespread belief that surgical success is essentially guaranteed by the technical sophistication of the CO$_2$ laser. Unhappily, but not unexpectedly, such beliefs are ill founded.

Certainly, because of the affinity of water for mid-infrared radiation, optical energy from the CO$_2$ laser displays several unique surgical properties: 1) disease volumes can be vaporized under precise visual control; 2) heat propagation to adjacent tissue can be minimal; 3) microorganisms at the impact site will be automatically destroyed; and 4) vessels smaller than 0.5 mm (arterioles) will be thermally sealed. Unfortunately, these surgical advantages are easily dissipated by unskilled use.

The CO_2 laser resembles the hot cautery, the electrodiathermy, and the cryosurgical probe, in that all are instruments of thermal destruction. With conventional devices, lateral heat propagation declines down a slow, linear gradient. Adjacent tissues must recover from the ill effects of a diffuse conduction burn or frostbite before the healing response can begin. In contrast with skilled use of the laser, thermal injury to adjacent tissues can be confined within a very narrow and sharply defined band.

Unfortunately, it is not sufficiently appreciated that unless strategies are employed to restrict heat conduction to adjacent tissues during photovaporization, the laser will produce the same kind of conduction burn as a hot cautery.[12] Few surgeons capitalize on the increased precision afforded by the rapid superpulse mode. Through a misdirected sense of caution, many use dangerously low power outputs and allow power densities to fall into the carbonization range. Surface ablation is often undertaken with a beam geometry suited only to thermal incision, thereby producing an array of ridges and gutters that must be flattened by a rastering technique, each sequential pass adding to the unnecessary thermal injury. Some surgeons still try to control the laser in delicate situations by turning down beam power, rather than through the strategy of prolonging reaction time with gated pulses. Particularly when operating on the thin, fragile epithelia of the vulva and vagina, such errors will rapidly squander the potential advantages that can attend laser surgery.[20]

As in other forms of surgery, success depends on both sound theoretic principles and skilled operative technique. Hence, besides selecting optimal physical parameters for each operation, a surgeon must also employ specific surgical strategies to ensure dexterous beam delivery, minimize heat injury to adjacent tissues, obtain hemostasis, facilitate exposure, delineate treatment margins, and confine the depth of thermal denaturation to the desired level. The application of these principles to CO_2 laser surgery within the vulva and vagina is discussed below.

PRINCIPLE 1: CHOICE OF AN APPROPRIATE BEAM DELIVERY SYSTEM

Laser energy always emerges from the optical resonance tube as a highly collimated beam. However, energy generated with medical lasers never reaches the tissue as a parallel beam, because the property of collimation is destroyed by the various delivery systems. This phenomenon of beam divergence within the delivery system exerts a major effect on the pattern of tissue destruction that occurs at the point of tissue impact. Hence, having selected the desired power and temporal mode, a gynecologist must give thought to whether the laser beam should be delivered through an operating microscope or with a hand–held probe.

Delivery Through an Operating Microscope

Expertise with a microscopically adapted laser capitalizes on the fact that the coherent radiation is transmitted through a separate set of lenses. When both the beam delivery system and the visual optics are equipped with 300-mm objectives, the point of sharp visual focus will produce a laser beam with the narrowest diameter attainable from a lens of that focal length (about 1 mm). At this point, the beam has a high power density and a peaked geometry, making it ideal for creating a deep incision. However, for the purpose of shallow epithelial ablation, the beam must be flattened by defocusing until a point is found at which the impact crater becomes approximately hemispheric. Hence, satisfactory ablation of vaginal and vulvar lesions absolutely requires a laser fitted with a microslad defocusing system.[12]

Delivery Through a Hand-Held Probe

Hand-held probes incorporate lenses of short focal length, as a means of attaining very narrow spot diameters and correspondingly high power densities. Unfortunately, this amplification of power density is achieved at the cost of a marked diminution in focal depth. Provided that the tip of the probe is kept in close focus, hand-held delivery systems are well suited to the creation of thermal incision. However, because of the apparent simplicity of the delivery system, novice surgeons are sometimes tempted to attempt vulvar ablations with the hand probe. This is always a serious mistake, for several reasons: *First,* the focal plane is so narrow that even slight variations in lens-to-target distance will have a dramatic effect on spot diameter, causing an exponential reduction in power density. *Second,* if the probe is angulated to allow a surgeon to assume a comfortable "pencil grip," the energy profile at the point of impact will have an oval (rather than circular) distribution. Creating an egg-shaped crater adds a further dimension to the difficulty of trying to ensure uniformity of power density. *Third,* failure to use the operating microscope robs a surgeon of the benefit of anatomic landmarks, making depth control a very haphazard affair. *Fourth,* the unaided eye has insufficient visual resolution to permit surgical control over beams of >750 watts/cm^2. In short, attempting to perform superficial ablation with a hand-held probe generally condemns a surgeon to making a series of nonuniform, poorly localized cuts, at a power density close to the carbonization range.[12]

PRINCIPLE 2: MINIMIZING THERMAL DAMAGE BY TISSUE COOLING

Despite the application of optimal physical principles, there will always be some heat conduction to adjacent tissues. The amount of lateral heat propagation while using the laser as a thermal knife is too small to matter. However, during vulvar laser ablation, limiting thermal spread by chilling the tissues with iced saline has greatly diminished postoperative pain and swelling and has contributed to a major reduction in healing time.[16]

Cooling is done with laparotomy packs soaked in a bowl of semifrozen saline slush. The tissues should be chilled before the initial laser impact and at frequent intervals during the operation. Precooling acts as a buffer against burning, in that diffused heat must first restore temperatures to the normal range before tissue injury can occur. Reapplication of the iced saline immediately after laser irradiation is also beneficial, probably because cooling antagonizes continued tissue damage by vasoactive peptides released at the time of the initial thermal injury.

Control of Intraoperative Bleeding

The easiest approach to this potentially frustrating problem is to prevent intraoperative bleeding by the use of vasoconstrictor injections, especially when making thermal incisions.

When hemorrhage is encountered, a surgeon must distinguish partial transection of a small vessel from laceration of a much larger artery or vein. Most intraoperative bleeding arises from a laser impact punching a hole in the side of a small vessel. Hence, relasing the bleeding point with a high-powered beam for about 2 to 3 seconds will usually secure hemostasis by transecting the perforated arteriole and sealing the cut ends. However, if this maneuver is not successful, a surgeon will have to either tamponade the bleeding point and coagulate the area at low power density or insert a hemostatic suture.

PRINCIPLE 3: ENSURING GOOD EXPOSURE AND A PERPENDICULAR BEAM IMPACT

Expert control over the CO_2 laser requires both good exposure and perpendicular beam delivery. Strategies for achieving these requirements vary according to specific surgical situations.

Laser Ablation Within the Vagina

The vaginal walls are most easily visualized by continuously rotating and withdrawing a bivalve speculum. If necessary, alignment can be further improved by traction with an iris hook or a tenaculum.

Lasing the vaginal vault after hysterectomy is more difficult than when the uterus is *in situ*. When confronted with the problem of being unable to locate and destroy the epithelium buried beneath the vaginal scar, a surgeon can attempt to evert any dysplastic epithelium with the lateral angles by traction with an iris hook. Exposure is sometimes further improved by using a bivalve speculum that has blades of equal length (e.g., Cusco's or Collin's speculum) (Fig. 10–5).

Laser Ablation of External Vulvar Skin

Exposure on external surfaces is generally simple. Although positioning either the laser or the target (so as to obtain a perpendicular impact) can be tedious, such difficulties can always be overcome. A surgeon must resist any temptation to trade the accuracy of the microscopically adapted laser for the easy maneuverability of hand-held delivery system. Finally, the importance of shaving needs emphasis, both as an aid to vision as well as to simplify postoperative dressings.

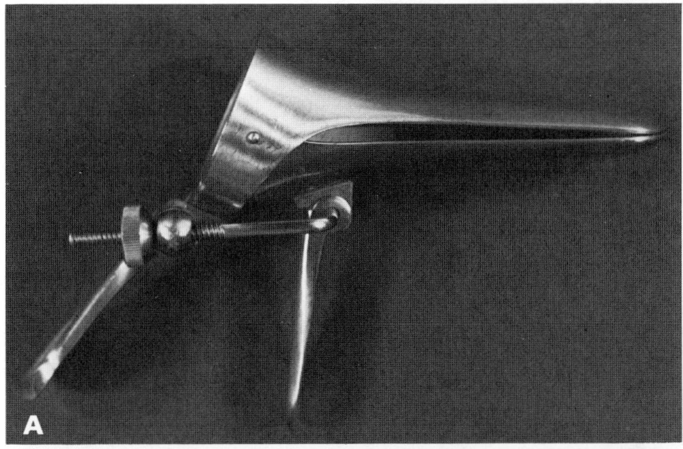

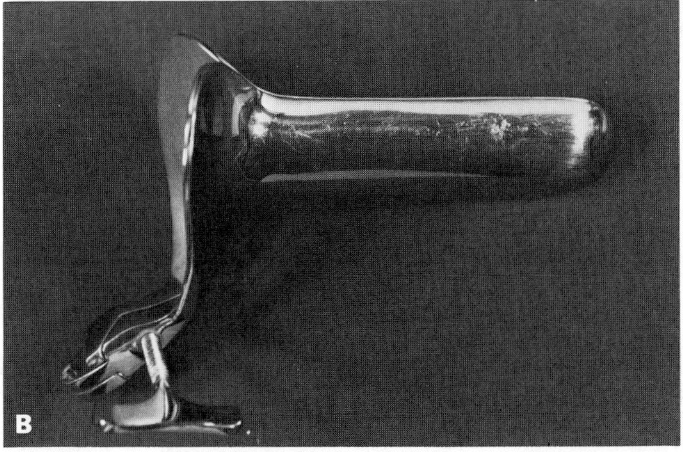

FIGURE 10–5. **(A)** A Cusco's speculum. **(B)** A Collin's speculum.

Laser Ablation Within the Distal Urethra and Anal Canal

Exposure within the distal few centimeters of the urethra is most easily achieved with a pediatric nasal speculum (Fig. 10–6) or by eversion with mucosal sutures. The anal canal is best visualized by use of a suitable anoscope (Fig. 10–7*A* and *B*).

PRINCIPLE 4: ACCURATE DELINEATION OF THE TREATMENT MARGINS

In all forms of surgery, an ability to set accurate margins for the excision or destruction of diseased tissue is an essential ingredient of success.

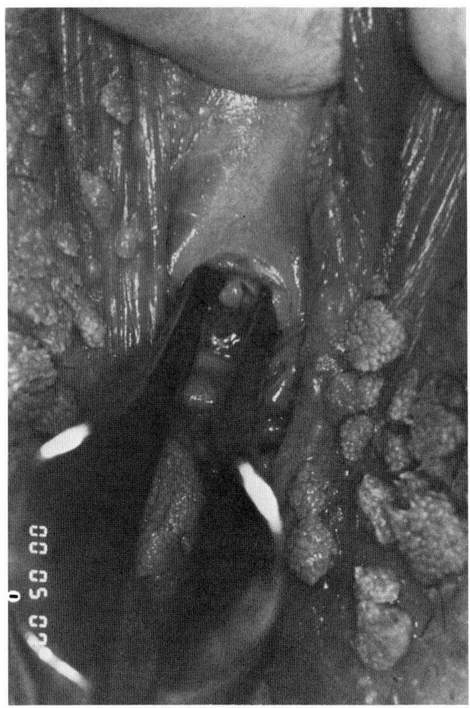

FIGURE 10–6. Exposure of the distal urethra with a pediatric nasal speculum.

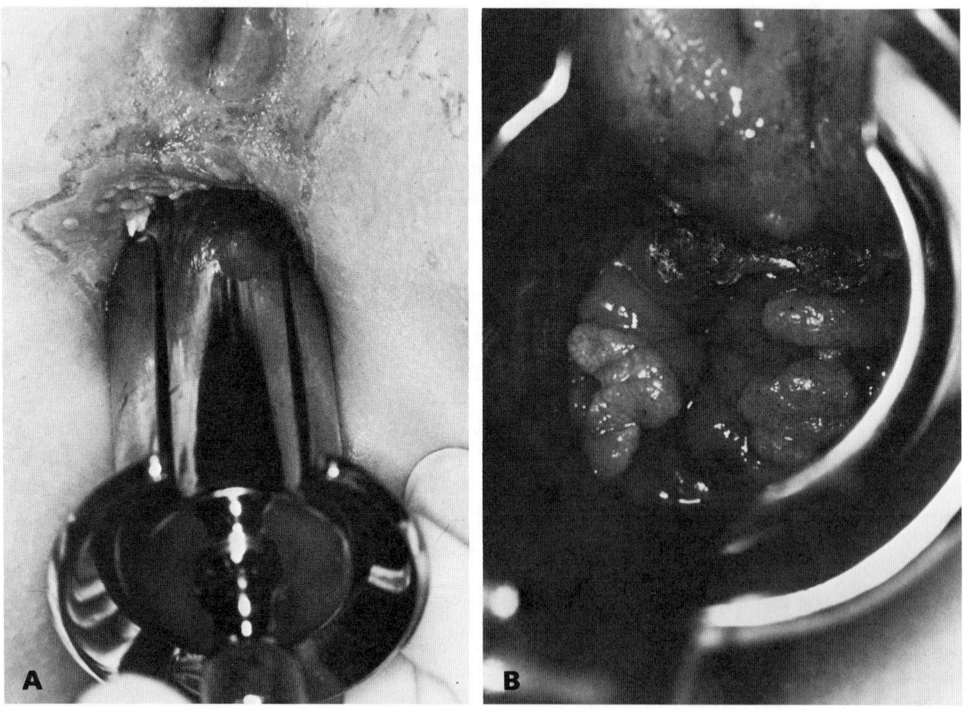

FIGURE 10–7. **(A)** Preparing to insert a fixed anoscope for exposure of the anal canal. **(B)** Extensive coalescent condylomata exposed and ready for laser destruction.

Margins for Vulvar Laser Surgery

Within the lower genital tract, exophytic condylomata and foci of obvious intraepithelial neoplasia are like the tip of an iceberg.

Soaking with 3 to 6% acetic acid will usually produce prominent acetowhitening of skin that had appeared normal to examination with the unaided eye (Fig. 10–8*A*). Such acetowhite epithelium generally contains the same type of viral DNA as demonstrable in biopsy specimens from the areas of principal pathology.[22] These observations suggest that macroscopically obvious lesions represent focal disease expression within a much wider field of inapparent papillomavirus infection. Nonetheless, clinical experience has taught that about 85% of patients will be cured by destruction of just the obvious lesions. However, the 15 to 20% of women with papillomavirus infections that are refractory to conventional office therapy constitute management problems. Failure to recognize the true extent of disease in this subset will adversely affect surgical outcome. Hence, it is not surprising that a randomized trial comparing laser "spot welding" with electrodiathermy reported control rates of only 9 of 21 in the laser group and 8 of 22 in the diathermy group.[3] These results are in keeping with the expectation that focal photovaporization should not offer any advantage over other forms of physical or chemical destruction.

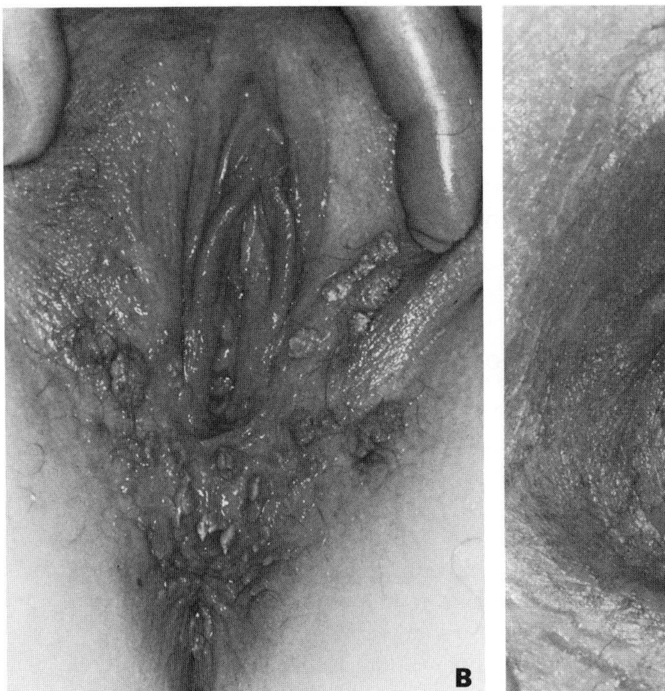
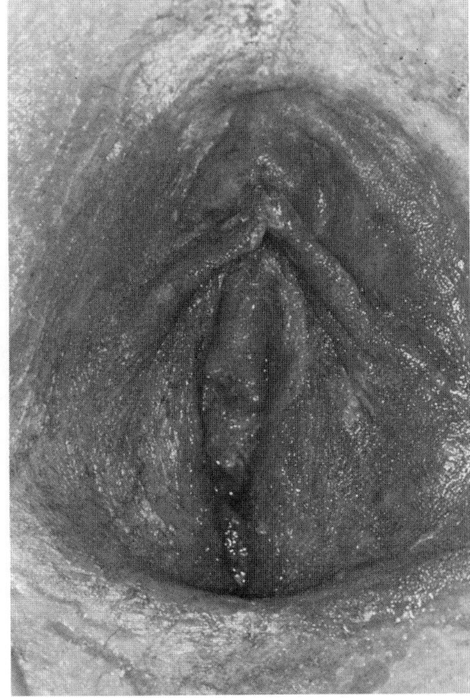

FIGURE 10–8. **(A)** Determining the extent of the adjacent subclinical papillomavirus infection, by soaking with 6% acetic acid. **(B)** A view at the conclusion of laser surgery, showing the extent of photovaporization.

The potential for better results with the laser hinges on a newfound capacity to ablate the entire field of papillomavirus-infected epithelium to a shallow depth (Fig. 10–8*B*). Healing occurs by epithelial regrowth from noninfected keratinocytes in the underlying skin appendages.[19] In contrast to the disappointing results of spot welding, this technique of superficial laser vulvectomy produced remission in 158 of the 160 (99%) most difficult patients referred to the authors between 1983 and 1987.[16]

PRINCIPLE 5: ACCURATE DEPTH CONTROL

Based on measurements of the average depth of the cervical crypts, most gynecologists destroy the transformation zone to a depth of 7 mm. The cylindrical nature of the resulting defect and the relatively large dimensions of the intended crater make it quite easy to control the depth of cervical ablation by actual measurement. In contrast, depths of destruction during vulvar and vaginal surgery are too shallow to control by measurement, particularly because the laser crater has no well-defined sides to act as points of reference.

Depth Control During Vaginal Laser Surgery

Because there are no epithelial crypts beneath the original squamous epithelium, vaginal lesions should be destroyed only to the level of the lamina propria (<1 mm). The most reliable method of depth control is to lase until submucosal stromal fibers can be seen through the operating microscope.[2] Infiltration with saline can be employed as an additional safeguard against injury to the bladder or bowel.

With the uterus *in situ,* laser destruction of VAIN is a straightforward exercise.[2] However, in patients who present with positive Papanicolaou smears after hysterectomy, thought should be given to excising the top of the vagina, in order to exclude occult invasion beneath the vault scar.[6,25] Of course, VAIN that does not involve the vault scar can still be managed safely by laser ablation.

Depth Control During Vulvar Laser Surgery

Satisfactory healing of vulvar wounds depends on the preservation of the skin appendages, a task that is too delicate to trust to crude measurement. Hence, a surgeon must learn to control depth according to the visual characteristics at the site of impact.[19]

From a surgical viewpoint, tissue destruction occurs through two distinct mechanisms: immediate photovaporization and delayed coagulation necrosis. The depth of photovaporization depends on hand-eye control. In contrast, thickness of the zone of coagulation necrosis varies widely, according to laser settings. Surgeons who use suboptimal laser settings must *understand* that necrotic tissue on the wound surface looks normal at the time of surgery, only to separate as an eschar after activation of the host inflammatory response. That is to say, when using low-powered continuous wave, any structures visible within the crater base will have already suffered irreversible thermal coagulation and will be sloughed off by the succeeding week. In contrast, with more optimal settings, visual appearances correspond closely to actual depth of destruction. Hence, the art of expert CO_2 laser surgery is to judge crater depth such that the zone of thermal necrosis (rather than the zone of photovaporization) lies at the intended depth of penetration. Visual orientation is preserved by continuously wiping away the surface char. Depth of destruction is inferred from anatomic landmarks in the crater base.[19] By means of this technique, four characteristic surgical planes are identifiable (Table 10–1) (Fig. 10–9).[15]

The First Surgical Plane. Destruction to the first plane removes only the surface epithelium to the level of the basement membrane. This plane is reached by putting the laser crater within the prickle cell layer. Penetration to the proper depth is accomplished by rapid oscillation of the micromanipulator, such that the helium-neon spot describes a roughly parallel series of lines. When done correctly, each pass of the laser beam reveals bubbles of silver opalescence beneath the charred surface squames (Fig. 10–10*A*), and the maneuver is accompanied by a distinctive crackling sound. Inadvertent penetration of the basement membrane is signaled by the loss of these two characteristic signs.

Lasing to the prickle cell layer shears the basal cells from the basement membrane, thereby producing a plane of cleavage. Hence, these detached basal cells are easily removed by wiping with moistened gauze, thus exposing the smooth, intact surface of the papillary dermis (Fig. 10–10*B*). Such wounds heal completely within 5 to 14 days, depending on temporal mode and the rapidity of energy delivery. The cosmetic appearance and functional qualities of the healed wound are entirely indistinguishable from normal vulvar skin.

The Second Surgical Plane. Destruction to the second surgical plane removes both the epidermis and the loose network of fine collagen and elastin

TABLE 10–1
Summary of the Salient Features of the Four Surgical Planes

	SURGICAL PLANE			
PARAMETER	First	Second	Third	Fourth
Target tissue	Surface epithelium	Dermal papillae	Pilosebaceous ducts	Pilosebaceous glands
Zone of vaporization	Proliferating layer of epidermis	Superficial papillary dermis	Upper reticular dermis	Midreticular dermis
Zone of necrosis	Basement membrane	Deep papillary	Midreticular	Deep reticular
Type of healing	Rapid and cosmetic	Rapid and cosmetic	Slower but usually cosmetic	Needs grafting
Visual landmark	Opalescent epidermis debris (shiny pink after wiping)	Yellowish and nonreflectant (chamois cloth)	Stark white with arcuate vessels and fibrous grain	Skin appendages visible as sand grains

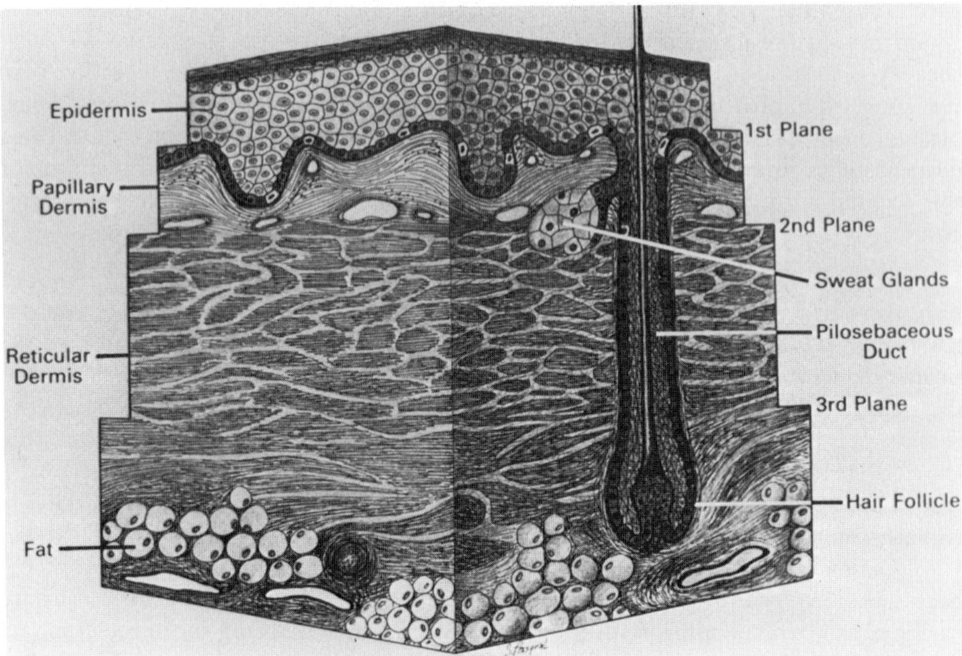

FIGURE 10–9. A diagram depicting the first three surgical planes. Reading from surface to base, the points of reference for each plane are indicated as stepwise expansions. The first surgical plane corresponds to the basement membrane, the second to the papillary dermis, and the third to the midreticular dermis. (Reproduced with permission from Reid R. Superficial laser vulvectomy. III. A new surgical technique for appendage-conserving ablation of refractory condylomas and vulvar intraepithelial neoplasia. Am J Obstet Gynecol 152:504–509, 1985)

fibers that compose the papillary dermis. This plane is reached by a similar set of rapid oscillations, moving the beam so quickly that the laser scorches (rather than craters) the exposed corium. When the procedure is done correctly, the scorched surface should show a finely roughened contour and a yellowish color, somewhat reminiscent of a chamois cloth (Fig. 10–11). This clinical appearance indicates that the zone of coagulation necrosis lies within the papillary dermis, with only minimal thermal injury to the underlying reticular dermis. The second plane is the preferred level of ablation for extensive condylomata. Such wounds heal rapidly and produce an end result indistinguishable from normal skin.

The Third Surgical Plane. VIN often extends into the pilosebaceous ducts (Fig. 10–12). Involvement is generally limited to the superficial portions of the ducts, making laser ablation to the midreticular level (the third surgical plane) an ideal treatment in most instances. Nonetheless, intended depth of destruction should be individualized by examining representative histologic sections. Foci of deep pilar extension are rare. However, any areas of deep pilar extension must be managed by surgical excision, reserving the laser for the ablation of adjoining superficial disease.

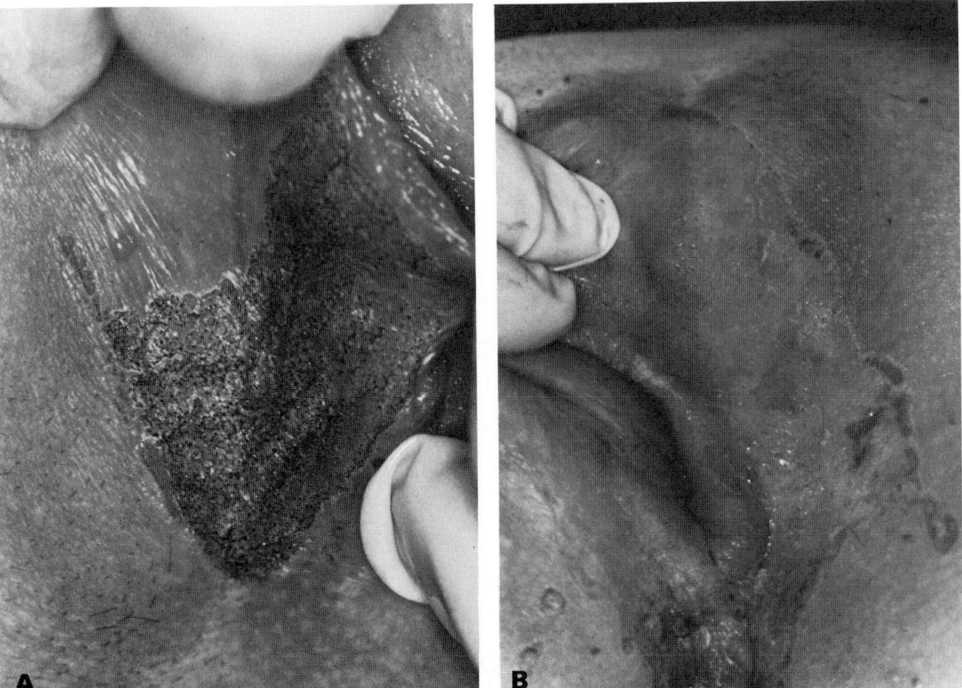

FIGURE 10–10. **(A)** First surgical plane. A view through the operating microscope after initial "brushing" with the laser. Beneath the charred remnants of the surface squames can be seen the refractile remnants of plump keratinocytes in the proliferating zone of the epidermis. **(B)** First surgical plane, after the epithelial debris has been wiped away with moist gauze. This maneuver exposes the intact surface of the underlying corium.

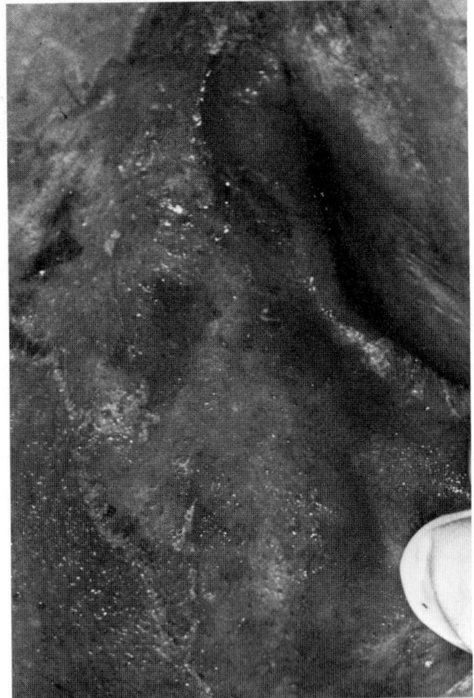

FIGURE 10–11. Second surgical plane. The exposed papillary dermis has been gently re-lased, sufficient to scorch (but not vaporize) the dermal surface.

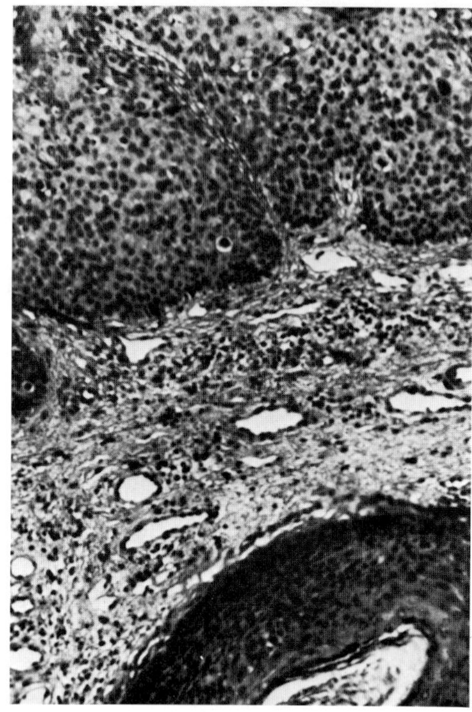

FIGURE 10–12. Extensive VIN 3 on the surface epithelium and within a skin appendage.

Destruction to the third surgical plane removes the epidermis, the upper portions of the pilosebaceous ducts, and a part of the reticular dermis. Ablation to the midreticular layer uncovers coarse collagen bundles that can be seen through the operating microsope as gray-white fibers resembling water-logged cotton threads (Fig. 10–13*A*). Wiping away the surface char then reveals a pattern of starkly white collagen plates, interspersed by a horizontally oriented network of deep dermal vessels (Fig. 10–13*B*).

The third plane is reached by lasing the exposed corium with slow, deliberate movements of the beam. Speed of cut is coordinated to the visual recognition of collagen bundles within the crater base. Moving the beam too rapidly will not expose these fibers, and moving the beam too slowly will uncover skin appendages within the deep reticular dermis. Such hair follicles and sweat glands are readily visible through the operating microscope, being seen as tiny refractile granules that resemble grains of sand. The rationale for limiting destruction to the third surgical plane is to allow re-epithelialization by regeneration from the keratinocytes within these skin appendages. Exposing these structures within the crater base signals the creation of a third-degree burn in that area. Hence, the third surgical plane represents the deepest level from which optimal healing will occur.

The Fourth Surgical Plane. Under rare circumstances, it may be necessary to produce a deliberate third-degree burn in order to destroy abnormal keratinocytes within the hair follicles or sweat glands. Because of its precision, the CO_2 laser can destroy the adnexal epithelium while still preserving a layer of colla-

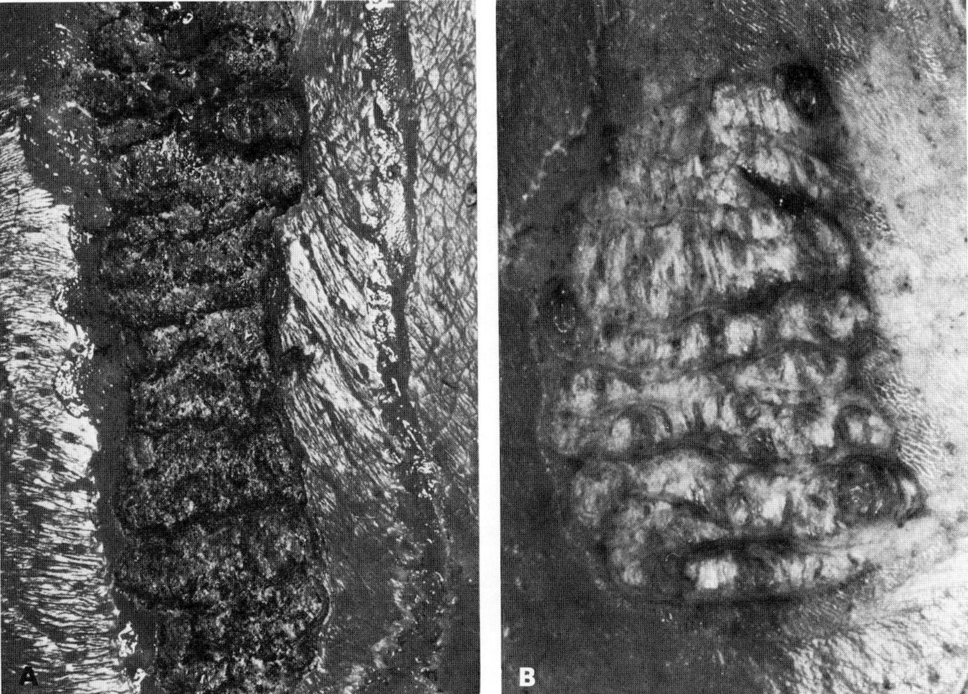

FIGURE 10–13. (A) Third surgical plane. A slower, more deliberate relasing of the exposed corium. This maneuver has vaporized the dermal surface, revealing the coarse collagen and elastic bundles of the reticular dermis. **(B)** After wiping, arcuate blood vessels at the base of the reticular dermis are visible against a background of starkly white collagen plates.

gen fibers within the deep reticular dermis. Dermal regeneration produces a much better bed for skin grafting than either subcutaneous fat or granulation tissue. Hence, cosmetic and functional results are vastly superior to those attainable by skinning vulvectomy (Fig. 10–14).

SUMMARY: THE NEED TO ABANDON POOR LASER TECHNIQUES

Although the physical principles governing the safe delivery of coherent radiation are well established, these rules are broken as often as they are followed. Of course, simply observing correct physical principles does not guarantee a successful outcome. Strategies are also required to ensure dexterous beam delivery and to oppose thermal injury within adjacent tissue. As in other forms of surgery, a gynecologist must learn how to control bleeding, gain exposure, delineate geographic margins, and control the depth of destruction.

When these lessons are assimilated, CO_2 laser treatment of HPV-associated disease within the male or female genital tract will carry a primary success rate of 85 to 95%. Wounds will heal rapidly, and the final result will be indistinguishable

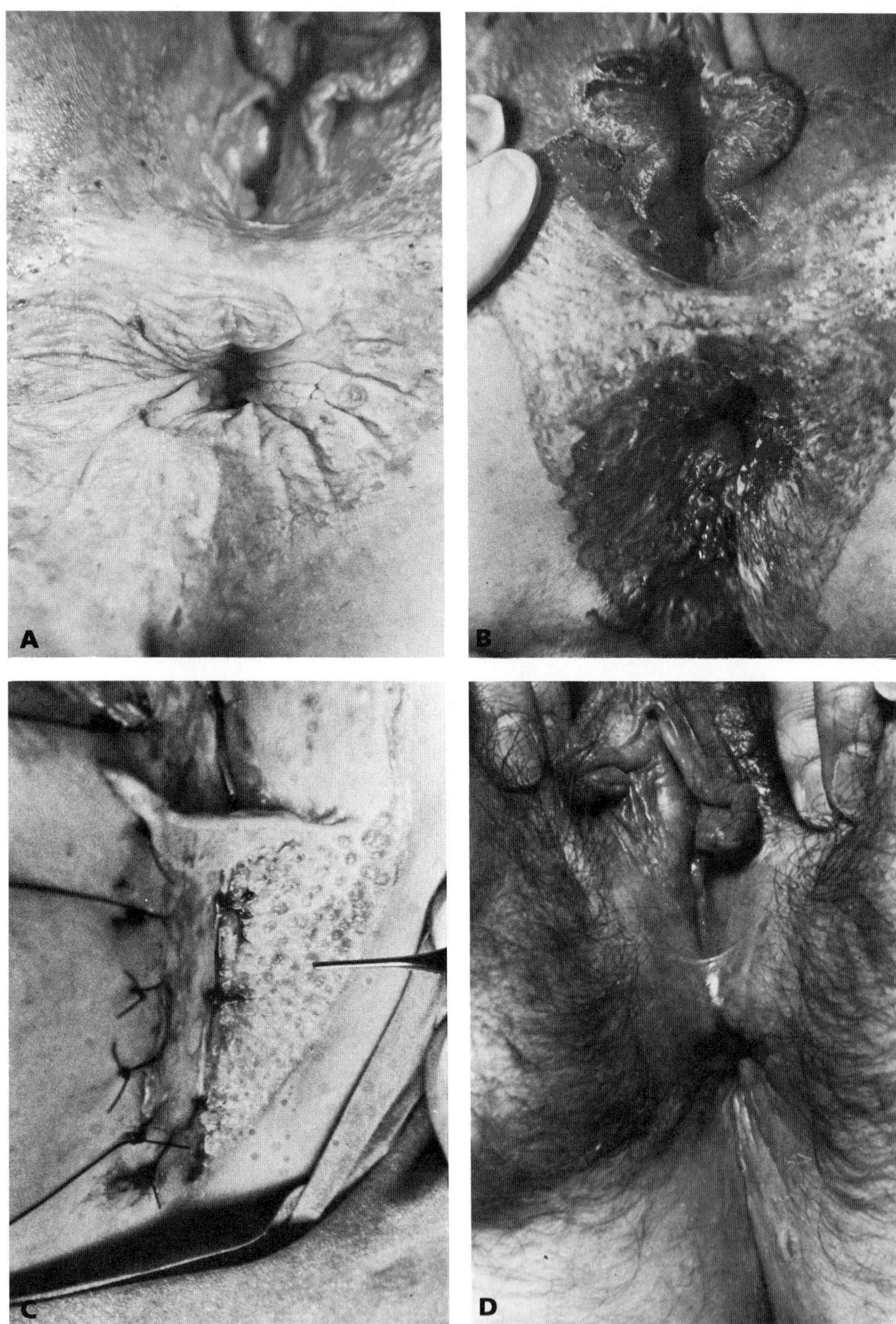

FIGURE 10–14. **(A)** An area of refractory perianal dysplasia that has failed three prior superficial laser vaporizations. **(B)** Vaporization of the perianal skin to the fourth plane. Each of the craters represents a site at which a skin appendage was destroyed, whereas the intervening areas represent viable collagen bundles within the deep part of the reticular dermis. **(C)** The same area 10 days later, showing the extent of dermal regeneration at the time of skin grafting. **(D)** The final result.

from normal tissue. Disease that is refractory to the initial therapy will usually respond to retreatment, especially if an antiviral regimen is prescribed within the early postoperative period.

REFERENCES

1. Buscema J, Woodruff JD, Parmley TH: Carcinoma in situ of the vulva. Obstet Gynecol 55:225–230, 1980
2. Dorsey JH, Baggish MS: Multifocal vaginal intraepithelial neoplasia with uterus in situ. In Sharp F, Jordan JA (eds): Gynecological Laser Surgery, pp 173–179. Perinatology Press, 1985
3. Duus BR, Philipsen T, Christensen JD et al: Refractory condyloma acuminate: A controlled clinical trial of carbon dioxide laser versus conventional surgical treatment. Genitourin Med 61:59–61, 1985
4. Friedrich EG: Intraepithelial neoplasia of the vulva. In Coppleson M (ed): Gynecologic Oncology. Fundamental Principles and Clinical Practice. London, Churchill Livingstone, 1981
5. Friedrich EG Jr: The vulvar vestibule. J Reprod Med 28:773, 1983
6. Jordan JA, Sharp F: CO_2 laser treatment of vaginal intraepithelial neoplasia. In Sharp F, Jordan AN (eds): Gynecological Laser Surgery, pp 181–188. Perinatology Press, 1985
7. Oriel JD: Natural history of genital warts. Br J Vener Dis 47:1, 1971
8. Pfister H: Relationship of papillomaviruses to anogenital cancer. Obstet Gynecol Clin North Am 14:349–361, 1987
9. Reid R: Editorial: Mass screening for cervical cancer. What have we learned? Colposcopy Gynecol Laser Surg 1:233–235, 1984
10. Reid R: Human papillomaviral infection. The key to rational triage of cervical neoplasia. Obstet Gynecol Clin North Am 14:407–429, 1987
11. Reid R: Laser therapy of human papillomavirus infections. In Keye W (ed): Laser Surgery in Obstetrics and Gynecology. Chicago, Yearbook Publishers, pp 46–99, 1989
12. Reid R: Physical and surgical principles governing expertise with the carbon dioxide laser. Obstet Gynecol Clin North Am 14:513–535, 1987
13. Reid R: Preinvasive cervical neoplasia. In Berek J, Hacker N (eds): Practical Gynecologic Oncology, pp 195–240. Baltimore, Williams & Wilkins, 1989
14. Reid R: Superficial laser vulvectomy. I. The efficacy of extended superficial ablation for refractory and very extensive condylomas. Am J Obstet Gynecol 151:1047–1052, 1985
15. Reid R: Superficial laser vulvectomy. III. A new surgical technique for appendage-conserving ablation of refractory condylomas and vulvar intraepithelial neoplasia. Am J Obstet Gynecol 152:504–509, 1985
16. Reid R, Greenberg MD, Lorincz AT et al: Superficial laser vulvectomy. IV. Extended laser vaporization and adjuvant 5-fluorouracil for HPV-associated vulvar disease. Obstet Gynecol (in press), 1990
17. Reid R, Campion M: Clinical diagnosis of cervical HPV infection. In Krebs H (ed): Clinical Obstetrics and Gynecology, pp 157–159. Philadelphia, JB Lippincott, 1989
18. Reid R, Campion MJ: The biology and significance of human papillomavirus infection in the genital tract. Yale J Biol Med 61:307–325, 1988
19. Reid R, Elfont EA, Zirkin RM: Superficial laser vulvectomy. II. The anatomic and biophysical principles permitting accurate control of the depth of dermal destruction with the carbon dioxide laser. Am J Obstet Gynecol 152:261–271, 1985
20. Reid R, Elson L, Absten G: A practical guide to laser safety. Colposcopy Gynecol Laser Surg 2:121–132, 1986
21. Reid R, Greenberg MD, Daoud Y et al: Colposcopic findings in women with vulvar pain syndromes. A preliminary report. J Reprod Med 33:523–532, 1988
22. Reid R, Greenberg M, Jenson AB et al: Sexually transmitted papillomaviral infections. I. The anatomic distribution and pathologic grade of neoplastic lesions associated with different viral types. Am J Obstet Gynecol 156:212–222, 1987
23. Reid R, Laverty CR, Coppleson M et al: Noncondylomatous cervical wart virus infections. Obstet Gynecol 55:476–483, 1980. Reviewed in Obstet Gynecol Survey 35:671–673
24. Skene AJC: Treatise on the diseases of women. New York, D. Appleton, 1889
25. Woodman C, Jordan JA, Wade-Evans T: The management of vaginal intraepithelial neoplasia after hysterectomy. Br J Obstet Gynecol 91:707, 1984
26. Woodruff JD, Parmley TH: Infection of the minor vestibular gland. Obstet Gynecol 62:609, 1983

Part Three

INTRA-ABDOMINAL LASER THERAPY

11

Laser Therapy for Endometriosis, Adhesions, and Tubal Disease

Joseph R. Feste

The carbon dioxide (CO_2) laser produces a highly directional, collimated light beam that may be precisely focused to a fine point. Microlaser surgery uses the laser as a scalpel. The spot size ranges from 2000 to 200 micrometers in diameter, with the small spot selected for fine dissection. Because the laser beam is used to vaporize tissue, small vessels are sealed and minimal damage is done to neighboring cells. Fewer sutures are required, and scar formation is usually less than with conventional surgery. Although the laser has been commonly used in recent years to treat lower genital tract pathology, its application to intra-abdominal surgery is still in its early phases. Special adaptations of the operative microscope and special accessory instruments are necessary for use of the laser within the abdominal cavity. The many procedures amenable to CO_2 laser treatment range from wedge resection of ovaries and ovarian cystectomy to myomectomy and metroplasty and include those discussed in this chapter: treatment of endometriosis, adhesiolysis, and tubal repair.

The major goal of gynecological surgeons treating infertile patients is to restore normal anatomy with the hope of enhancing the chances for a successful pregnancy. As with most surgical procedures, the first attempt is usually the most successful. As a microsurgical tool, the laser should be used in accordance with the guidelines established for successful microsurgery.[18] In addition, the following rules for reproductive surgery should be observed:

1. Atraumatic techniques with special instruments should be used.
2. Sponges and powder should not be used.

3. The area should be frequently irrigated with heparinized lactated Ringer's solution.
4. Because blood is known to contribute significantly to the formation of adhesions, hemostasis should be optimized.
5. Cautery should be used judiciously in order to minimize the amount of necrotic tissue for adhesion formation.
6. Complete excision of pathologic tissue is important, particularly for salpingitis isthmica nodosum and endometriosis.
7. Precise alignment of tissue planes and reperitonealization should be attempted whenever possible.
8. Magnification should be used because it allows the use of fine suture and defines the exact border of pathologic tissue in order to facilitate complete removal.
9. Copious pelvic lavage with heparinized lactated Ringer's solution should be used to remove necrotic debris.

If properly used, the laser, which is essentially a light scalpel, offers several advantages over conventional surgery. The advantages that have been clearly demonstrated include the following:

1. Reduction in operating time.
2. Attainment of excellent hemostasis in order to reduce the postoperative formation of adhesions.
3. By using flat-surfaced rhodium or molybdenum mirrors, the capability of reaching operative sites otherwise inaccessible.

Despite the advantages that the laser offers, it is not a panacea for all pelvic pathology. A laser is no better than the gynecological surgeon using it, and it is not indicated when traditional techniques would provide better results.

Because the use of the laser in microsurgery is relatively new, its efficacy will not be apparent for several years, and significantly increased pregnancy rates have not yet been reported. However, documentation by early second-look laparoscopies after laser surgery has shown the degree of adhesion reformation to be decreased, and subsequent adhesions are usually filmy.[26,29]

INSTRUMENTATION

The major requirements for microlaser surgery are a laser with a hand piece or coupled to a microscope by a micromanipulator, titanium or quartz rods, atraumatic pickups, molybdenum or rhodium mirrors, and fine 6-0/8-0 sutures.

Hand Piece

The laser hand piece, like a scalpel, is easily held in the hand; however, the depth of insertion into the pelvis is limited by the knuckles of the laser's articulating arm. The ability for the laser to be rapidly focused and defocused gives the hand piece a wide range of power density changes during pelvic surgery. Control is adequate for ablation, incision, or coagulation. However, because with the hand–held instrument a change of a few millimeters in the focal length causes significant change in the power density, extra caution is required to prevent unnecessary tissue damage. Most hand pieces use a 125-mm lens producing a spot size of 0.22 mm; they produce a power density of 26,000 watts/cm^2. Rapid changes in power densities may be achieved by barely defocusing. Thus, the hand–held unit is quite versatile but somewhat dangerous, in that too large a decrease in power density increases the tissue necrosis, resulting in greater ischemia and fibrosis. With the microscope, in contrast, power density change is controlled by adjusting the variable spot size adapter on the micromanipulator. This maneuver is more precise.

The use of the mirror in conjunction with the hand–held unit should be avoided because maximal steadiness is required to keep the mirror and unit from moving in opposite directions and thus resulting in possible inadvertent injury to other pelvic viscera. The use of backstops helps prevent the laser from injuring other vital pelvic structures. Backstops commonly used are soaked non–woven sponges, irrigating solutions, and titanium or quartz rods. The tissue itself may be used as a backstop during lysis of adhesions. The adhesions should be excised rather than incised; thus, there will be a lased area on both ends of the adhesion attachments. For vessels greater than 1.2 to 1.5 mm in diameter, the CO_2 laser generally stops the bleeding by defocusing to decrease the power density. However, in order to avoid more fibrosis and necrosis, it is preferable to use bipolar microcautery to control the bleeding from larger vessels.

Micromanipulators (Microscope)

A micromanipulator with a variable spot size adapter is more versatile, as it provides a greater depth of field, better cutting control, and therefore a sharper and more precise incision. A surgeon is able to defocus more precisely and thus potentially cause less necrosis due to a rapid decrease in the power density using the hand piece. Micromanipulators control the laser's energy by a joystick that allows for greater control in aiming the beam, and thus they are safer to use than a hand piece.

The main disadvantage of using the microscope is that the entire field is not visible at all times. The resulting difficulty in maintaining orientation requires that a surgeon be familiar with the techniques of conventional microsurgery before attempting to use the laser. Safety precautions are the same as for use of a hand–held laser.

Mirrors

Used in conjunction with a microscope, front–surfaced rhodium or solid molybdenum mirrors are very helpful in dealing with inaccessible areas deep in the pelvis, but several precautions should be observed. Rhodium mirrors crack very easily if they are not in fact front–surfaced and also crack if superpulses rather than continuous or repeated single pulses are used. Because molybdenum mirrors are made from a solid slug of metal, etching or cracking of the surface does not occur. Back–surfaced glass dental mirrors should not be used. Moreover, extreme care must be taken not to allow other organs, instruments, or fingers of the assisting or operating surgeons to migrate into the field between the mirror and the laser energy.

Quartz and Titanium Rods

During the process of vaporizing diseased or abnormal tissue, a backstop is required to prevent damage to adjacent normal tissue. Quartz rods may be used, but because of their limited heat tolerance, laser energy may cause them to crack or break. To prevent this problem, titanium rods 3 to 6 mm in diameter have been used to absorb the energy of the CO_2 laser. They also offer the advantage that tissue rarely sticks to them as it does to quartz rods. Both round and flat surface rods are available and may be used.

LASER SURGERY FOR ENDOMETRIOSIS

The etiology of endometriosis remains ambiguous. Among the many causes postulated are retrograde menstruation, coelomic metaplasia, and lymphatic or hematologic spread. Reflux menstruation is currently considered the most likely cause of endometriosis, and animal studies seem to confirm this theory.[21] Endometriosis is thought to account for approximately 25% to 30% of laparoscopy procedures and up to 15% to 20% of laparotomy procedures to promote fertility.[21]

Endometriosis is a condition that is particularly amenable to laser surgery because it develops on the surface of the peritoneum. It is possible to vaporize the surface of the lesion, penetrate to deeper tissues where the endometriosis is embedded, and vaporize to normal tissue. Because there is a very thin layer of retroperitoneal fat throughout the peritoneum, the water vapor created by vaporization of this thin layer is an indication of complete removal of the lesion. In treatment of endometriotic implants, the vaporized glandular layer has a brownish appearance; the deeper layer or stroma is white and appears curdy. It is important to vaporize a margin of 1 to 2 mm around each lesion to eradicate any remaining microscopic disease.

Before laser surgery for endometriosis, preparation of the patient is important. Patients who have endometriomas more than 3 cm in diameter receive danazol (Danocrine) or leuprolide (Lupron) to reduce the endometrioma to its minimum size. Subsequent vaporization is usually easier, and it is often possible to preserve a greater amount of normal ovarian tissue. The duration of medical treatment depends on the size and response of the lesion. Treatment for 3 months is adequate to suppress most endometriomas. If medical suppression is not needed, the surgery is often scheduled in the proliferative phase of the patient's cycle to avoid ovarian surgery with a fresh corpus luteum.

The laser beam may either be delivered by a hand piece or by a micromanipulator in conjunction with an operating microscope. Magnification, using either loupes or the microscope, assures a surgeon of complete vaporization of the endometriosis. Because magnification may be increased to outline the margins of each lesion by using the microscope, many pelvic surgeons prefer it instead of the loupes.

The treatment for endometriosis varies according to its location, as discussed in the paragraphs that follow.

Peritoneal Endometriosis. Endometrial implants along the uterosacral ligaments, lateral pelvic wall, and bladder peritoneum may be vaporized with continuous or repeat-pulse modes. In areas where there are no vital structures, a continuous mode may be used safely. Power densities between 1000 and 3000 watts/cm^2 using a spot size of 0.8 to 1.0 mm are adequate to debulk these lesions. While moving the joystick rapidly, one can easily vaporize the lesion from the surface of the peritoneum to normal retroperitoneal fat (Fig. 11–1). However, if vaporizing over ureters, bladder, and blood vessels, it becomes necessary to switch to single- or repeat-pulse modes to limit the amount of penetration of the laser beam through the peritoneum. The single- or repeat-pulse modes vaporize the lesion 100 to 300 micrometers at a time. Defects greater than 1 to 2 cm should be closed with fine suture, such as 6-0 Vicryl, PDS, or nylon. Experience has shown that if two lased areas are not in close proximity to each other, adhesion formation is unlikely. Hemostasis is excellent, as blood loss is almost nonexistent.

Tubal Endometriosis. When lesions involving the fallopian tubes are vaporized, it is necessary to use a much smaller spot size, a faster exposure time, and a power density in the range of 2000 to 3000 watts/cm^2. In this way, penetration through the delicate muscularis of the tube is prevented as control of the laser is more precise. Frequent irrigation is important after vaporization to provide a cooling effect and thus decrease thermal damage to adjacent tissue. Defects in the tube, particularly if they are in close proximity to another lased area, should be closed with 6-0 to 7-0 interrupted suture.

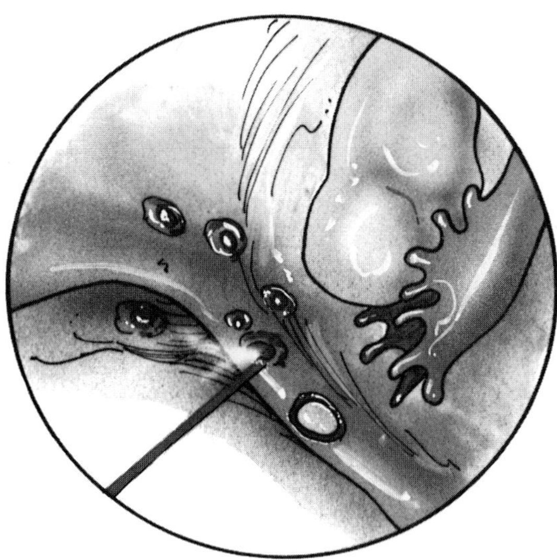

FIGURE 11–1. Laser vaporization of endometriosis on parietal peritoneum.

Ovarian Endometriosis. Laser vaporization of ovarian endometriosis may vary according to the size of the endometrioma and the presence of adhesions. Periovarian adhesions are best vaporized with a single-pulse mode, particularly when a front-surfaced rhodium or molybdenum mirror is used to visualize the adhesions. Because the adhesions are inaccessible to direct vision, they are vaporized by reflecting the laser beam from the mirror to the adhesion. Whenever possible, titanium or quartz rods are interphased between the adhesion and pelvic sidewall to prevent vaporization of the normal lateral pelvic walls. After the ovary is detached from the sidewall, the endometriomas are treated using any of three techniques: (1) Endometriomas less than 3 cm in diameter can be vaporized with the continuous mode using the ovary itself as a backstop. (2) The larger endometriomas, greater than 3 to 4 cm in diameter, are opened by excising an elliptical portion of the ovarian cortex with a continuous-pulse mode of 3000 to 4000 watts/cm². The chocolate material is drained from the endometrioma, and the cyst lining is thoroughly irrigated. With a defocused beam of 1.5 to 2 mm and a power setting of 20 to 30 watts, the entire lining of the endometrioma is vaporized down to normal ovarian tissue. (Unless the glandular and stromal components are completely removed, future recurrence of the endometrioma is very likely.) (3) Endometriomas 3 to 6 cm or greater in diameter can be removed either by entering the capsule of the ovary and enucleating the ovarian cyst or by vaporizing the capsule. The deep layer may be closed with interrupted suture of 3-0 Vicryl, and the capsule carefully approximated with 6-0 PDS suture (Fig. 11–2). Both of these procedures preserve most of the compressed ovarian cortex and result in little loss of ovarian tissue.

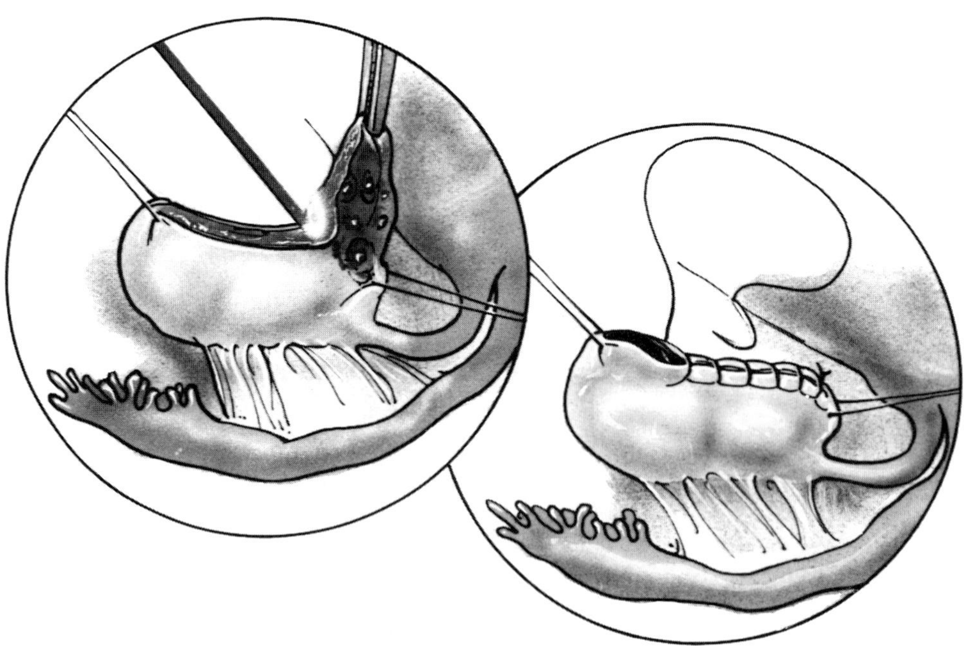

FIGURE 11–2. Laser excision of an ovarian endometrioma.

Endometriosis on the Colon. Small endometriomas involving the serosa and muscularis of the colon may be vaporized with repeat- or single-pulse modes using a defocused beam 0.8 to 1.0 mm in diameter to limit the degree of penetration of the laser. Use of 1/20 to 1/10 of a second exposure allows removal of endometriomas at the rate of 100 to 200 micrometers down through the lesion to the normal muscularis or mucosa. All patients with colon disease should have bowel preparation in case of inadvertent entry into the colon or the unforeseen presence of lesions. After complete vaporization of the lesion, the muscularis and serosal surface can be approximated loosely with interrupted suture of 2-0 to 3-0 permanent suture. Treating the small lesions this way can eliminate the need for wedge or segmental resection of the colon or rectum. However, in cases of large endometriomas involving the mucosa or lying circumferentially around the rectum, the wedge or segmental resection is mandatory. In these cases, it is important that hemostasis be achieved after resection and that all peritoneal defects be closed without tension on the suture closure line.

Follow-up and Results

In all patients treated for endometriosis, heparinized lactated Ringer's solution (1000 units of heparin, 1000 ml of Ringer's) is used as an irrigating solution, and an optional 100 to 200 ml of 32% dextran-70 (Hyskon) is instilled into the pelvic cavity before closure of the abdomen. All patients are kept on danazol for a period of 4 to 6 weeks to prevent ovulation until healing is adequate. In cases of large endometriomas, patients are kept on danazol for 90 days.

During the past 5 years, few publications have reported pregnancy rates following laser surgery. Chong and Baggish[9] reported a pregnancy rate of 50% in patients with stage I to stage III endometriosis. The duration of follow-up has been less than 1 year in 45 infertile women treated for endometriosis. Friedlander[17] reported that reduction of pelvic pain and visible amelioration of endometriosis can be expected in 40% of patients treated with danazol. Dmowski and Cohen[14] and Greenblatt and Tzingounis[19] report a 50% response rate. Regression of disease after conservative surgery has been reported in 30% to 94% of patients following conservative surgery using a combination of sharp dissection and needle cautery. Buttram,[8] correlating success of surgical treatment with severity of disease, reported an 84% pregnancy rate with mild stages of endometriosis and 75% and 56%, respectively, with moderate or severe endometriosis.

In the author's series of 108 patients observed for more than 1 year, there were 79 pregnancies (73%); of these, 69 (87%) reached term and 9 (11%) ended in spontaneous abortions; one pregnancy was ectopic (Table 11–1). Additionally, almost 67% of those who became pregnant conceived within 12 months of the surgery (Table 11–2), a figure that is consistent with other reports. When patients with either ovulatory dysfunction or partners with sperm abnormalities were excluded from evaluation, the pregnancy rates improved for all stages of disease (Table 11–3). If only those patients with male or female factors are included, the pregnancy rates are essentially the same during an extended period of time (Table 11–4). Life table analysis of all three endometriosis states clearly demonstrates the pregnancy trend

TABLE 11-1
Pregnancies Following Laser Laparotomy for Endometriosis in Infertility Patients

STAGE	TOTAL PATIENTS	TOTAL PREGNANCIES	TERM	ABORTION	ECTOPIC
I	0	0	0	0	0
II	49	38 (78%)	35	3	0
III	40	30 (75%)	26	3	1
IV	19	11 (58%)	8	3	0
	108	79 (73%)	69 (87%)	9 (11%)	1 (1%)

TABLE 11-2
Time Between Laser Laparotomy for Endometriosis And Pregnancy

STAGE	TOTAL PREGNANCIES	<6 MONTHS	6-12 MONTHS	>12 MONTHS
I	0	0	0	0
II	38	13	13	12
III	30	11	9	10
IV	11	4	3	4
	79	28 (35%)	25 (32%)	26 (33%)

TABLE 11-3
Pregnancies Following Laser Laparotomy for Endometriosis in Patients Without Male or Female Factors

STAGE	TOTAL PATIENTS	TOTAL PREGNANCIES
I	0	0
II	14	11 (79%)
III	9	8 (89%)
IV	5	2 (40%)
	28	21 (75%)

TABLE 11-4
Pregnancies Following Laser Laparotomy for Endometriosis in Patients With Male or Female Factors

STAGE	TOTAL PATIENTS	TOTAL PREGNANCIES
I	0	0
II	35	27 (77%)
III	31	22 (71%)
IV	14	9 (64%)
	80	58 (73%)

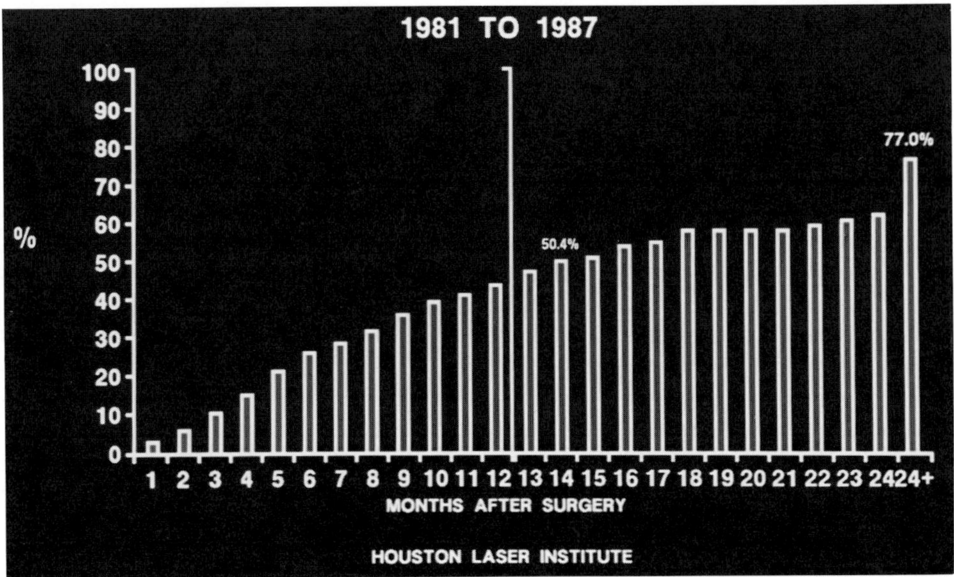

FIGURE 11–3. Life table analysis of all stages of endometriosis treated with CO_2 laser at laparotomy, both with and without male and female factors.

during a period of years. The maximum pregnancy rate should eventually reach 77% (Fig. 11–3).

In summary, the CO_2 laser offers some strategic advantages over conventional operative methods for conservative management of endometriosis. Improved hemostasis and precision are two major benefits. The ability of the laser beam to reach into recessed or otherwise poorly visible areas such as between the pelvic sidewall and severely adhesed endometriomas represents a significant technological advance. The follow-up period is yet too brief to allow meaningful comparisons between results of laser treatment and treatment by conventional methods. Second-look laparoscopy should be performed in most, if not all, patients to assess the results of conservative surgery as well as to provide treatment (vaporization) of any residual adhesions. However, many women whose symptoms have been more or less ameliorated may object to this additional operative procedure.

ADHESIOLYSIS

During the past several years, little clinical information has been gathered concerning the results of CO_2 lasers in the treatment of postoperative or postinfection pelvic adhesions. Initial studies in animals have shown no significant difference in adhesion formation when results of laser surgery were compared with those of conventional electrosurgery.[16,25] Multiple reports have described the ideal techniques for vaporizing pelvic adhesions,[13,20] but the efficacy of laser surgery in preventing formation of new adhesions postoperatively and the pregnancy rates achieved subsequent to surgery are currently being evaluated. Potentially, evaluation of results will be complicated by variations in surgeons' skills, in techniques used, and in the degree of tubal damage and interpretation of findings. In a study published by Kelly and Roberts,[20] five pregnancies occurred in 21 patients.[24] The majority of the pregnancies occurred in those patients with stage Ia and IIa adhesions. After 1 year, the pregnancy rate was 46.2%, with 32.6% carrying to term.

A recent study by Diamond and colleagues[13] showed no significant difference between postoperative formation of adhesions in patients who had laser surgery and those treated with the micro-electrode needle. The 106 patients evaluated showed no significant decrease in adhesions except in the areas over the colon and cul-de-sac. There appeared to be increased tubal patency at the time of second-look laparoscopy in patients who had undergone neosalpingostomies. However, the number of adhesions at second-look laparoscopy was shown to be similar to the number in the group treated with microelectrocautery.

Another series reported 26 patients treated for adhesions with laser surgery and followed for 2 or more years. Ten of 26 patients (38.5%) conceived.[5] Several other researchers have reported that pregnancy rates did not differ significantly between those patients treated with laser and those treated with electrosurgical techniques.[4,28,29]

Laser surgery does offer several advantages over standard microelectrocautery for the treatment of postoperative adhesions[3,4]:

1. The laser can be reflected through front-surfaced silver rhodium or molybdenum mirrors to vaporize adhesions between the ovaries and tubes that are inaccessible with the microelectrode needle under direct vision.
2. Adhesions that developed after laser surgery have been shown to be finer and much easier to deal with at second-look laparoscopy. This suggests that the amount of thermal damage to the tissues is less with laser than with the microelectrode needle.
3. If the laser is used in conjunction with the microscope, the control is exact because the laser can be focused to a very fine point for precise surgical direction.
4. Because the laser beam is focused from a distance, it does not occupy additional space and thereby allows unobstructed vision.
5. The laser heat is so intense that microorganisms are destroyed. It seals lymphatics and blood vessels and thus prevents contamination and infection.
6. The time from surgery to conception may be shorter with the use of the CO_2 laser.

CLINICAL TECHNIQUES

When dense adhesions between the ovary and tube are vaporized, the development of a plane between these two structures can be carefully dissected with a CO_2 laser. With single-pulse, repeat-pulse, or low-power superpulse modes, small segments of adhesions can be vaporized slowly and directly. This method separates the two structures with little change of normal anatomy. The amount of thermal damage at the higher power densities (more than 5000 watts/cm^2) produces as little as 100 micrometers of irreversible thermal damage to the tubal or ovarian surface. Higher magnifications allow performance of this procedure with precise control; the tube and ovary can be virtually dissected with minimal thermal effect on either structure. If vessels that are more than 1.2 to 1.5 mm in diameter are encountered, either they must be sealed with microbipolar cautery or the lumen must be occluded and coagulated with the laser.

In cases of adhesions between the ovary or tube and the lateral pelvic wall, a carbide-tipped Babcock clamp is used to grasp the tube or ovary and put tension on these structures. The adhesion can then be vaporized using a mirror to reflect the beam (Fig. 11–4). Single-pulse modes, repeat-pulse modes, and occasionally continuous-pulse modes should be used for this technique. It may be difficult to learn to move the mirror in the right direction while looking through the microscope, thus creating difficulty in controlling the point of laser beam impact. Because the ovary or tube usually is densely adhered to the pelvic wall, only occasionally is it feasible to insert a titanium rod behind the adhesion. In these instances, mirror vaporization of adhesions themselves frees up the ovary or tube and leaves an area of thermal effect not more than 100 micrometers deep. Once the ovary and tube are freed of their

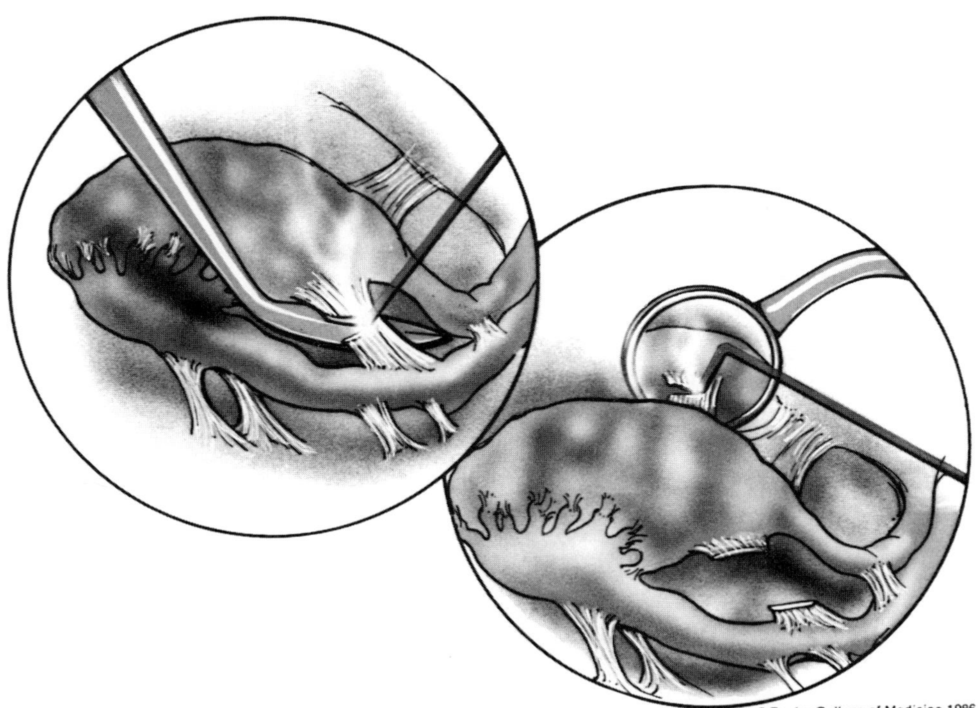

FIGURE 11–4. Laser vaporization of adhesions with a titanium rod as a backstop and with a front-surfaced rhodium mirror to reflect the laser beam.

adhesions, the pelvic cavity can be packed with a lint-free Kerlex pack and the adhesions "picked" off the ovary and tube with higher magnification and single-pulse modes. This technique of adhesion removal is preferred over the blatant "painting" of the entire ovarian surface with a defocused beam.

Adhesions overlying the bladder, ureter, rectum, or even large vessels are best removed by vaporization with single-pulse or repeat-pulse modes. This technique prevents penetration of the laser beam to more than 100 to 200 micrometers and makes it possible for the attachment of the adhesions to be vaporized rather than incised.

Many techniques are used to prevent adhesion recurrence after laser vaporization. Hyskon, heparinized lactated Ringer's solution, and biodegradable peritoneal grafts have been used. An important element in irrigation with heparinized lactated Ringer's solution is the removal of the greatest possible amount of carbon and fibrin, which may cause postoperative adhesions. It is best not to wipe off the carbon with a cotton pledget because microscopic bleeding may ensue and thus defeat the purpose of using the laser as a collimated light scalpel that seals small vessels. Proper hemostasis and irrigation are two of the most important factors in successful laser vaporization of adhesions.

Confirmation of the hypothesized advantages of the laser over the microneedle requires further studies with laser superpulses or megapulses. It is important to note, moreover, that many of the reported cases of adhesive disease treated by laser surgery have been severe. Many of these cases might have been treated by hysterectomy in the past. Therefore, it is important when comparing results to stage adhesions in the manner described by Raj and Hulka[26] and to evaluate effects of surgery by second-look laparoscopy.

LASER SURGERY OF THE FALLOPIAN TUBES

Endometriosis accounts for 25% to 30% of infertility, but tubal disease is equally responsible. Tubal disease is most commonly associated with infection, particularly with *Neisseria gonorrheae, Chlamydia,* and *Mycoplasma.* Tubal surgery is also performed frequently for reversal of sterilization requested because of separation, divorce, or death of an infant. Needless to say, whether the tubal procedure is performed by laser or conventional technique, careful preoperative evaluation of the patient is extremely important. The laser is particularly useful for cornual isthmic anastomosis required for interstitial disease of the proximal fallopian tube.

Isthmic and Ampullary Disease

During the past 6 years, a significant amount of experience has been accumulated in the use of the CO_2 laser for tubal reanastomosis. Animal studies have shown no difference in adhesion rates, patency rates, or pregnancy rates when comparing results of CO_2 laser surgery with those of conventional electrosurgical techniques.[1] Numerous reports have suggested that laser incision of the tube in preparation for anastomosis requires significantly less time and achieves greater hemostasis than standard techniques of microsurgery. However, other studies have shown neither decrease in operating time nor a measurably reduced amount of blood loss. Within the realm of presently available technology (10,000 watts to 200,000 watts/cm^2 and the TEM mode 00 with a 0.2-mm spot size), the results of reanastomosis are comparable to those achieved by other microsurgical techniques.[23]

The preparation of the tubes for reanastomosis apparently can be performed equally well by either laser or microelectrode.[23] Advocates of the use of the unipolar microelectrode say that in the hands of experienced surgeons it decreases operating time. The transection can be precise, with tissue surrounding the tubal lumen showing neither combustion nor charred debris. For these surgeons, handling the microelectrode is easier and probably safer than using the laser. However, advocates of the use of the laser consider it equally safe.

For surgeons familiar with the laser technique, the process of preparation of the tube consists of three steps:

1. The serosal layer is vaporized with a power density greater than 10,000 watts/cm^2 with a very small spot size.
2. The muscular layer is then incised to the mucosa with a power density of 20,000 watts/cm^2 with a repeat-pulse mode of 5/100 of a second exposure time.
3. The mucosa is divided with a knife or iris scissors.

In some instances, it has been reported that the tube can be repaired by incising through the full thickness and the mucosa can be freshened with a pair of scissors or a sharp knife. This method eliminates the problem of fibrosis. Pregnancy rates with this technique have been as good as those with microelectrode,[32] and in the hands of a competent laser surgeon, the operating time has been cut significantly. Kelly and Roberts[20] reported use of a CO_2 laser in treatment of 20 patients with tubal endometriosis. Twelve of these patients had previously had tubal ligation, and after reanastomosis, a pregnancy rate of 71.4% was reported. Baggish and Chong[2] reported that in their series of 52 cases there were 17 pregnancies, of which 5 terminated as abortions or ectopic pregnancies. Twenty-nine of the 52 showed tubal patency in postoperative hysterosalpingography. This series included diseased tubes, with no differentiation made between the diseased tubes and unipolar or bipolar cautery-induced tubal occlusion.

Interstitial or Cornual Obstruction

The most significant use of the laser for reanastomosis is for cornual or interstitial disease. A technique borrowed from lower genital tract surgery provides hemostasis as an adjunct to laser surgery. This technique takes advantage of the laser's excellent hemostatic properties and leaves mucosal architecture normal at 500 micrometers from the laser impact zone. A 1:20 vasopressor solution injected via a 1-mm tuberculin syringe through a 27-gauge needle produces considerable vasoconstriction. The vasoconstriction causes larger vessels (those greater than 1 mm) that would otherwise be severed to undergo spasm. The traversing laser beam can then seal these larger vessels. As the cornu is opened, small oozing vessels may be sealed by defocusing the beam. Use of the laser precludes the need for clamping vessels and applying ligatures or cautery coagulation. The laser can completely outline the tube

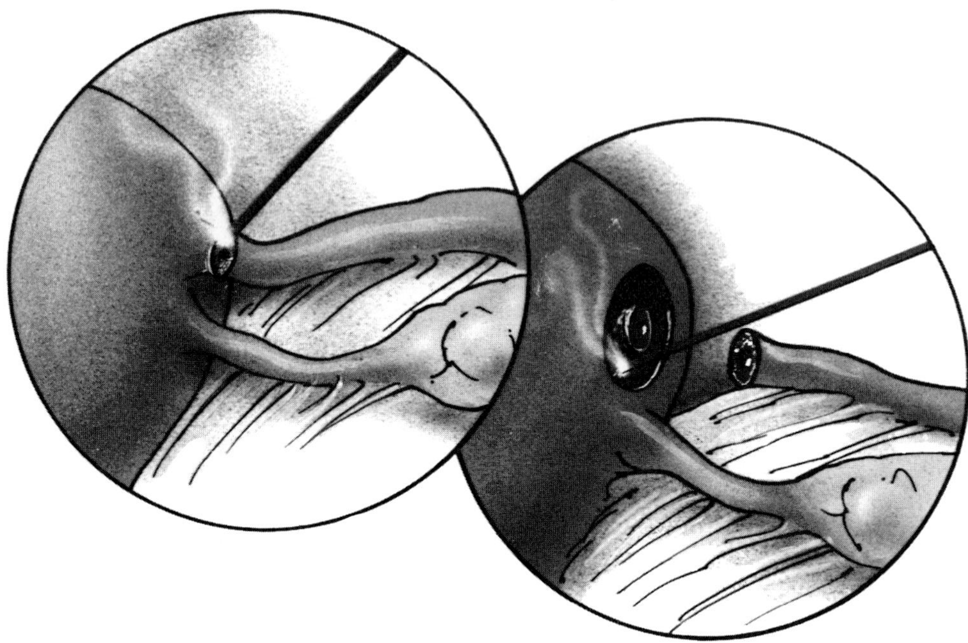

FIGURE 11–5. Vaporization around the interstitial portion of the fallopian tube in preparation for an interstitial anastomosis.

at the serosal area through the interstitial portion of the tube to within 2 mm of the endometrial cavity as needed. This hemostatic technique provides a "lip" on which to sew and makes the reanastomosis less difficult (Fig. 11–5).

Tubal Reconstruction: Distal Occlusion of the Fallopian Tube

Reconstruction for distal tubal patency may be achieved by either fimbrioplasty or neosalpingostomy. Fimbrioplasty includes those procedures in which the tubal fimbriae are agglutinated or adhered but not completely closed (*i.e.,* clubbed). This lesion usually results from postoperative adhesions, endometriosis, and sometimes from mild tubal infections. In contrast to the techniques used for saccular hydrosalpinges that result from gonococcal endosalpinges or other overt infections of the tube, the techniques used to treat these cases are basically comparable to those used with the microelectrode. In the past 3 years, reports of patency rates have been few but the pregnancy rates have been as good with the CO_2 laser. Initial studies in animals showed no significant differences between the use of the conventional microelectrosurgical technique and microlaser techniques.[2] Bruhat and Mage[7] reported salpingostomies in 30 patients treated with electromicrosurgery and 28 patients treated with CO_2 laser surgery. They reported a term pregnancy rate of 16.6% in the electrosurgical group and 23.7% in the laser microsurgical group. Similar results were reported by several other investigators as well.[11,15,30,31] In 1984, Tulandi[28] reported that 23 patients treated with CO_2 lasers for hydrosalpinx showed a 21.7% pregnancy rate as compared with 22.7% with conventional microdiothermy. In the author's series of 24 patients observed for a period of 24 months, 16 had a postoperative second-look laparoscopy or hysterosalpingogram with 27 tubes evaluated for patency. Two closed tubes and 25 open tubes were noted, resulting in a patency rate of 93%. This success rate is not only comparable, but is higher than those reported in series using microelectrocautery techniques.

The technique of fimbrioplasty by laser surgery consists of magnification with single-pulse or repeat-pulse modes to vaporize the adhesions between the fimbriae. It is advisable to use a titanium or quartz rod as a backstop inside the ostium of the fimbria or to transilluminate whenever possible. Transillumination with the fiberoptic bundle provides a clear view of the adhesions between the fimbria walls. With a small spot size, 0.2 to 0.5 mm, the adhesions can be easily vaporized to create normal anatomy.

Laser neosalpingostomy with a completely distended hydrosalpinx is begun by injecting the tube with indigo carmine dye to distend its distal portion. The point of "puckering" is noted. The location of the incisions for the laser is outlined with single- or repeat-pulse modes in order not to penetrate into the lumen of the hydrosalpinx until the markings are completed. In this way, when the hydrosalpinx is entered and the fluid within is released, boundaries for creating the four flaps can be easily identified. When the hydrosalpinx is entered, a 3-mm titanium rod is placed into the lumen. With continuous or superpulse mode at a high power density (greater than 20,000 watts/cm^2), the four flaps are created by incising through the serosa, muscularis, and mucosa for a distance of approximately 1.5 cm. Any bleeding encountered is treated with bipolar microcautery.

After the four flaps are developed, a Bruhat maneuver[7] (flowering technique) is performed with a lower power density (200 to 300 watts/cm^2). Moving this defocused 2-mm beam rapidly across the peritoneal surface actually coagulates and retracts the edges of the serosa, everting the tube toward the proximal ampulla (Fig. 11–6). Fine suture of 7-0 or 8-0 Vicryl usually is preferred to stabilize the edges and to prevent retraction later. In the cases of much thicker hydrosalpinx, these flaps are more difficult to create and the flowering technique is nearly impossible. Nevertheless, the pregnancy rate usually is higher with this type of tube because there is less damage to the mucosa. The size of the hydrosalpinx, the presence or absence of mucosal folds or adhesions, and the thickness of the tubal wall are important factors to evaluate in determining the success of the repair. Kelly and Roberts[20] reported a pregnancy rate of 11% in 28 patients with neosalpingostomies observed for a period of 1 year. The same series was updated to include 61 patients observed for 1 or more years resulted in a term pregnancy rate of 22%. The pregnancy rates reported by others have ranged from 13.8% to 29%.[20,30] Follow-up of at least 3 to 5 years will be required for comparison of pregnancy rates after neosalpingostomy with laser versus standard microsurgical techniques. Assuming that the mucosa is the limiting factor, use of the laser might be expected to improve the outcome significantly over standard microsurgery by leading to a higher tubal patency rate and fewer postoperative adhesions.

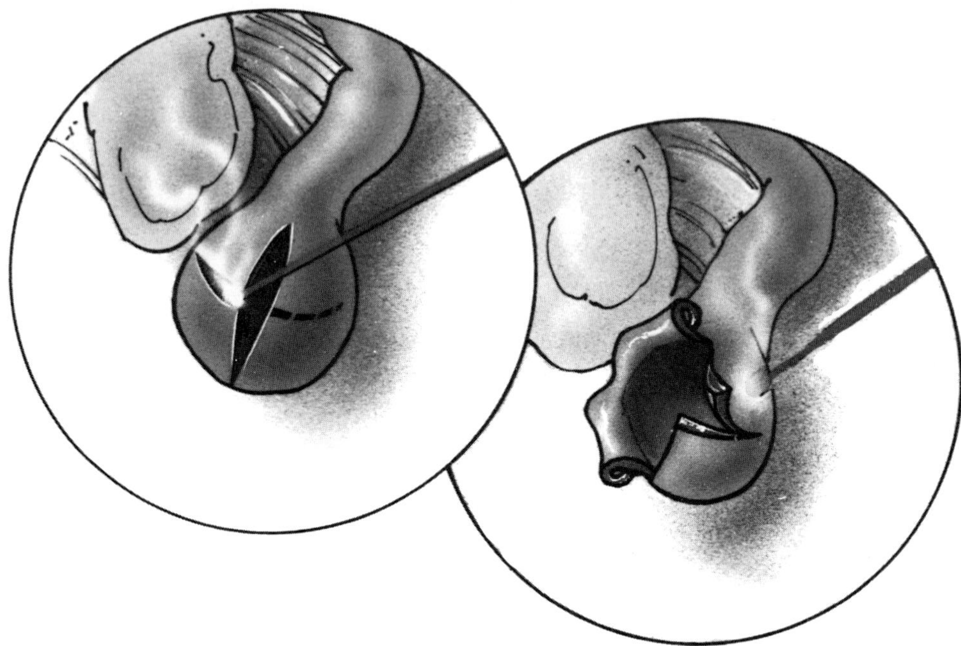

FIGURE 11–6. Incision of a hydrosalpinx with a CO_2 laser and Bruhat maneuver to evert its edges.

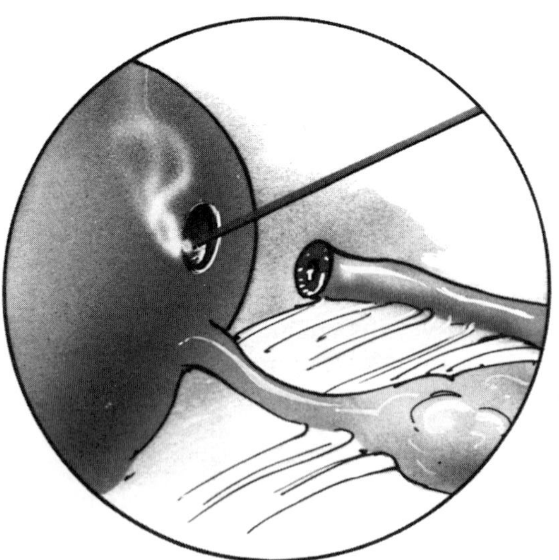

FIGURE 11–7. Preparation of the uterus with a CO_2 laser for tubal implantation.

Tubal Implantation

Tubal implantation is rarely performed because the preferred technique, interstitial isthmic anastomosis, is associated with a better prognosis for pregnancy. However, it may be indicated when there is no remaining interstitial tube. If this procedure is undertaken, the following steps should be followed. After injection of a dilute solution of vasopressin (1 : 20) or epinephrine into the myometrium, a defocused beam at the maximum controllable power density should be used to quickly and rapidly drill a hole into the endometrial cavity (Figure 11–7). To prevent damage to the opposite side of the intrauterine cavity, it is important that dye distend the cavity while laser vaporization is being performed. The size of the opening can easily be adjusted according to the size of the tube to be implanted. The only disadvantage of this technique is that when a vessel larger than 1.5 mm is encountered with the laser, there will be an obvious welling of blood, which will absorb the energy and prevent adequate penetration. In most instances, however, this situation should be prevented by the use of vasopressin.

After preparing the orifice, the isthmic portion of the tube is prepared either by bivalving the distal isthmic portion of the tube or by splitting the antimesenteric border as described by Gomel.[18]

Cornual Polyps

Cornual polyps have been reported as a cause of infertility for several years. The first reports were those by Phillip and Huber[24] in 1939. The incidence of polyps detected by hysterosalpingogram varies from 1.2% to 2.77%.[27] Polyps of various sizes have been described but most commonly are approximately 5 mm in diameter. They may be unilateral or bilateral. Treatment success with medication has been extremely limited.[12] In most instances, surgeons have elected to correct the problem with excision of the polyps and a uterotubal implantation. However, experience with uterotubal implantations suggests a poor prognosis.

The first to report microsurgical tubal implantation after excision of cornual polyps were Boeckx and associates.[6] They reported no pregnancies in their series. Others have suggested microsurgical linear salpingostomies to preserve the integrity and physiology of the uterotubal junction as well as to maximize tubal length. In 1984, McLaughlin reported a successful outcome following removal of bilateral cornual polyps by microsurgical linear salpingostomy with the aid of the CO_2 laser.[22] This technique appears to be the most efficacious for dealing with such tubal disease.

The usual technique includes injection of dilute vasopressin, one ampule per 20 ml of normal saline, into both cornua as well as into the base of the area of the polyps. With a small spot size of 0.2 mm and power density greater than 15,000 watts/cm^2, a linear incision is made into the cornua. The polyps are excised at the base with single-pulse and repeat-pulse modes. The tubal muscularis is reapproximated with 8-0 Vicryl, nylon, or PDS suture and the serosa with a similar suture.

Significant benefits of linear salpingostomy are that a waiting period is not required before pregnancy is attempted, and if pregnancy is achieved, a cesarean section is not mandatory. Therefore, until new techniques are developed, salpingostomy as performed by McLaughlin appears to be the most effective means of dealing with this unusual problem.

Salpingostomy for Ectopic Pregnancy

With the early use of vaginal ultrasonography and beta-human chorionic gonadotropin evaluation, early unruptured ectopic pregnancies can now be diagnosed. It is often possible to incise the tube by laser laparoscopic linear salpingostomy. If not, laparoscopic salpingectomy is often attempted before laparotomy. Laparotomy is necessary, however, if the ectopic pregnancy is too large for a laparoscopic procedure to be performed safely or if excessive bleeding is encountered. A laser linear salpingostomy can usually be performed using a bloodless technique. A 27-gauge needle is used to inject the serosa and mesosalpinx of the tube with dilute vasopressin (1 : 20); the larger vessels are constricted, and the cushion of the fluid absorbs the laser beam's heat and protects the surrounding oviductal tissue. The operative microscope with micromanipulator is used to direct the beam with power densities ranging from 10,000 to 20,000 watts/cm^2 using a continuous mode. The products of conception can then be very easily teased out through this small defect (Fig. 11–8). Generally the edges of the incision are adequately sealed because of the coagulating properties of the laser. Should bleeding occur, microbipolar forceps coagulation can be applied. It is not usually necessary to close the salpingostomy incision; it can be allowed to heal by secondary intention. Croop and colleagues[10] reported one case of failure of tubal closure after laser salpingostomy for an ampullatory tubal ectopic pregnancy.

Baggish and Chong[3] reported six cases treated with this technique, and tubal patency of the surgically treated tube was demonstrated postoperatively in all pa-

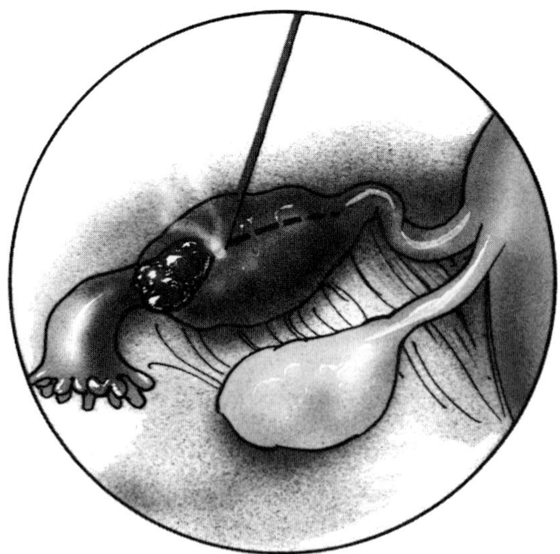

FIGURE 11–8. Salpingostomy for ectopic pregnancy with a CO_2 laser.

tients. Voros and colleagues[32] also cited six ectopic pregnancies managed conservatively with a CO_2 laser. Within 6 months after surgery, 33% of the patients had conceived intrauterine pregnancies.

CONCLUSION

It is apparent that lasers are playing an increasingly important role in treatment of infertility-related disorders. As clinical experience and investigative protocols are reported, these important developments will almost surely validate the necessity for surgeons to become knowledgeable about laser surgery, if not proficient in its use. Even if the pregnancy rates do not surpass those achieved after conventional microsurgery, the other advantages of using the laser in microsurgery cannot be ignored.

As newer wavelengths become applicable for surgical procedures, further major advances may be expected in the treatment of endometriosis, adhesions, and tubal disease.

REFERENCES

1. Badaway ZA, ElBakry M, Baggish MS: Comparative study of continuous and pulsed CO_2 laser on tissue healing and fertility outcome in tubal anastomosis. Fertil Steril 47:843, 1987
2. Baggish MS, Chong AP: Carbon dioxide laser microsurgery of the uterine tube. Obstet Gynecol 58:111, 1981
3. Baggish MS, Chong SP: Intra-abdominal surgery with the CO_2 laser. J Reprod Med 28:269, 1983
4. Barbot J, Parent B, Dubuisson J et al: A clinical study of the CO_2 laser and electrosurgery for adhesiolysis in 172 cases followed by early second-look laparoscopy. Fertil Steril 48:140, 1987
5. Bellina J: Microsurgery of the fallopian tube with the carbon dioxide laser: Analysis of 230 cases with two-year follow-up. Lasers Surg Med 3:255, 1983
6. Boeckx W, Brosens I, Gordts S et al: Tubal cornual polyps: Microsurgical polypectomy and cornual anastomosis (abstr), p 147. Presented at the Fifth European Congress on Sterility, Venice, October, 1978
7. Bruhat MA, Magee G: Pregnancy following salpingostomy: Comparison between CO_2 laser and electrosurgery procedures. Fertil Steril 40:472, 1983
8. Buttram VC Jr: Surgical treatment of endometriosis in the infertile female: A modified approach. Fertil Steril 32:635, 1979
9. Chong AP, Baggish MS: Management of pelvic endometriosis by means of intra-abdominal carbon dioxide laser. Fertil Steril 41:14, 1984
10. Cropp CS, Cowell PLD, Rock JA: Failure of tube closure following laser salpingostomy for ampullary tubal ectopic pregnancy. Fertil Steril 48:887, 1987
11. Daniell JF, Diamond MP, McLaughlin DS et al: Clinical results of terminal neosalpingostomy with the use of CO_2 laser: Report of the intra-abdominal laser study group. Fertil Steril 45:175, 1986
12. David MP, Ben-Zwi D, Langer L: Tubal intramural polyps and their relationship to infertility. Fertil Steril 35:526, 1981
13. Diamond MP, Daniell JF, Martin DC et al: Pelvic adhesions at early second-look laparoscopy following carbon dioxide laser surgical procedures. Fertil Steril 7:39, 1984
14. Dmowski WP, Cohen ME: Treatment of endometriosis with an antigonadotropin, Danazol: A laparoscopic and histologic evaluation. Obstet Gynecol 46:147, 1975
15. Fayez JA, McComb JS, Harper MA: Comparison of tubal microsurgery with the CO_2 laser and the unipolar microelectrode. Fertil Steril 40:476, 1983
16. Filmar S, Gomel V, McComb PF: The effectiveness of CO_2 laser and electromicrosurgery in adhesiolysis: A comparative study. Fertil Steril 45:407, 1986
17. Friedlander RL: The treatment of endometriosis with Danazol. J Reprod Med 10:197, 1975
18. Gomel V: Clinical results of infertility microsurgery. In Crosignani PG, Rubin BL (eds): Microsurgery in Female Infertility, p. 77. Academic Press, London, 1980

19. Greenblatt RB, Tzingounis V: Danazol treatment of endometriosis: Long term follow up. Fertil Steril 32:518, 1979
20. Kelly RW, Roberts DK: Experience with the carbon dioxide laser in gynecologic microsurgery. Am J Obstet Gynecol 146:585, 1983
21. Kistner RW: Endometriosis in infertility. In Kistner RW, Behrman SJ (eds): Progress in Infertility, 2nd ed. Boston, Little, Brown & Co, 1975
22. McLaughlin DS: Successful pregnancy outcome following removal of bilateral cornual polyps by microsurgery with the aid of the CO_2 laser. Fertil Steril 42:939, 1984
23. McLaughlin DS, Bonaventura LM, Jarrett JC II: Tubal reanastomosis: A comparison between microsurgical and microlaser techniques. Microsurgery 8:78, 1987
24. Phillip E, Huber H: Cause of endometriosis with contribution on the pathology of the interstitial portion of the tube. Zentralbl Gynakol 67:7, 1939
25. Pittaway DE, Maxson WS, Daniell JF: A comparison of the CO_2 laser and electrocautery on postoperative intraperitoneal adhesion formations in rabbits. Fertil Steril 40:366, 1983
26. Raj SG, Hulka HF: Second-look laparoscopy in infertility surgery: Therapeutic and prognostic value. Fertil Steril 38:325, 1982
27. Strangel J, Chervenak FA, Mouradian-Davidian M: Microsurgical resection of bilateral fallopian tube polyps. Fertil Steril 35:580, 1981
28. Tulandi T: Salpingo-ovariolysis: A comparison between laser surgery and electrosurgery. Fertil Steril 45:489, 1986
29. Tulandi, T: Adhesion reformation after reproductive surgery with and without the carbon dioxide laser. Fertil Steril 47:704, 1987
30. Tulandi T, Farag R, McInnes R et al: Reconstructive surgery of hydrosalpinx with and without the carbon dioxide laser. Fertil Steril 42:839, 1984
31. Tulandi T, Vilos G: A comparison between laser surgery and electrosurgery for bilateral hydrosalpinx: A 2-year follow-up. Fertil Steril 44:841, 1985
32. Voros JI, Bellina JH, Moorehead ME et al: Management of ectopic pregnancy by carbon dioxide laser. J La State Med Soc 135:9, 1984

12

Uterine and Ovarian Laser Surgery

David S. McLaughlin

Lasers were first introduced in gynecological practice by Bellina in 1974.[4] From that initial report, which primarily described external application of the carbon dioxide (CO_2) laser, much controversy evolved regarding the application of lasers for fertility-promoting procedures.[2] Healthy skepticism regarding the true benefits of intra-abdominal laser surgery initially was founded on a lack of long-term scientific studies, along with the lack of familiarity with laser equipment and the new, no-touch technique. During the past decade, published scientific data regarding the laser's use for fertility-promoting procedures have accumulated. The CO_2 laser was initially used freehand or coupled to an operating microscope at laparotomy. Surgical techniques improved with experience in conjunction with the evolution of improved surgical laser delivery systems. Many pathologic processes primarily treated only by laparotomy are now approached primarily endoscopically—either by laser laparoscopy, pelviscopy, or laser hysteroscopy.[16] Despite newer medical treatment options (*e.g.,* gonadotropin agonists for uterine myoma and endometriosis, pure follicle-stimulating hormone for polycystic ovarian disease) and alternative reproductive therapies (*in vitro* fertilization and gamete intrafallopian transfer), indications remain that require laparotomy for appropriate laser therapy. These include excision of large myomas, the reunification of a bicornuate uterus, excision of large ovarian cysts, and ovarian wedge resection. The laser's advantages of precision, hemostasis, and the ability to reach previously inaccessible areas may be maximized to preserve or enhance reproductive potential.

OPERATING ROOM SETUP AND INSTRUMENTATION

Although freehand delivery of the laser (CO_2, argon, KTP, and Nd:YAG laser with contact tips) in conjunction with optic loupes or the operating microscope is slightly easier to learn, the author prefers the enhanced precision of microlaser technique. This method uses the CO_2 laser coupled to the dual-headed operating microscope (Fig. 12–1) by a micromanipulator. A 300-mm laser lens is used in conjunction with a 300-mm optic objective for the operating microscope. These lenses offer adequate working distance along with precision and light. A sterile angiocath cover is used over the joystick (Fig. 12–2), but no sterile microscope drape is used over the microslad, as the laser energy would melt the plastic as it passes the exit port. Shortened, ebonized instruments are used to reduce the possibility of contamination from the nonsterile microslad and reduce the risk of reflection of the laser's beam to vital intra-abdominal structures. Rhodium mirrors to reflect the laser's beam to inaccessible areas and quartz rods to absorb the laser's energy are used as well (Fig. 12–3). To further insulate vital intra-abdominal structures, moistened non-woven packs are used.[25] A high power density, in excess of 18,000 watts/cm^2, using superpulse mode whenever possible, is preferred to reduce heat transfer to normal remaining tissue. Dilute vasopressin (Pitressin) (10 units/30 cc) is used for uterine surgery to enhance hemostasis, as opposed to using tourniquets or rubber-shod clamps. (Note: The author has encountered one patient who had severe peripheral vasoconstriction for rapid absorption of nondilute vasopressin, which had accidentally been mixed 20 units/30 cc.)

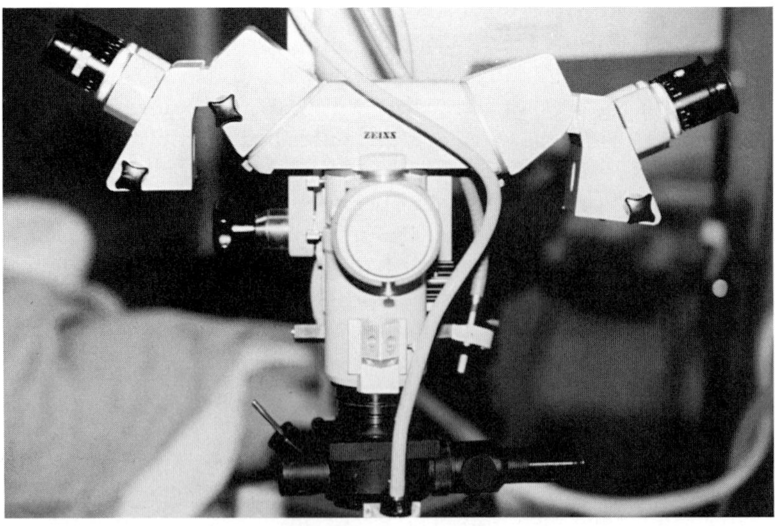

FIGURE 12–1. Dual-headed operating microscope showing attachment of the microslad to the operative objective.

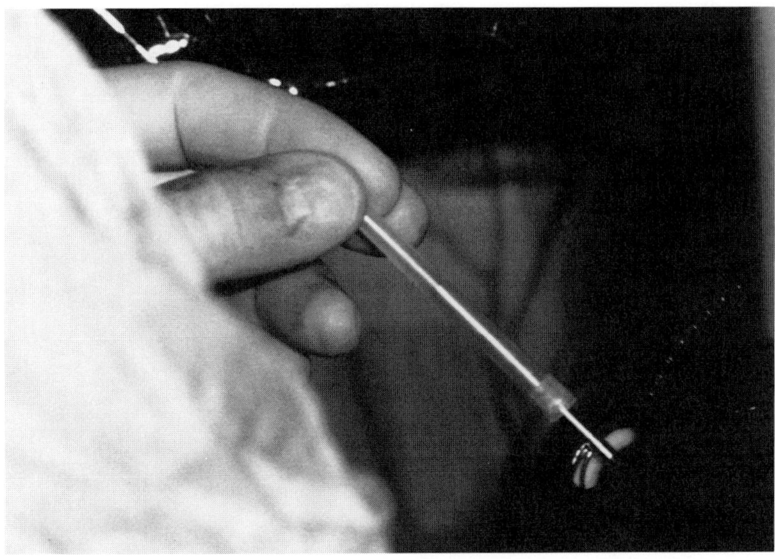

FIGURE 12–2. Sterile angiocath cover over a joystick.

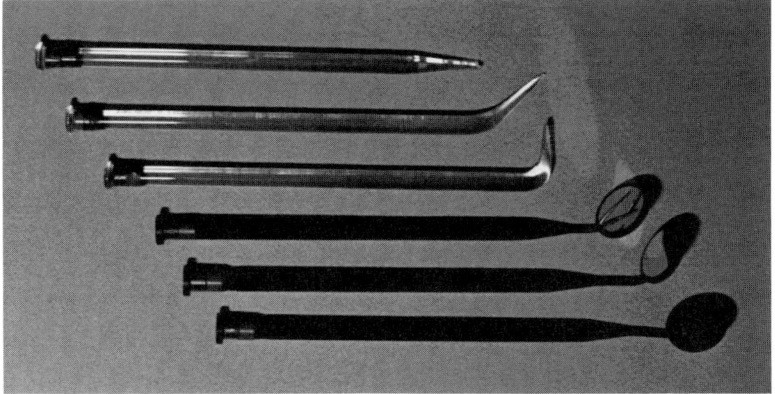

FIGURE 12–3. Quartz rods and rhodium mirrors. The mirrors and rods are angled at 90 degrees, 60 degrees, and 0 degrees.

MYOMECTOMY

Technique

Small fibroids may be excised (Figs. 12–4 and 12–5), or vaporized directly or indirectly by reflecting the laser's energy off the surface of a rhodium mirror to strike the target perpendicularly (Figs. 12–6 through 12–9). Although suturing the uterine defect to facilitate serosal coaptation is usually desired, early second-look laparos-

(*text continued on page 175*)

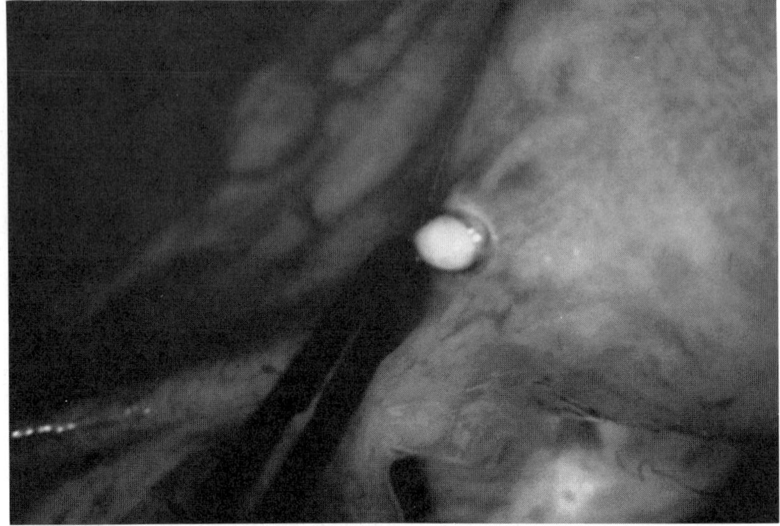

FIGURE 12–4. Small cornual fibroid. A laser incision is made using the joystick to direct the laser's energy over the myoma.

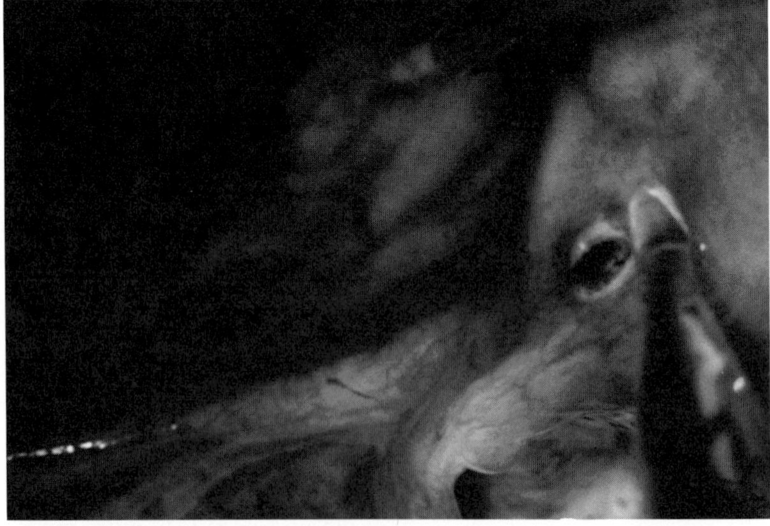

FIGURE 12–5. Small fibroid removed. The fibroid was dissected free using laser and blunt dissection.

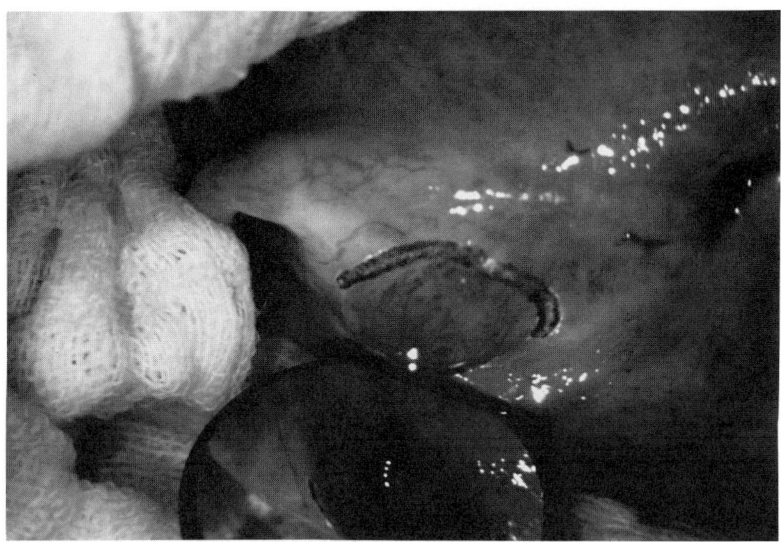

FIGURE 12–6. Larger posterior-cornual fibroid partially circumscribed by direct application of the laser's energy.

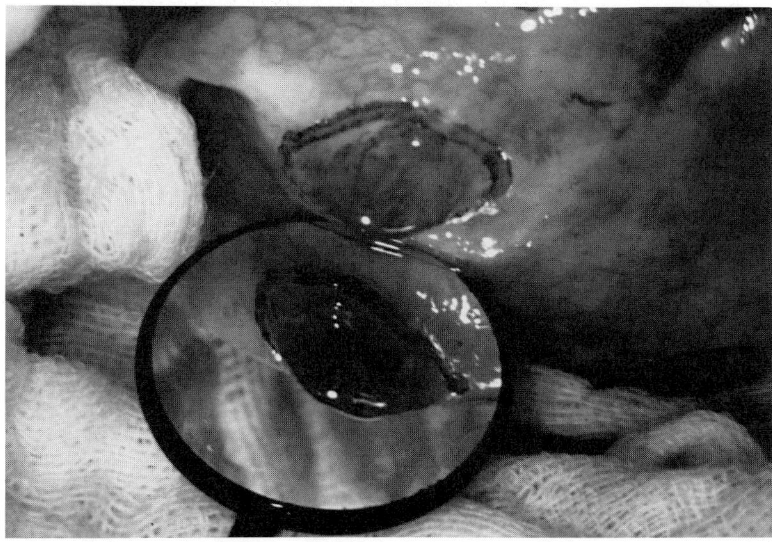

FIGURE 12–7. Indirect myoma vaporization. The laser's energy is fired into the rhodium mirror to reflect back on the myoma at a 90-degree angle.

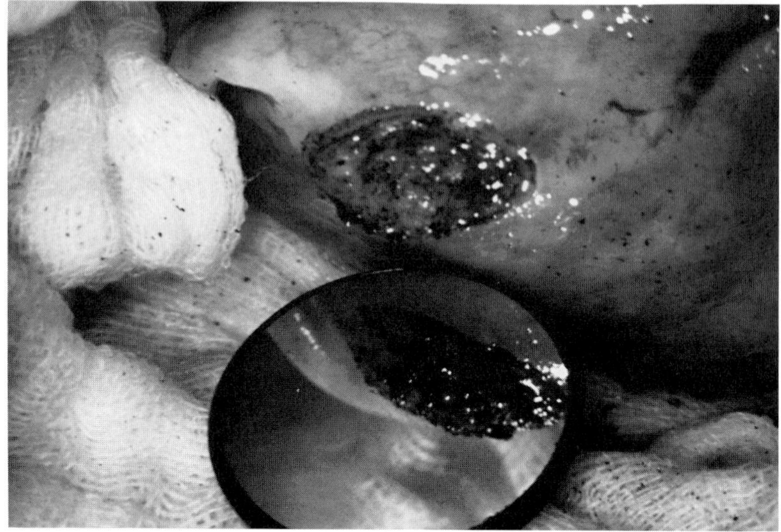

FIGURE 12–8. Myoma nearly completely vaporized directly and indirectly. Note the lack of bleeding and the moistened non-woven gauze sponge placed in the cul-de-sac to insulate the pelvic viscera.

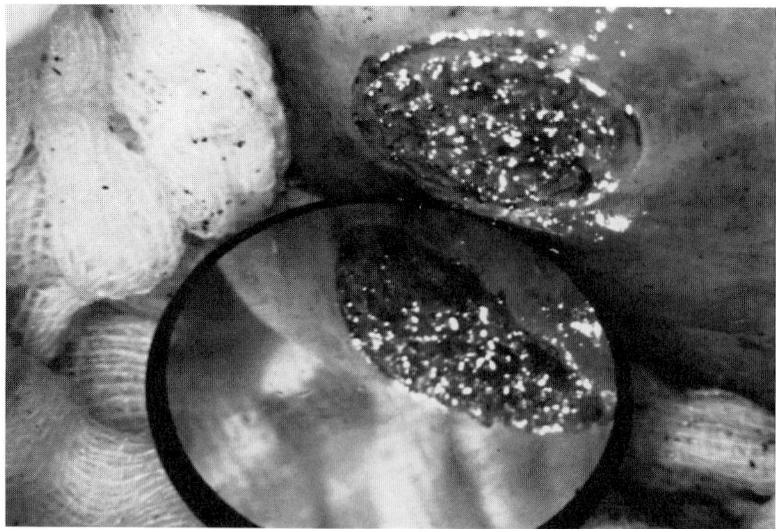

FIGURE 12–9. Myoma completely vaporized.

copy demonstrated excellent healing with no adhesion reformation 6 weeks postoperatively (Fig. 12–10).

The base of a medium-sized fibroid (Fig. 12–11) is injected with dilute vasopressin (10:30), grasped with an ebonized towel clamp, and a traction suture is placed into the uterine fundus for countertraction. The laser is fired directly at the base of the myoma, as seen through the microscope (Fig. 12–12). The inferior portion of the myoma is approached by reflecting a laser beam off a rhodium mirror (Fig. 12–13). This technique is continued until the entire myoma is removed, taking care to preserve as much of the normal uterus as possible. The uterine defect is closed with 2-0 Surgilon (siliconized, braided nylon) and 4-0 Surgilon superficially to join the serosal layer. Early second-look laparoscopy shows an absence of recurrent adhesions, which is usually the case when hemostasis is meticulously maintained (Fig. 12–14).

Large myomas, which would exceed the field of view of the microscope (Fig. 12–15), are approached using the hand piece attached to the articulating arm (*i.e.,* freehand). The base of the myoma is injected with vasopressin (Fig. 12–16) and circumscribed with a marking pen to delineate the intended laser incision (Fig. 12–17). (Note: Plan to leave a slight excess of superficial uterine tissue in order to facilitate coverage of the uterine defect after myomectomy.) The laser's energy is directed along the uterine marking with traction by a blackened towel clip placed into the myoma. Straight quartz rods are inserted between the myoma and the uterus to act as backstops and facilitate dissection as the laser is fired at the fibroid capsule's attachments, until the myoma is completely excised (Fig. 12–18). The defect is closed with layered 2-0 Surgilon, finishing the serosal layer with 4-0 Surgi-

(*text continued on page 180*)

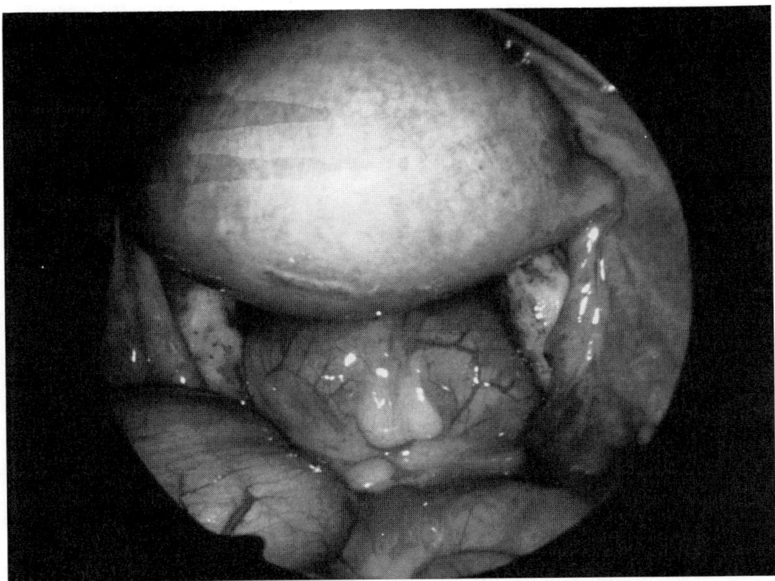

FIGURE 12–10. Early second-look laparoscopy showing no adhesions to the myoma vaporization site.

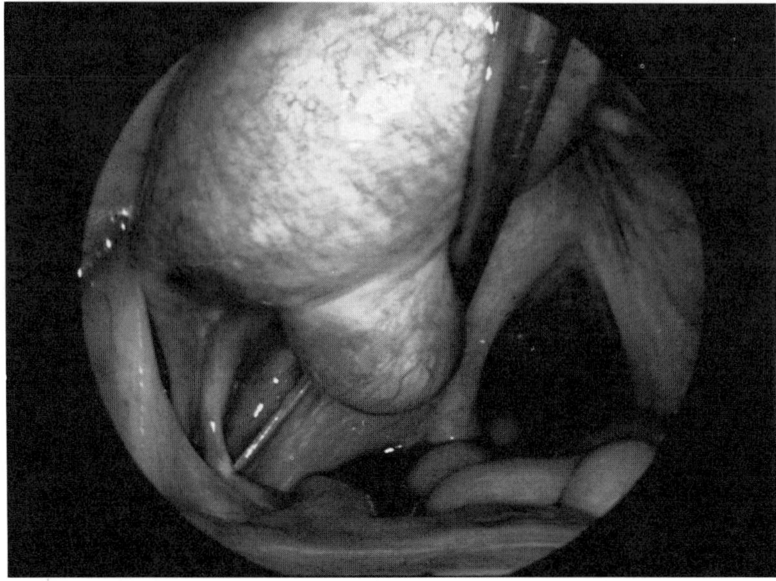

FIGURE 12–11. Moderate myoma encountered at the posterior lateral aspect of the uterus as viewed through the laparoscope.

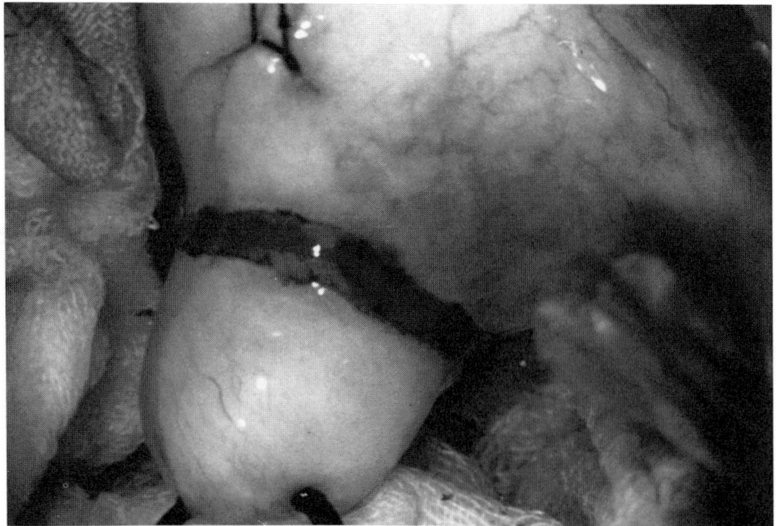

FIGURE 12–12. Myoma at the time of microlaser myomectomy. Laser energy has been applied directly to the base of the fibroid after injection of dilute vasopressin (10 units/30 ml). Note the traction suture on the uterine fundus and the ebonized towel clip grasping the myoma.

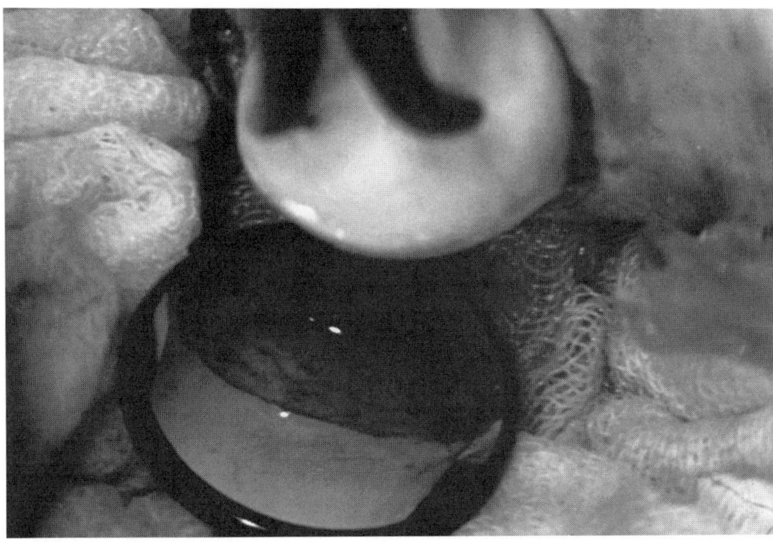

FIGURE 12–13. Indirect vaporization of the myoma base. High power densities are applied by reflecting the beam off a rhodium mirror to the base of the fibroid.

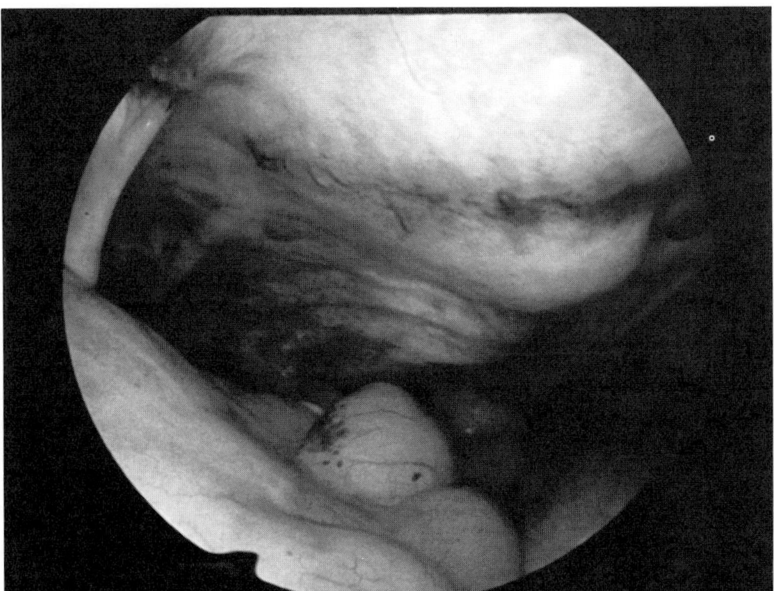

FIGURE 12–14. Early second-look laparoscopy from the suture site following microlaser myomectomy. The 4-0 Surgilon suture has no adhesions, although the epiploic fat occasionally attaches to the suture line. These adhesions are usually lysed bluntly, with minimal effort.

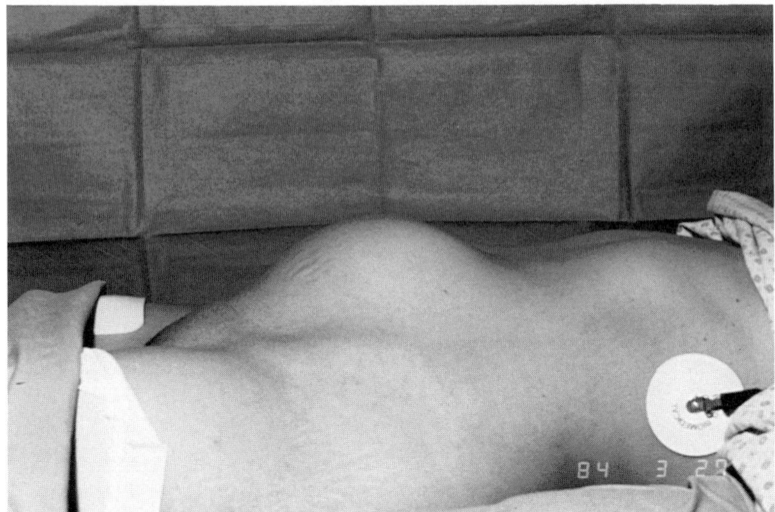

FIGURE 12–15. Large myoma. This patient had previously had midtrimester intrauterine fetal demise of twins and had been offered hysterectomy in her country for the preceding 5 years.

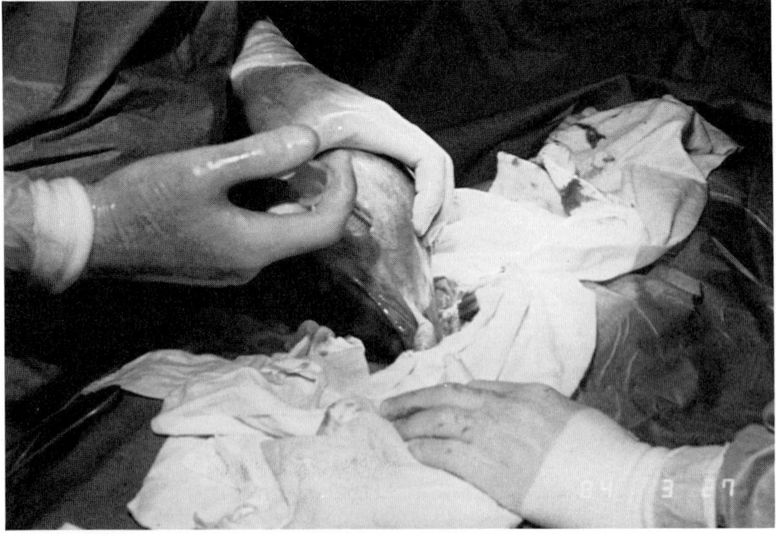

FIGURE 12–16. Dilute vasopressin injected into the base of the myoma.

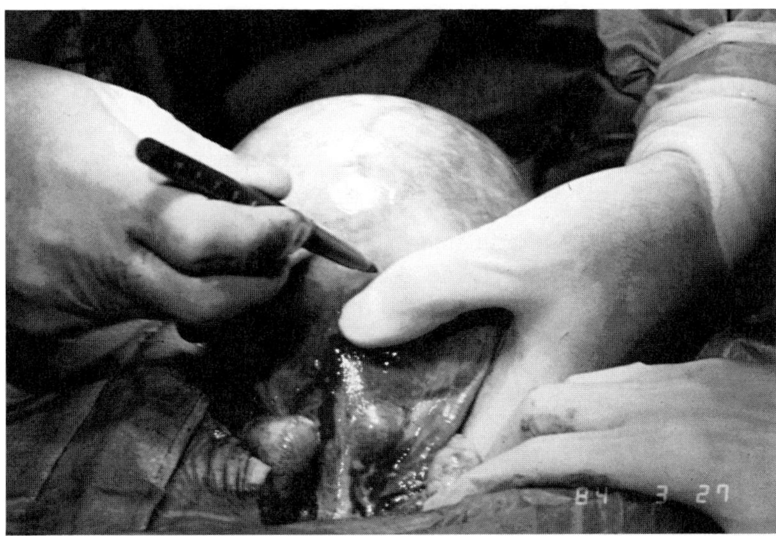

FIGURE 12–17. The myoma is circumscribed with a sterile marking pen. It is important to orient one's approach to preserve the maximum of normal uterine tissue.

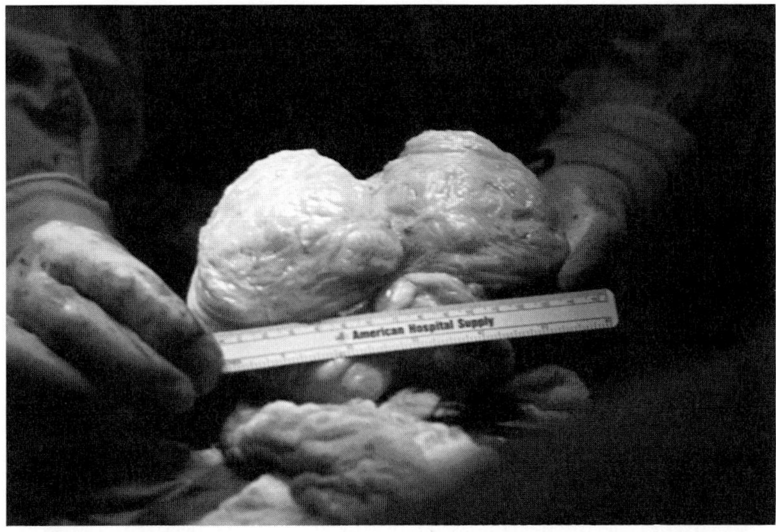

FIGURE 12–18. Large myoma removed. This fibroid weighed more than 800 g.

lon. No omental or peritoneal grafts are used, and 200 ml of 32% dextran 70 (Hyskon) is instilled before closure. Cesarean section is usually advised after removal of a large myoma, particularly if greater than 50% of the myometrium was penetrated.

Discussion

The most commonly encountered uterine neoplasms, myomas, have a reported incidence of 4% to 11%.[10] Many patients may spontaneously conceive and deliver healthy infants at term. Others may have difficulty conceiving and, if they do, have their pregnancies complicated by spontaneous abortion, premature labor, fetal malpresentation, postpartum hemorrhage, or delayed uterine involution.[10] In infertile patients, if myoma is the only abnormal finding, more than half of these patients will conceive after myomectomy, usually within the first year postoperatively.[1,7]

Although the technique of myomectomy was first reported in 1842 by Augusta[11] and later by Bonney,[5] because of the complications of hemorrhage and sepsis it did not gain in popularity until after World War II. Microlaser technique, to enhance hemostasis and preserve more normal uterine tissue, was initially reported in 1982 by the author.[12] In that preliminary report, 60% of the patients conceived within the first year, and in a subsequent report one-third did likewise.[14] Further studies have reported similar success with this new technique.[19,21] Of special note is the improvement in hemostasis when employing the microlaser technique for myomectomy over conventional surgical technique. The author noted that on the average, those patients who underwent myomectomy with conventional surgical technique lost nearly 50% more blood than those who had microlaser myomectomy (311 ml per patient versus 200 ml per patient).[15] Thus, microlaser technique for myomectomy should be considered for removal of myoma in infertile patients wishing to enhance their reproductive potential or gynecological patients wishing to preserve it.

METROPLASTY

Technique

Although suspected on the basis of hysteroscopy or hysterosalpingography, a septate uterus (which could be reunified by laser hysteroscopy) should be ruled out and true bicornuate uterus should be confirmed by laparoscopy (Fig. 12–19) before scheduling a microlaser metroplasty. At the time of laparotomy, traction sutures should be initially placed at each uterine horn and dilute vasopressin injected immediately into both horns (Fig. 12–20). A non-woven, moistened laparotomy sponge should be placed into the posterior cul-de-sac before activating the laser. Using superpulse, at 25 to 35 watts, with a small spot (0.2 to 0.5 mm), a medial incision is made into each horn until each uterine cavity is entered. A quartz rod is placed into each cavity to further delineate the exact boundaries of each cornu as the incision is extended, stopping short of impinging on the tubal ostia (Fig. 12–21). Two layers of continuous 2-0 Surgilon are placed, one anteriorly and the other posteriorly (Fig.

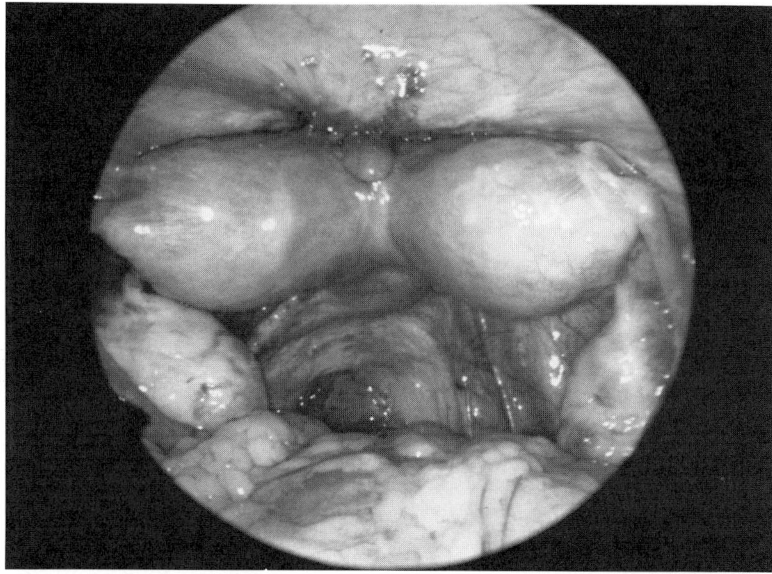

FIGURE 12–19. True bicornuate uterus. This patient also had pelvic adhesions secondary to endometriosis in the anterior and posterior cul-de-sac, along with adhesions.

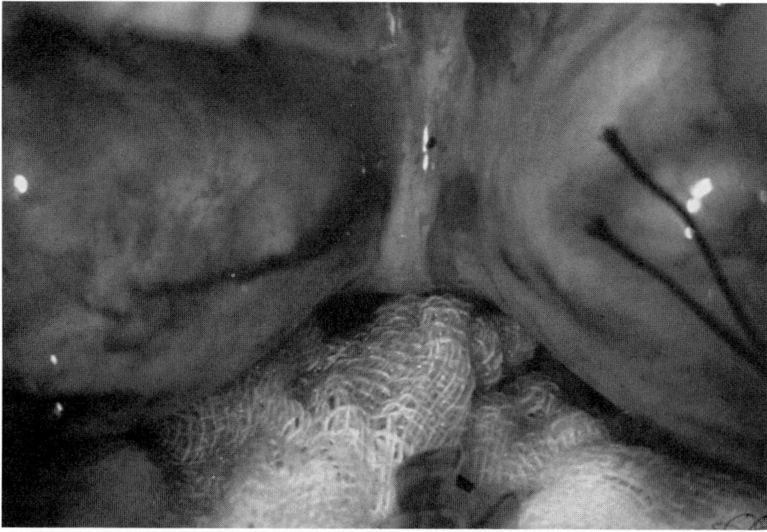

FIGURE 12–20. At the time of microlaser metroplasty, both uterine horns are fixed with traction sutures and the posterior cul-de-sac is insulated with moistened, non-woven laparotomy sponges. Dilute vasopressin is injected into the medial aspect of both uterine horns, and the laser energy is applied.

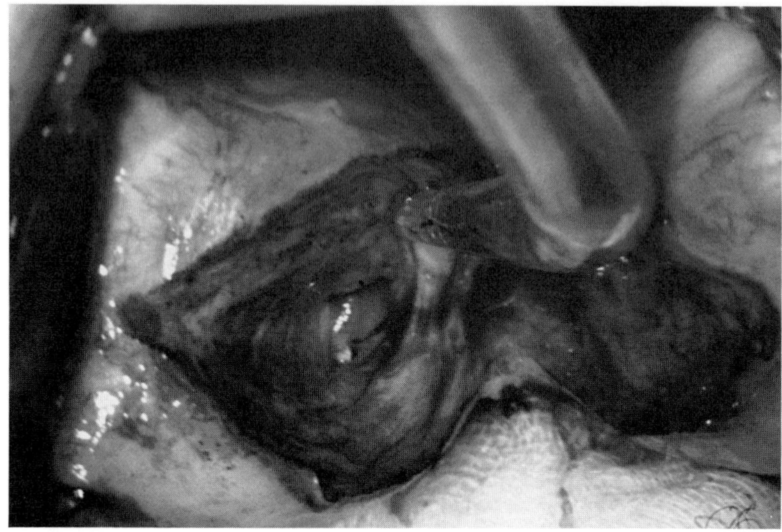

FIGURE 12–21. The uterine cavities are usually entered superior to the internal cervical os, and an angled quartz rod is placed into the endometrial cavity to help further delineate the entire medial border of the uterine horn. Note that minimal bleeding is encountered, with marked hemostatic action of the laser.

12–22). Uterine horns are joined in two layers (one deep and one more superficial), taking care not to include the endometrium in the suture line (Fig. 12–23). Upon completion of the myometrial layer, 4-0 Surgilon is used to approximate the serosa (Fig. 12–24). Hemostasis is assured before closure, and no omental graft is used, which would increase the likelihood of adhesion reformation. Although early second-look laparoscopy demonstrates excellent healing 6 weeks postoperatively (Fig. 12–25), pregnancy should be delayed for approximately 3 to 6 months. Delivery should be scheduled by cesarean section as soon as fetal maturity has been established.

Discussion

From 0.1–0.4% of the general female population[8] and up to 14% of infertile women[22] have congenital uterine malformations such as a septate uterus (due to failure of septum resorption) or a bicornuate uterus (due to failure of fusion).[10,23] Although congenital uterine defects may be suspected by a history of habitual abortions, premature labor, or fetal malpresentations, the exact extent of uterine developmental anomalies should be confirmed by hysterosalpingography, hysteroscopy, and laparoscopy. The reported live birth rate improves from 7% to 57% to 70% to 88% after pelvic reconstructive surgery to unify the uterus.[6,9,10,20,22] It has been recommended that none, or a minimum, of the tissue be removed during uterine reunification surgery. Baggish and Chong[3] initially reported the advantage of a bloodless field while excising a septum using a laser hand piece. The author[15] later

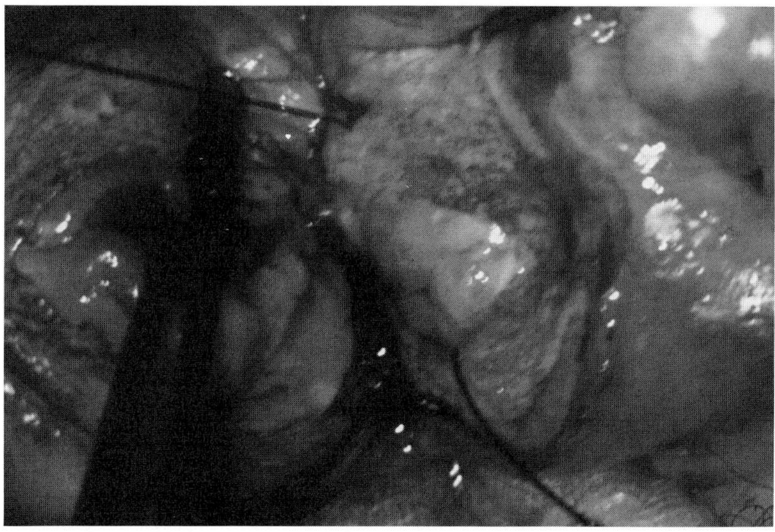

FIGURE 12–22. Note the lush endometrium overlying the uterine incision as Surgilon sutures are placed anteriorly and posteriorly. These sutures are angled into the deeper part of the myometrium, and a tag is left. It will be used to tie to the opposing suture once the superficial layer has been completed.

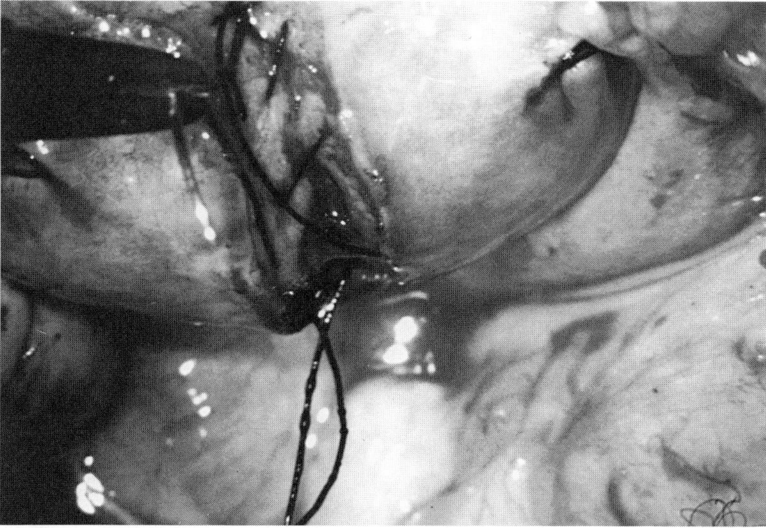

FIGURE 12–23. The uterine cavities are reapproximated as each suture line meets in the midline of the fundus and continues in the same direction superficially until it is tied at the anchor suture.

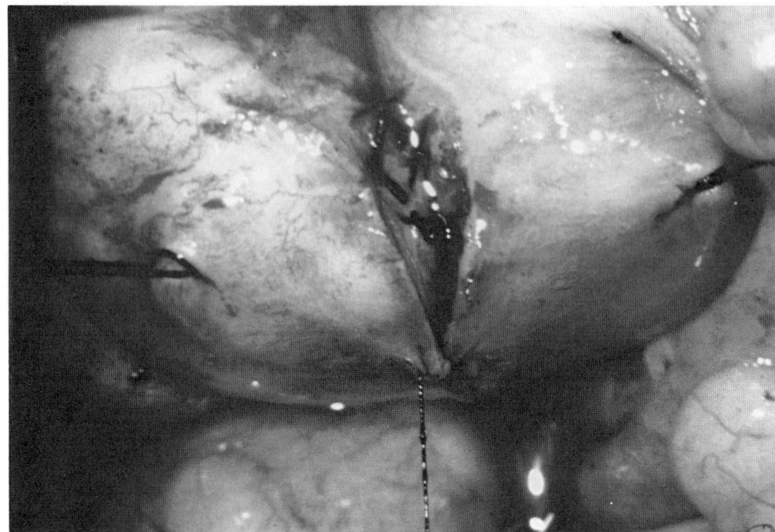

FIGURE 12–24. The uterine cavity is nearly closed, with 4-0 Surgilon used to approximate the serosa.

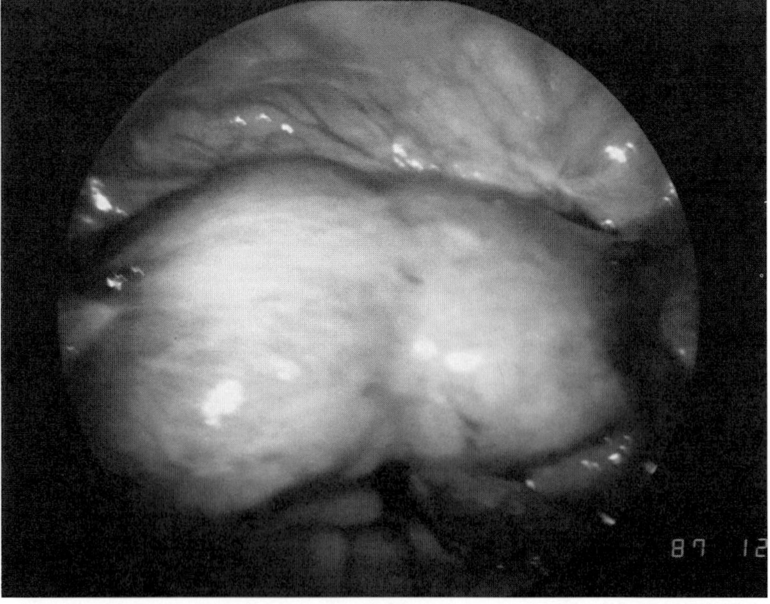

FIGURE 12–25. Early second-look laparoscopy shows excellent healing of the myometrium.

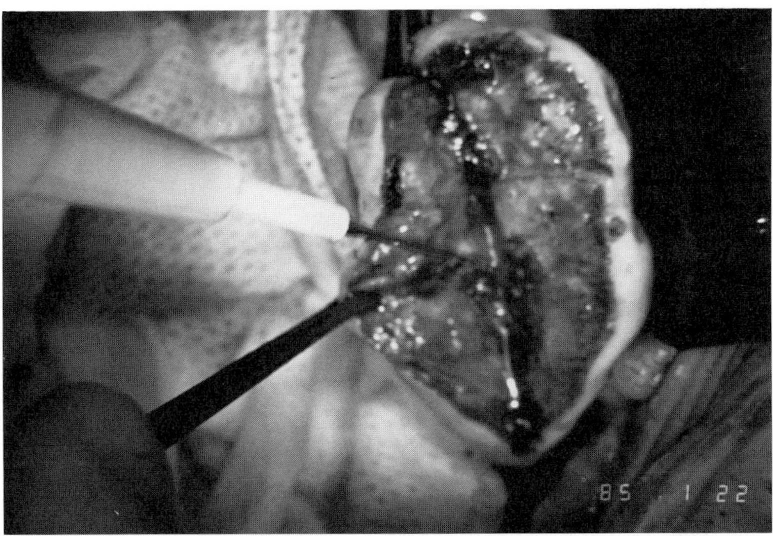

FIGURE 12–37. Using a needle electrode, bleeders at the base of the ovary are cauterized. There is usually a minimum of bleeding following laser surgery.

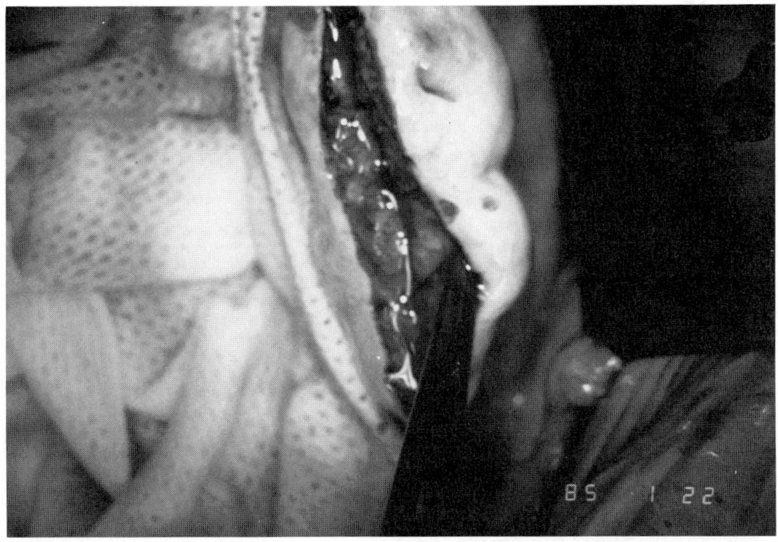

FIGURE 12–38. A deep layer of 4-0 Surgilon is continuously placed to join each side of the ovary.

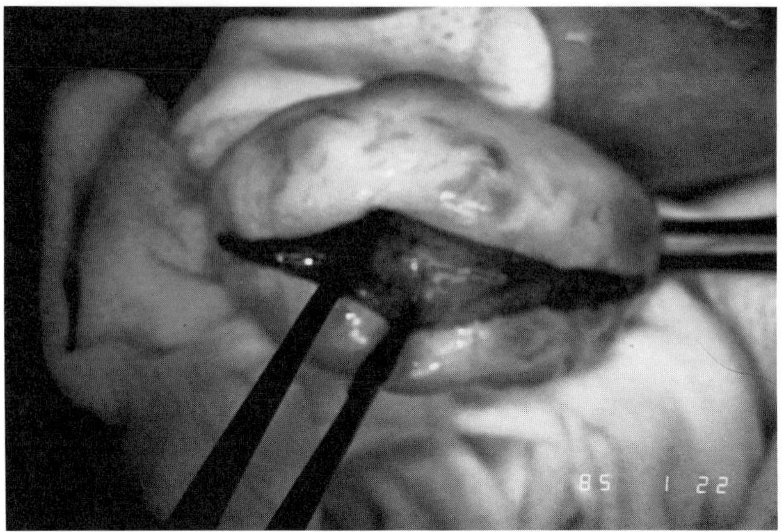

FIGURE 12–39. A subcortical layer of 4-0 Surgilon is placed.

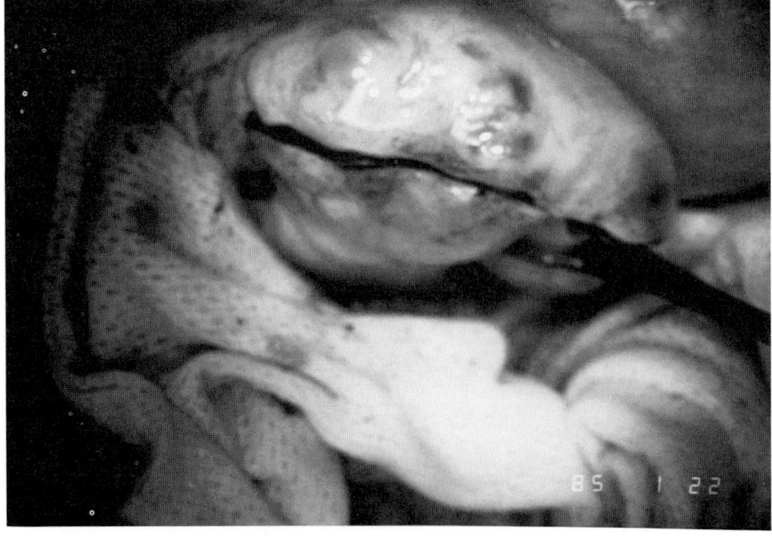

FIGURE 12–40. The cortex is approximated, and the 6-0 Surgilon suture is initiated.

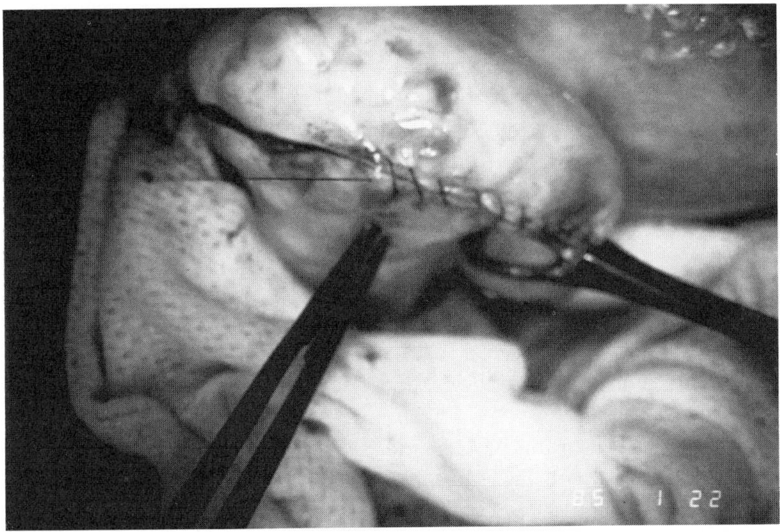

FIGURE 12–41. A continuous cortical 6-0 nylon suture is placed.

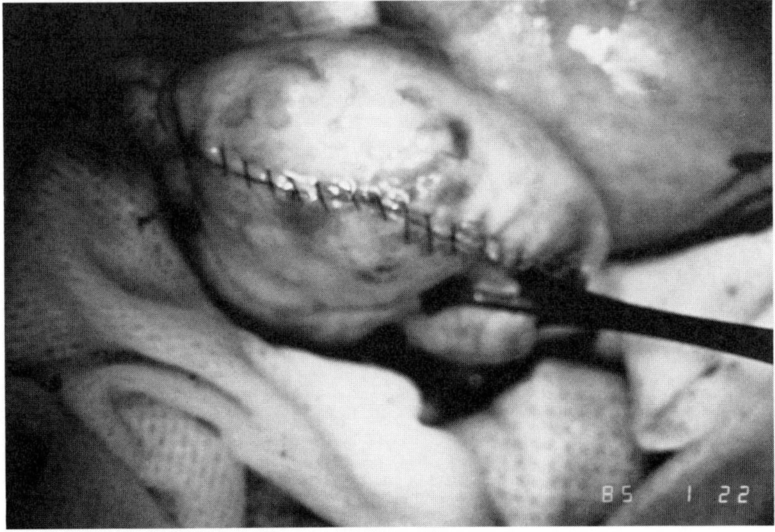

FIGURE 12–42. The cortex is completely approximated.

Discussion

Ironically, mechanical sterility may result because of subsequent adhesions reforming after conservative pelvic reconstructive surgery. This is particularly true for patients undergoing ovarian surgery without the aid of magnification and laser energy at the time of laparotomy (Fig. 12–43). Endometriosis has been encountered in as many as 21% of infertile patients.[24] Baggish and Chong[3] initially reported five patients whose endometriosis was treated by laser therapy and who subsequently underwent early second-look laparoscopy with no adhesions encountered and a pregnancy rate of 60%. The author[13] later reported a pregnancy rate of 60% for infertile patients undergoing microlaser excision of ovarian endometriomas or wedge resection for polycystic ovarian disease. In that same study, adhesions were seen in 37% of the ovarian suture lines; 83% of these adhesions were mild and filmy (Fig. 12–44) and were easily lysed by blunt laparoscopic dissection (Fig. 12–45). The majority of the patients studied had no adhesions to the ovarian suture line (Fig. 12–46). A subsequent multicenter study demonstrated no adhesions in 63% of the Surgilon-sutured ovaries as opposed to only 6% of the Vicryl-sutured ovaries.[18] Another disadvantage of using Vicryl to close the ovarian defect was loss of suture integrity with subsequent ovarian dehiscence at the time of adhesiolysis at early second-look laparoscopy.

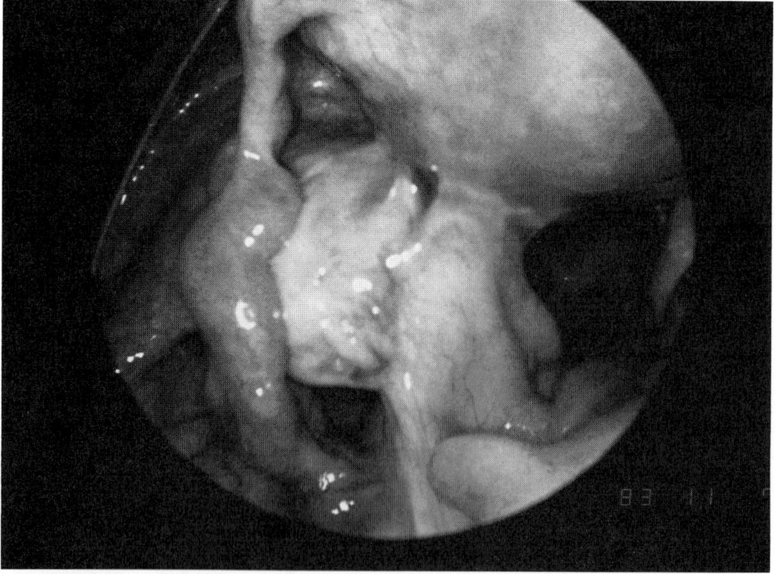

FIGURE 12–43. Early second-look laparoscopy showing dense adhesions 6 weeks after *non*-laser wedge resection performed without magnification.

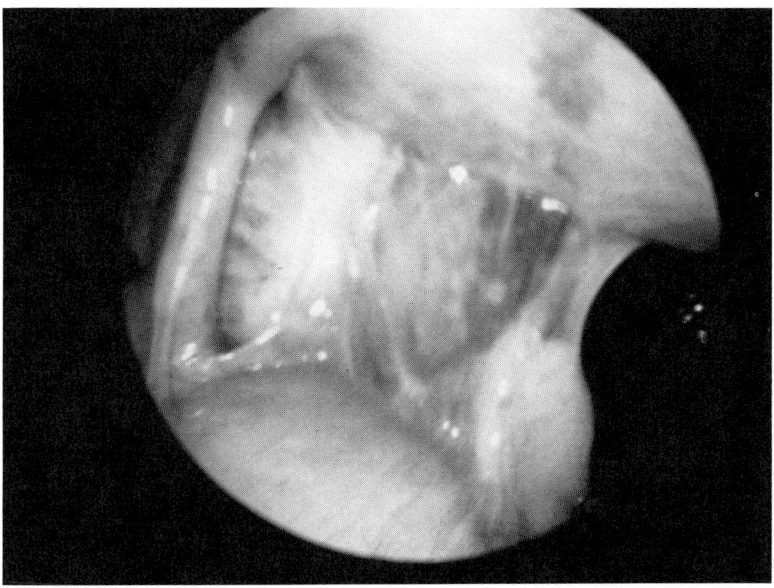

FIGURE 12–44. Mild, filmy adhesions encountered at the time of early second-look laparoscopy 6 weeks after microlaser wedge resection.

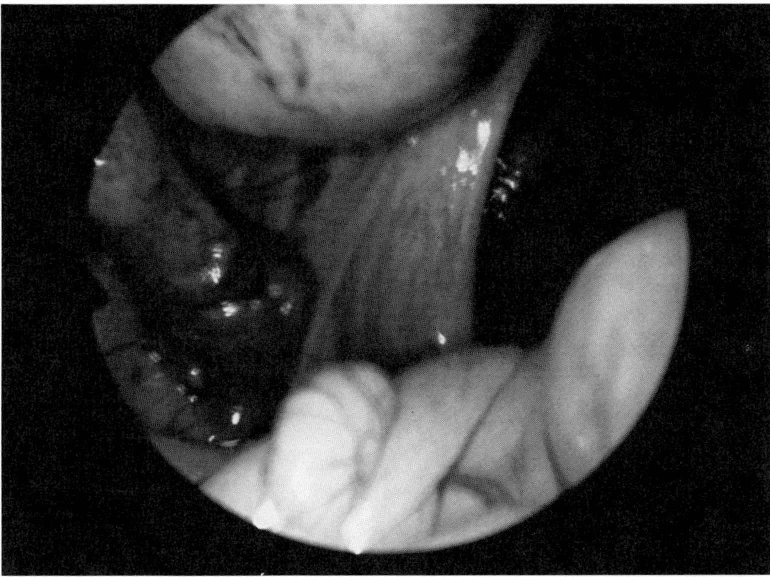

FIGURE 12–45. Adhesions are lysed bluntly with restoration of the normal anatomy at the time of early second-look laparoscopy after microlaser surgery.

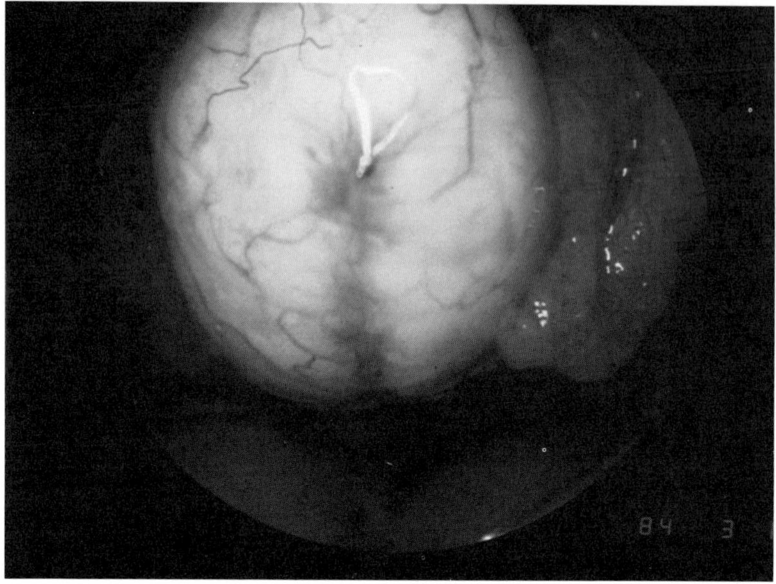

FIGURE 12–46. Excellent healing is seen at the time of early second-look laparoscopy. No mechanical cause of sterility is noted.

CONCLUSION

When performing uterine and ovarian surgery, the use of the CO_2 laser in conjunction with the operating microscope (*i.e.,* microlaser technique) appears to have the advantages of improved precision, enhanced hemostasis, the ability to reach previously inaccessible areas, preservation of more normal reproductive tissue, and a probable reduction of adhesion reformation. When employing this technique, it is important to use high power densities (25 to 35 watts), 0.2- to 0.5-mm spot size, superpulse mode, and rapid movement of the laser beam on tissue stretched by traction and countertraction whenever possible. With proper training, organization, and forethought, one should be able to effectively and safely offer this technique to women who wish to enhance or preserve their reproductive potential.

REFERENCES

1. Babaknia A, Rock JA, Jones HW Jr: Pregnancy success following abdominal myomectomy for infertility. Fertil Steril 30:644, 1979
2. Baggish MS: Status of carbon dioxide laser for infertility surgery. Fertil Steril 40:442, 1983
3. Baggish MS, Chong AP: Intra-abdominal surgery with the CO_2 laser. J Reprod Med 28:269, 1983
4. Bellina JH: Gynecology and the laser. Contemp Obstet Gynecol 4:24, 1979
5. Bonney V: The technique and results of myomectomy. Lancet 2:171, 1931
6. Buttram VC Jr: Mullerian anomalies and their management. Fertil Steril 40:159, 1983
7. Finn WF, Müller PF: Abdominal myomectomy: Special reference to subsequent pregnancy and to the reappearance of fibromas in the uterus. Am J Obstet Gynecol 60:109, 1959

8. Green LK, Harris RE: uterine anomalies, frequency of diagnosis and associated obstetric complications. Obstet Gynecol 47:427, 1976
9. Heinonen PK, Saarikoski S, Pystynen P et al: Reproductive performance of women with uterine anomalies: An evaluation of 182 cases. Acta Obstet Gynecol Scand 61:157, 1982
10. Jewelewicz R, Husami N, Wallach EE: When uterine factors cause infertility. Contemp Ob/Gyn 16:95, 1980
11. Malone LJ, Ingersoll FM: Myomectomy in infertility. In Behrman SJ, Kistner RW (eds): Progress in Infertility. Boston, Little, Brown & Co, 1975
12. McLaughlin DS: Microlaser myomectomy technique to enhance reproductive potential: A preliminary report. Lasers Surg Med 2:107, 1982
13. McLaughlin DS: Advanced surgical instrumentation needed for intra-abdominal application of the carbon dioxide laser in reproductive biology. Lasers Surg Med 2:241, 1983
14. McLaughlin DS: Evaluation of adhesion reformation by early second-look laparoscopy following microlaser ovarian wedge resection. Fertil Steril 42:531, 1984
15. McLaughlin DS: Metroplasty and myomectomy with the CO_2 laser for maximizing the preservation of normal tissue and minimizing blood loss. J Reprod Med 30:1, 1985
16. McLaughlin DS: Current uses of the laser for fertility-promotion procedures. Lasers Surg Med 5:539, 1985
17. McLaughlin DS: Instruments necessaires pour une microlaser de surete. Rev Fr Gynecol Obstet 81:47, 1986
18. McLaughlin DS: Miomectomia e Metroplastica. In Bandieramonte G, Gagna G (eds): Testo Atlante di Laser Chirurgia. Turin, utet (in press)
19. McLaughlin DS, Diamond MP, Daniell JF et al: Laparoscopic assessment of ovarian healing following CO_2 laser microsurgery: Vicryl vs. Surgilon. Microsurgery 8:99, 1987
20. Musich JR, Behrman SJ: Obstetric outcome before and after metroplasty in women with uterine anomalies. Obstet Gynecol 52:63, 1978
21. Reyniak JV, Corenthal L: Microsurgical laser technique for abdominal myomectomy. Microsurgery 8:92, 1987
22. Rock JA: Diagnosing and repairing uterine anomalies. Contemp Ob/Gyn 17:43, 1981
23. Sobrero AJ, Silverman CJ, Post A et al: Tubal insufflation and hysterosalpingography. Obstet Gynecol 18:91, 1961
24. Strathy JH, Molgaard CA, Coulam CB et al: Endometriosis and infertility: A laparoscopic study of endometriosis among fertile and infertile women. Fertil Steril 38:667, 1982
25. Swolin K, Gendz A, Larsson B et al: Traumatization of the abdominal serosa: A comparison between non-woven and cotton abdominal sponges. Acta Chir Scand 140:203, 1974

13

Carbon Dioxide Laser Laparoscopy

Gordon D. Davis
Dan C. Martin

Although Bruhat and colleagues[6] and Tadir and colleagues[42] published the first description of laparoscopic instruments that would effectively direct the laser beam, Daniell and Pittaway[12] first began laparoscopic use of the carbon dioxide (CO_2) laser in the United States. Operative laparoscopy using the CO_2 laser gained popularity as endoscopic use of the CO_2 laser beam was shown to be predictably feasible and safe.[32] Laparoscopic use of the CO_2 laser continues to expand; instrumentation allowing its use continues to evolve from the initial direct coupling of the articulating laser arm to the laparoscope, through a closed–tube micromanipulator, to a CO_2 laser wave guide.

Advantages of the Carbon Dioxide Laser

At power densities greater than 4750 watts/cm^2, the depth of coagulation created by the impact of the CO_2 laser beam may be limited to 0.1 to 0.4 mm for "what you see is what you get" vaporization. The power density may be decreased to 420 to 4750 watts/cm^2 for increased hemostasis with a coagulation of 0.2 to 0.7 mm.[43] Increased coagulation is useful for myomas but is generally undesirable for other pelvic pathology. Pulsed mode with manual control or a superpulsed mode can increase control while maintaining high power densities with decreased thermal effect.[32,43]

In contrast, coagulation with the argon, KTP, and Nd:YAG lasers is variable and determined by the intrinsic penetration of the laser, the time of exposure, the power density, and the tissue type. Although the maximal depth of coagulation of the argon and KTP lasers appears to be about 2 mm for endometriosis, the

Nd:YAG laser coagulates 1.0 to 4.4 mm when cutting liver with a non-contact fiber. But with high power densities, the argon, KTP, and Nd:YAG lasers are vaporizing lasers. Vaporizing with the Nd:YAG laser, using sapphire tips, decreases the lateral coagulation to 0.3 to 0.8 mm.[28] The equivalent depth of coagulation for the CO_2 laser is at 500 watts/cm^2 in continuous and repeat pulse modes.[43]

Lenses used in CO_2 laser surgery focus the collimated laser beam and allow surgeons a varied range of spot sizes. Small spot sizes (0.1 mm) create very high power densities. Lenses with a longer focal length and laparoscopic transmission interaction[32,41] produce spot sizes of 0.6 to 1.2 mm, with lower but sufficient power densities and an extended depth of field (Fig. 13–1).

Operative Laparoscopy

An average reduction of 49% in overall hospital costs has been observed when laparoscopic surgery has replaced open laparotomy.[29] However, laparoscopic operations may require increased operating time. Endurance and patience on the part of the surgeon are absolute requirements. Operating room personnel, as well as other surgeons on the hospital staff, must understand that operative laparoscopy can commonly require from 1 to 3 hours and uncommonly require 4 to 5 hours.

Three and four puncture laparoscopy sites are commonly used, although five punctures may be required. If second-puncture laser probes are used, they need to be placed low in the abdomen but high enough to allow access to retrouterine tissue. When placed higher in the abdomen, they may interfere with the laparoscope (so-called "clashing of swords"). Single-puncture laparoscopy has the advantage of directing the laser beam through the channel of the operating laparoscope. This advantage, however, may be negated by the need for higher power densities and backstop probes of the second-puncture delivery systems (Fig. 13–2).

Accessory instruments include a uterine cannula for manipulation of the uterus and transmission of dye, bipolar, or thermal coagulators for control of bleeding, and

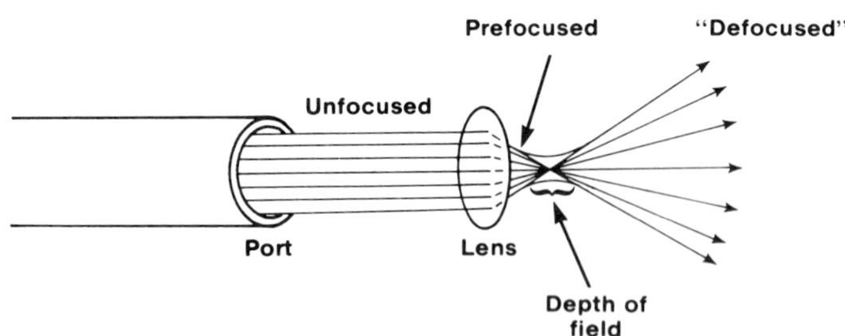

FIGURE 13–1. The CO_2 laser beam is focused to a theoretical focal point. In use, the spot size at the focal length is usually larger than predicted and is held over a longer length, which may be referred to as the depth of field. This depth of field increases with increasing focal length, with the use of complex lens systems for focusing, and on interaction with the laparoscopic barrel. (From Martin DC [ed]: Intra-abdominal Laser Surgery, 2nd ed. Memphis, Resurge Press, in preparation)

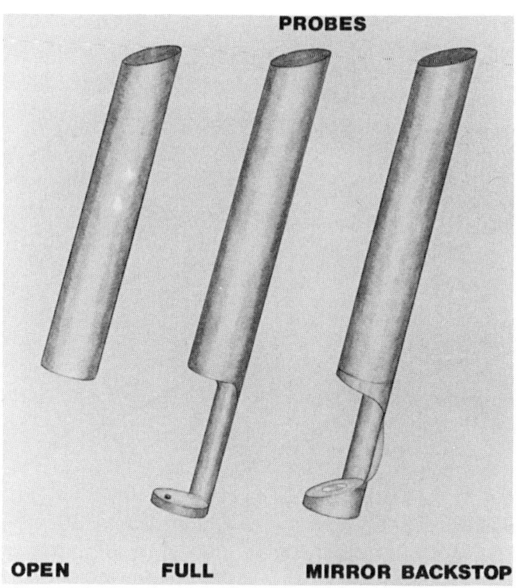

FIGURE 13–2. The second puncture probe for the CO$_2$ laser may have a backstop or mirror placed on it. The backstop probe is useful in lysing adhesions. Mirror backstops appear interesting but have not been clinically useful. (From Martin DC [ed]: Intra-abdominal Laser Surgery, 2nd ed. Memphis, Resurge Press, in preparation)

a lavage cannula for irrigation, suction, and dissection. Constant pressure, high flow, and recirculating insufflators are also required.

The articulating arm of the CO$_2$ laser is coupled to the operating laparoscope and fired on a moistened tongue blade to check for coaxial alignment of the helium-neon and CO$_2$ beams. The laser usually makes an impact spot on the testing field from 0.6 to 2.0 mm in diameter. An operator must adjust the power output for a comfortable power density.

Long operations produce considerable strain on a surgeon's musculoskeletal system. It is important to place the patient in a modified Trendelenburg position and have the operating table raised to the level of the surgeon's chest, minimizing the amount of time spent bending. Intermittent use of video monitors is preferred over relying solely on these devices for identification of endometriosis.

Safety

The cul-de-sac may be flooded with solution for peritoneal lavage and as a backstop for the laser beam. Great care is taken to keep all areas of adjacent tissue moist and all vital reproductive areas covered with fluid when the laser is used near them. When more than 20 to 80 ml is placed in the pelvis, some of the solution flows into the upper abdomen (Fig. 13–3). The fluid that accumulates in the upper abdomen can be

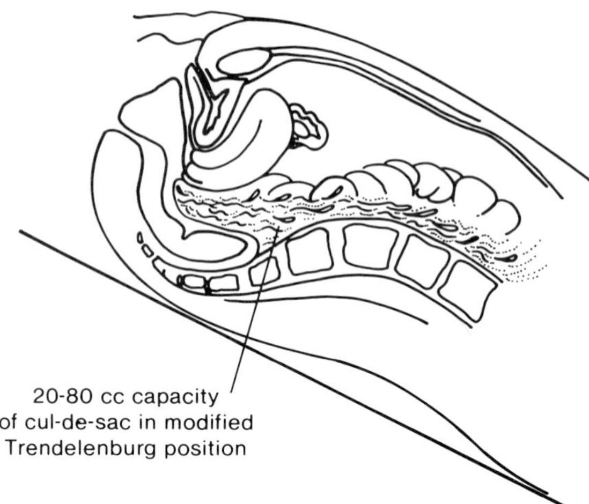

FIGURE 13–3. When more than 20 to 80 ml of solution is placed in the cul-de-sac, it spills into the upper abdomen. If an abscess or dermoid cyst is opened, the position must be reversed rapidly to avoid carrying this material into the upper abdomen. (From Martin DC [ed]: Intra-abdominal Laser Surgery, 2nd ed. Memphis, Resurge Press, in preparation)

removed at the end of the operation by reversing the patient's position, allowing the fluid to run down into the pelvis.

Prolonged operating time can also strain patients. Positioning the legs comfortably while the patient is awake, the use of leg padding, and allowing no one to apply pressure to the patient's thighs are precautions in decreasing the chance of leg injury or footdrop.

Suprapubic punctures should be performed by transillumination of the abdomen and direct visualization of the penetrating trocar. Punctures in the inguinal region should be directed medially to avoid the common iliac and other large vessels. Surface veins and penetrating musculofascial arteries may produce hematomas in the abdominal wall, and the inferior epigastric artery may bleed sufficiently to require a transfusion. If the artery is severed, coagulation generally controls bleeding, but a hemostatic suture may be required.

Patients who have had previous laparotomies are at increased risk for bladder or bowel damage at the time of trocar insertion. This hazard should be discussed with the patient preoperatively, and adequate preparations should be made. These may include surgical consultation, bowel preparation, and autologous blood donation. After catheterization, observation of the dome of the bladder while inserting the midline suprapubic trocar helps avoid trocar penetration.

Absorption or dispersion of the laser beam as it penetrates tissue during excision should be accomplished by using backstops. Proper control of the laser should take into consideration the path and intensity of the beam. Some second-puncture probes have a backstop that disperses the laser beam over a treated surface. Open second-puncture probes and single-puncture techniques require additional protection distal to the intended laser impact zone. Such backstops may include aqueous solutions or titanium or glass-beaded metal rods. In addition, tissue serves as its own backstop, such as the wall of a hydrosalpinx, the undersurface of penetrating endometriosis, or peritoneum lining the abdominal cavity.

Because the CO_2 beam itself is invisible, the coaxial helium–neon beam serves as the aiming beam. The laser should never be fired unless the helium–neon beam is adequately seen. Helium–neon beams may appear faint because of low power output of the helium–neon component of the surgical system, damaged halide laser lenses, or excessive laser plume. A less common but more dangerous cause is the presence of bowel in the intended pathway of the laser. When using second-puncture probes, particularly, a surgeon should view the intended impact site and the distal laser probe in the same viewing field. Again, do not activate the laser unless you can clearly see the helium–neon aiming beam!

The laser plume created during CO_2 laser laparoscopy is malodorous, and it may cause bronchitis, pneumonitis, and long-term health problems.[1,2,22,23,36,44] Venting the plume directly into the operating room creates a safety hazard. Therefore, proper evacuation intervals, adequate suction, appropriate filters, and external venting should be used to evacuate the plume so that it does not directly enter the operating room environment. Using higher power densities, superpulse mode, and excisional techniques, when possible, minimizes the amount of laser plume created and thus helps protect the operating room personnel and the patient.

ENDOMETRIOSIS

The lesions of endometriosis, which have a high water content, may be surrounded by a fibromuscular matrix clinically resembling neoplastic growth into soft tissue. They may be superficial or penetrating. The endometriotic implants may appear as cystic accumulations of blackish-brown blood surrounded by glands and stroma. Additionally, the condition may be associated with invaginations, infoldings, and puckering of the pelvic peritoneum. The characteristics of these lesions relate to the surface of the reproductive viscera as well as to the serosal surface of the uterus. The large or small bowel may be involved, and the lesions characteristically penetrate the musculature and often are associated with a dense fibromuscular matrix. The implants usually penetrate the peritoneum and remain confined to the areolar space just below the mesothelial surface. In these areas, lesions commonly appear as pleomorphic changes in the surface peritoneum.[27,40] These implants often appear to be within the peritoneum and, occasionally, only on the peritoneal surface. However, apparently superficial lesions may actually be the surface of deep penetrating lesions. Additionally, there may also be deep lesions, which may be found best by palpation, as well as lesions that are not usually recognized with current laparoscopic techniques.[32]

Surgeons should be careful to avoid traumatizing the peritoneum, as subperitoneal hemorrhage may mask endometriosis or be confused with endometriosis. Magnifying the peritoneum with near-contact laparoscopy may be useful to identify peritoneal lesions.[32,40] Examine all the tissue under the uterosacral ligaments, under both ovaries, and between the ovaries and fallopian tubes, as subtle lesions are easy to overlook in these regions.

Therapeutic Options

Nonsurgical Therapy

Hormonal suppression, analgesics, pain therapy, and other nonsurgical methods of managing endometriosis will not be discussed in this chapter. However, any treatment of endometriosis designed for an infertile patient requires a complete workup with treatment of all the other causes of infertility as well.[32] Pain management frequently requires a comprehensive approach, as endometriosis may not be the only cause of a patient's pain.

Vaporization

Using continuous or pulsed laser energy, endometriotic implants may be removed by vaporization to a depth at which no further pigment or scar is seen or until retroperitoneal fat is encountered. To ensure adequate vaporization of the implants, the surgical goal should be to destroy all identifiable lesions by creating a "punched-out" defect. When the CO_2 laser is used as a continuous wave at 10 to 30 watts with a spot size of 0.6 to 1.2 mm (power density of 900 to 11,000 watts/cm^2), a zone of thermal necrosis 0.2 to 0.8 mm in diameter[43] creates hemostasis sufficient to allow relatively bloodless vaporization of peritoneal and ovarian lesions. This zone of thermal injury, however, does not produce significant tissue blanching, which allows a surgeon to see the tissue at the floor and walls of the crater produced.

Frequently, however, a surgeon wishes to minimize the zone of thermal coagulation, particularly when dissecting endometriotic implants from the surface of the bowel, ovary, or fallopian tube or from peritoneum overlying the ureter or other vital structures. Cleaner vaporization can be produced with less char by using superpulse mode at 10 to 30 watts. The laser produces a peak power of 250 to 500 watts; with a 0.6- to 1.2-mm spot, the peak power density is 22,000 to 175,000 watts/cm^2 while the average power density is 900 to 11,000 watts/cm^2. The high peak power densities create a clean incision, whereas the low average power density slows the rapidity of vaporization, making the beam more controllable and allowing the tissue to cool. This mode is appropriate for cutting tissue while simultaneously sealing small capillaries, venules, arterioles, and lymphatics.

Excision

Adequate excision of penetrating endometriotic implants depends on proper recognition of the normal layers of pelvic anatomy. The implants should be grasped to tent the peritoneum so that small lesions may be undercut and excised. When larger peritoneal implants are encountered, the surgeon should identify an area of normal peritoneum, in order to place this area on traction and enter the retroperitoneal areolar space. A circumferential incision is usually needed in order to delineate the exact margins of the lesion before excision. Blunt dissection using traction and countertraction may also be helpful. Appropriate mobilization of the peritoneum allows adequate inspection of both sides of the endometriotic nodule. This technique permits delineation of the entire depth of penetration and lateral spread of each individual endometriotic implant. Direct visualization of the retroperitoneal space, using medial traction on the peritoneal surface, helps identify and avoid significant vessels, nerves, and the ureter as well. Implants near large vessels are more commonly coagulated with bipolar coagulation than vaporized because of the possibility of perforation of the vessels. Lesions near the ureter are usually excised or vaporized in order to avoid thermal damage. Peritoneal implants less than 5 mm in diameter are usually vaporized.

Since 1982, laser excision has been used more frequently to treat endometriosis. This technique was initiated when residual endometriosis was found in association with carbon from previous vaporization attempts.[32] The technique gained in popularity as a result of the increased recognition of all the endometrial lesions[33,40] and also because of the ability to excise larger and deeper lesions[31] (Fig. 13–4). Reperitonealization has not been used, as the excision of progressively larger areas did not result in an increase in postoperative adhesions, although adhesions may occur after any technique. This premise is consistent with other clinical observations that adhesions are usually caused by ischemic tissue rather than by healthy non-reperitonealized tissue.[3,4,13,15,16,17,34,38]

Pockets

Invaginations of the peritoneum have been reported in 4.6% of patients with pelvic pain and were pathologically positive for endometriosis in 68% of those patients.[7] The most common sites of pocket formation are the pararectal space, the uterosacral ligaments, and the broad ligaments. To excise the pocket, the base of the peritoneum is grasped, the pocket is everted, and the peritoneum is dissected free of the retroperitoneal areolar and fatty tissue. Alternatively, the pocket of peritoneum may be coagulated or vaporized. The rim of the pocket should also be excised or vaporized, as it is a frequent site of endometriosis as well.

Ovarian Lesions

Ovarian endometriosis may be superficial or deeply penetrating. Superficial lesions may be coagulated or vaporized (Fig. 13–5). The same power densities are used for vaporization of superficial ovarian endometriosis as are used for vaporization of peritoneal lesions. Keep in mind that ovarian surface endometriotic implants may appear as pleomorphic in color and texture as the peritoneal lesions. In addition, adhesions should be coagulated, vaporized, or excised because they frequently contain lesions.[27,40]

Penetrating endometriotic implants of the ovary are much more difficult to eradicate than penetrating implants of the peritoneum. The technical difficulty arises in developing a surgical plane by which a surgeon can completely ensure that all the lesions have been destroyed. The capsule of the implant may be thick and reddish and have irregular borders as the lesions invade the ovary. The technical approach by laser laparoscopy is similar to that performed at laparotomy. The ovary is incised in the thinnest portion of the capsule; the contents are evacuated by lavage; and the

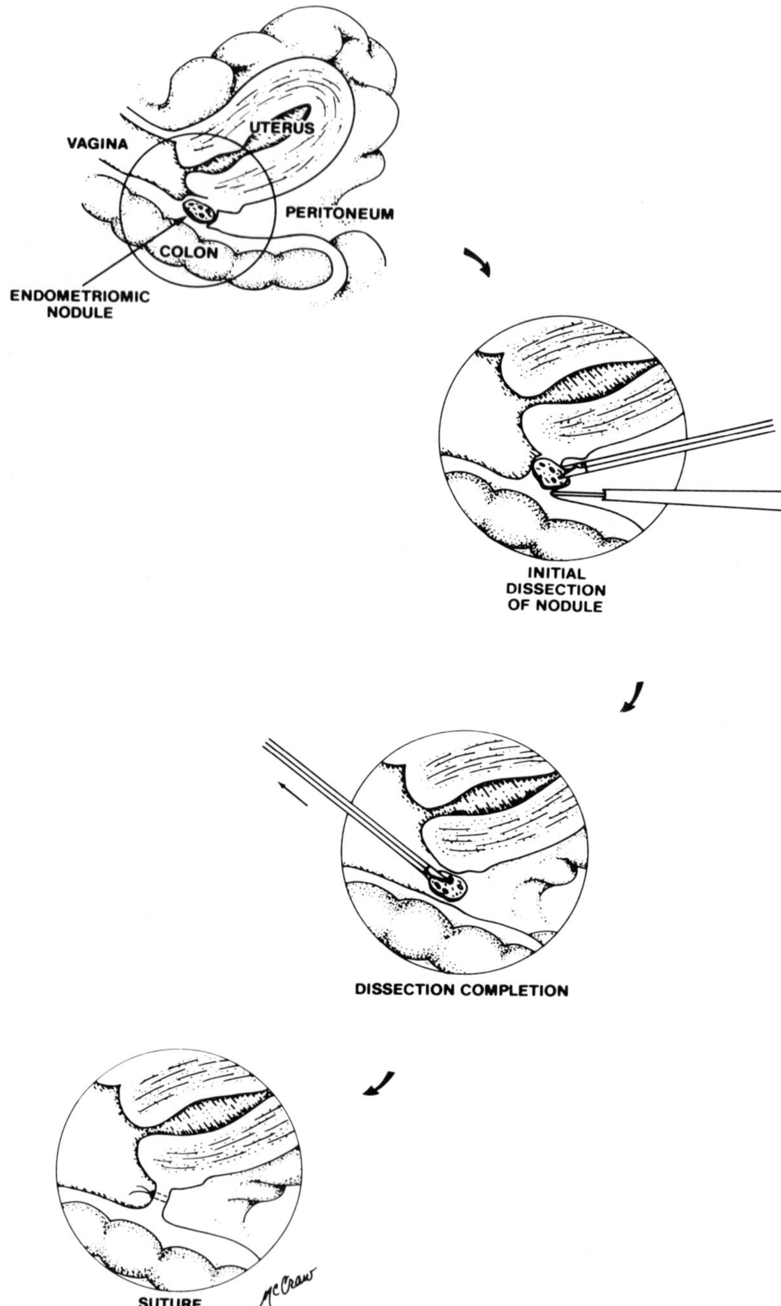

FIGURE 13–4. A vaginal colpotomy for infiltrating endometriosis is performed by cutting through healthy tissue on either side of the deep nodule. This incision is extended down to the level of the vagina. The vagina is entered, the lesion pulled through, and the colpotomy sutured. Vaginal and rectal probes help identify these areas. (From Martin DC: J Reprod Med 33:806, 1988)

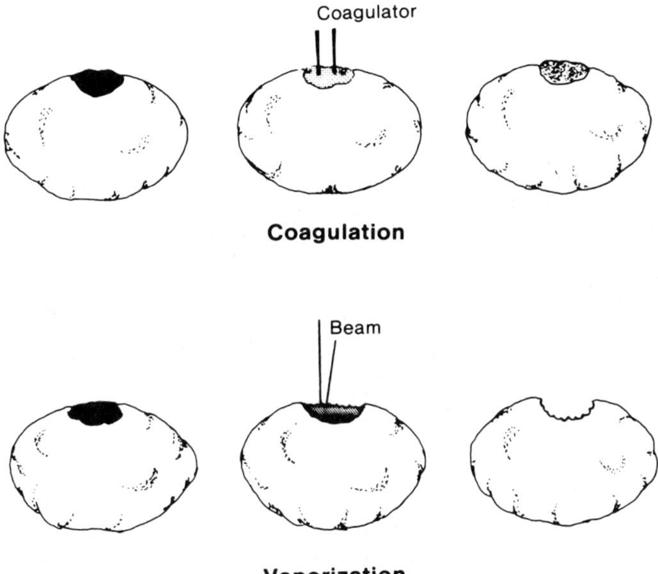

FIGURE 13–5. Both coagulation and vaporization are effective for superficial lesions. However, the depth of a lesion is frequently hard to determine until vaporization demonstrates the depth. Except for the most obvious superficial lesions, vaporization is preferred. (From Martin DC [ed]: Intra-abdominal Laser Surgery, 2nd ed. Memphis, Resurge Press, in preparation)

ovary is subsequently opened. If the capsule can be identified, it is stripped, peeled, and rolled away from normal ovarian cortex and stroma and removed *in toto* to ensure complete excision (Fig. 13–6). However, if fragmentation of the capsule occurs or if the ovarian cortex cannot be identified, the operator may not be sure that all of the endometriosis is removed from the ovary. Vaporization and coagulation of the base of the endometriotic capsule should complete the process, although such landmarks may be difficult to ascertain. Some laser laparoscopists leave the ovary open to heal without suture material,[32] whereas others place sutures to approximate the ovaries.[39]

Bowel Lesions

Endometriosis of the intestinal tract is generally not treated with the CO_2 laser at laparoscopy. Although superficial serosal implants on bowel can be safely treated by pulsed vaporization, these seemingly superficial implants are often the surface of deep palpable nodules.[39,44] When there is pain or other clinical indication for bowel surgery, these lesions are usually removed at laparotomy after general surgery consult and bowel preparation.

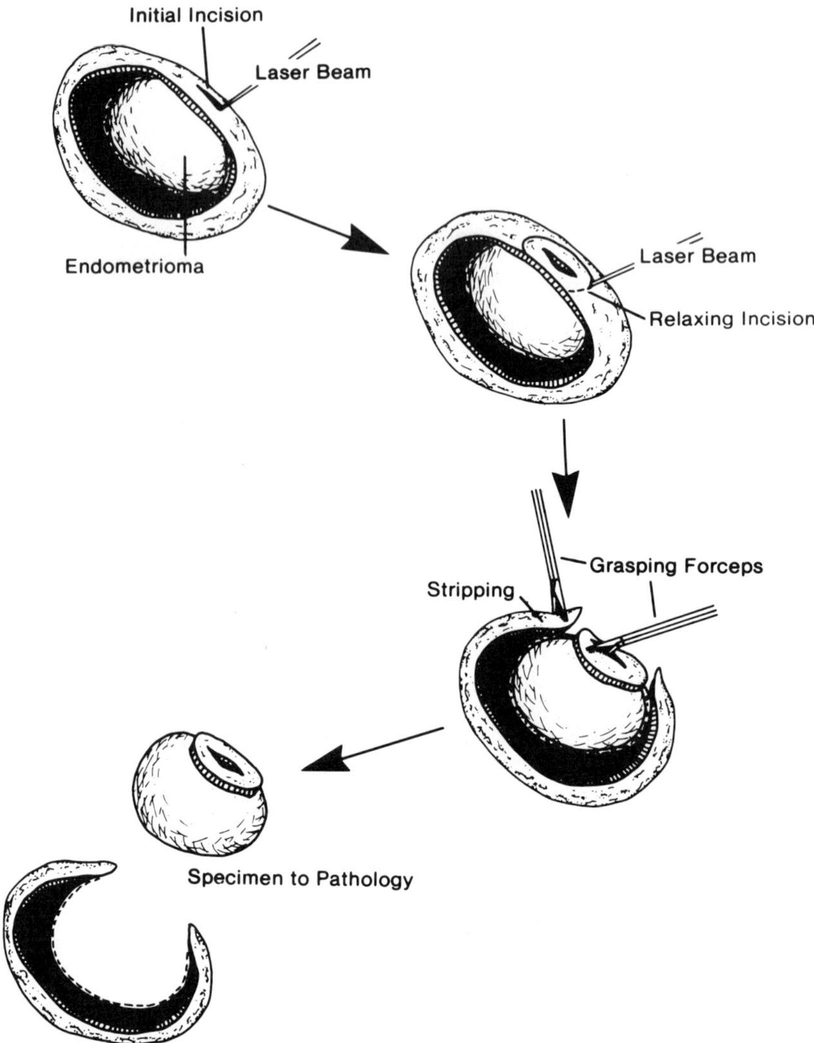

FIGURE 13–6. After an ovarian endometrioma is opened and drained, a relaxing incision is made so that grasping forceps can be placed on a healthy rim of tissue. A second set of forceps is placed on the remnant ovary, and tension is used to develop a plane of dissection. Pressure is slowly applied to strip the wall of the endometrioma out of the ovary. The entire wall is then sent to pathology. Histologic examination is needed to confirm endometriosis. (From Martin DC [ed]: Intra-abdominal Laser Surgery, 2nd ed. Memphis, Resurge Press, in preparation)

Postoperative Pregnancy Rates

After laser treatment of endometriosis, the pregnancy rates for eight reported series containing a total of 841 patients were 58% in minimal, 51% in moderate, and 52% in patients with severe endometriosis.[32] The overall pregnancy rate was 55%. When these data were analyzed and endometriosis was the only identifiable factor, the overall pregnancy rate was 69%. Olive and Martin[37] used life table analysis and compared these data with other reported series. They concluded that the pregnancy rates after laser treatment for mild and moderate disease were equal to those in other studies, and for advanced disease were comparable to or better than other techniques reported. Although the overall cure rate appeared equivalent to that achieved by laparotomy, patients conceived more rapidly.

ADHESIOLYSIS

Gomel's reported 57% pregnancy rate following laparoscopic lysis using electrical coagulation and scissors[25] has been compared with similar pregnancy rates following laser adhesiolysis.[10,11,19,20,32] For many adhesions, scissors and coagulation are adequate. However, for dense adhesions, the laser has been superior to bipolar cautery for developing planes in delicate areas. Using the CO_2 laser, one may safely dissect the fallopian tube from the ovary or the adnexae from the ureter if dense adhesions are present. Saline may occasionally be injected beneath the peritoneum overlying vital structures to enhance safety, as the fluid stops the CO_2 laser's energy before it damages the ureter or underlying blood vessels. Paraovarian or peritubal adhesions may be coagulated, excised, or vaporized. A backstop is usually used for incising pelvic adhesions, although adhesions may be placed on end for laser ablation, and thus the adhesion becomes its own backstop. It is usually preferable to excise the entire adhesion whenever possible. For salpingolysis, the fallopian tube is placed on traction. Higher power densities using 25 to 30 watts of superpulse are often needed to dissect the tube away from its attachment with a minimum of char. If the fallopian tube adheres to the peritoneum, it is sometimes easier to place the peritoneum on traction to free the peritoneal margin and then remove the peritoneum from the fallopian tube.

Ovariolysis may be facilitated by applying traction or torsion to the utero-ovarian ligament with grasping forceps. The ovary should be elevated and rotated medially while laser pulses lyse the adhesions that hold the ovary to the pelvic sidewall. A titanium rod or an ebonized or glass-beaded probe may be inserted behind the adhesions to serve as a laser backstop. If the ovary is encased in adhesions but not densely adhered to the pelvic sidewall, an incision is made into the superficial adhesions to produce a defect through which Ringer's solution may be injected. The adhesions may then be vaporized, although attempts should be made to excise the adhesions, as many may contain endometriotic implants.[27] If densely adherent to the pelvic sidewall, the ovary may be approached through a retroperitoneal dissection that is started by incising the superior peritoneum between the round ligament and infundibulopelvic ligaments. The round ligaments and infundibulopelvic ligaments are placed under tension, and a blunt probe or an irrigation cannula is inserted into the retroperitoneal space. Dissection with the blunt probe or by the irrigation cannula with or without flowing irrigant should help identify the ureter and allow laser incision of the peritoneum superior to the ureter but inferior to the ovary. Thus, to prevent ureteral damage, a retroperitoneal approach is advised when the adnexa is densely adherent.

SALPINGOSTOMY

In 1977, Gomel reported the technique of laparoscopic cuff salpingostomy using scissors and unipolar cautery.[26] The resulting intrauterine pregnancy rate was 44%. Fayez[18] used a similar technique and found a 10% tubal pregnancy rate with no intrauterine pregnancies. The earliest reports of the use of the CO_2 laser to perform laparoscopic salpingostomies were by Daniell.[8,9] He noted an 18% intrauterine pregnancy rate following a laparoscopic cuff salpingostomy technique. His basic technique was similar to that described by Bruhat[5] (Fig. 13–7). Following transcervical hydrotubation, Daniell used high power densities of 4,000 to 12,000 watts/cm^2

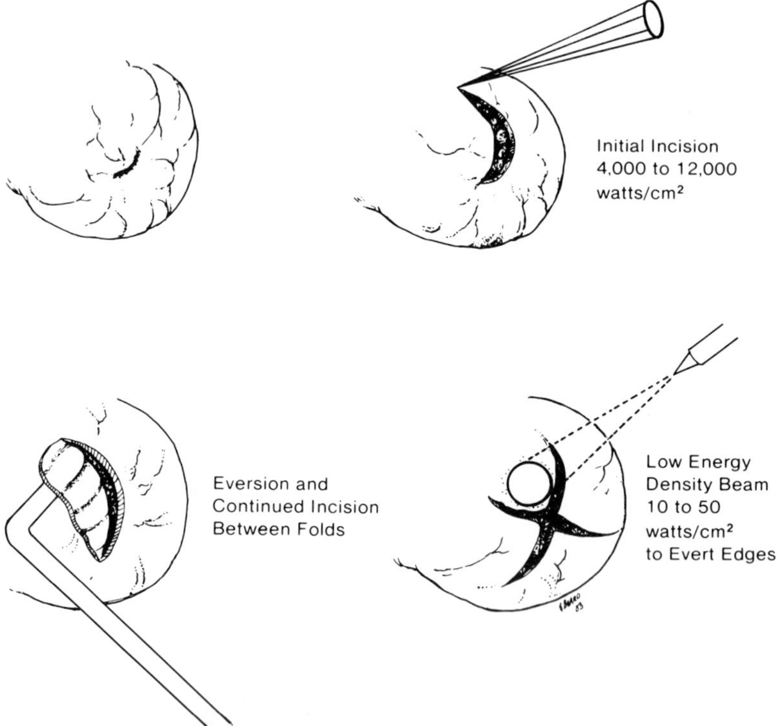

FIGURE 13–7. The Bruhat maneuver of distal cuff salpingostomy uses high power density radial and linear incisions to open the tube. Subsequent low power density surface coagulation of the tubal serosa everts the edges. (From Martin DC, Absten GT, Levinson CJ et al [eds]: Intra-Abdominal Laser Surgery. Memphis, Resurge Press, 1986)

to make an initial incision into the tube. The incision was then carried along avascular lines in radial and linear fashions to complete the opening of the tube. With the tube open, a beam of 10 to 200 watts/cm^2 was used along the external serosal surfaces to contract the serosa and evert the tube, exposing the endosalpinx. The contracture that is produced is soft and tends to relax over time. Tubal patency with minimal or no scarring has generally been observed at second-look laparoscopy.

ECTOPIC PREGNANCY

Conservative surgery for ectopic pregnancy may be performed using any of several techniques, such as lasers, unipolar or bipolar cautery, or sharp dissection with scissors. Before undertaking a laser laparoscopic linear salpingostomy, a gynecological surgeon should feel comfortable performing a laparoscopic salpingectomy using conventional pelviscopic surgical techniques. Most early unruptured tubal pregnancies can be diagnosed 23 to 27 days after ovulation. A high index of suspicion coupled with judicious use of quantitative beta-human chorionic gonadotropin (HCG) titers and vaginal ultrasonography should help gynecologists select those cases that can usually be managed conservatively. The technique consists of injecting dilute vasopressin (10 units/30 cc) by a spinal needle placed transabdominally, into the tubal portion containing the ectopic. The CO$_2$ laser is fired, using 20 to 30 watts superpulse through a single- or double-puncture probe, to the tubal area containing the ectopic. The ectopic is then shelled out using the grasping forceps. Hemostasis may be ensured by unipolar or bipolar cautery. The defect is usually left open. The patient should be admitted overnight to observe for delayed hemorrhage. Serial quantitative beta-HCG titers should be monitored to rule out a persistent ectopic. These complications may occur whether the procedure is performed at laparoscopy or laparotomy.[32]

MYOMAS

When myomectomies are performed through the CO$_2$ laser laparoscope, the myomas should be pedunculated. Bleeding from the pedicle base may occasionally be extensive, and unipolar or bipolar cautery may be needed. The power density should be low (400 to 800 watts/cm^2) in order to increase the thermal coagulation, resulting in improved hemostasis.

POLYCYSTIC OVARIAN DISEASE

Laparoscopic aspiration and drainage of microcystic follicles in polycystic ovarian disease have been previously reviewed.[24,32] Drainage of the microcysts produces ovulation and a decrease in androgen similar to that following a wedge resection, but the results appear to last only 12 to 24 months. It is also possible to perform a laparoscopic wedge resection using the CO$_2$ laser, although deep hemostasis with unipolar or bipolar cautery is sometimes necessary. The small number of second-look laparoscopies performed suggests that adhesion formation is less than that noted after previous microsurgical closures of wedge resections. Either technique appears to produce fewer adhesions than 3-0 chromic or 4-0 Vicryl ovarian closures following wedge resection.[35]

UTEROSACRAL TRANSECTION

Transection of the uterosacral ligament using the CO_2 laser laparoscope is similar to the paracervical denervation reported by Doyle.[14] Satisfactory pain relief in up to 70% of patients with dysmenorrhea has been reported following use of the CO_2 laser[11,19–21] or scissors and coagulation (LUNA).[30] The superior portion of the uterosacral ligament as it inserts into the uterus is vaporized using 20 to 25 watts superpulse to the level of the vagina. This junction may be easily identified by placing a sponge in a ring forceps into the vagina and displacing the uterus anteriorly up toward the operating field in order to better visualize attenuated ligaments. Identify the ureter before lasing, and apply the laser's energy medially to avoid bleeding from the blood vessel that is commonly found laterally. Should bleeding occur, unipolar cautery usually controls it more rapidly than bipolar cautery.

SUMMARY

CO_2 laser laparoscopy offers an excellent new technique for vaporizing or excising endometriosis with considerably less morbidity and cost than by laparotomy. The magnification possible with the laparoscope and the predictable precision of the CO_2 laser beam make this modality excellent for the treatment of even moderate to severe endometriosis. Excision of endometriosis provides histologic documentation and allows more complete removal of penetrating disease, although vaporization is easier and is satisfactory for superficial disease. Note: What appears to be superficial may only be the tip of the iceberg of the lesion, which may only be determined by complete dissection.[39,45] For other pelvic pathology, CO_2 laser laparoscopy has been shown to be precise and predictable. Treatment of adhesions, small fibroids, polycystic ovarian disease, and unruptured ectopic pregnancies by this new modality appears to be cost-effective and, with further studies, perhaps the treatment of choice.

REFERENCES

1. Baggish MS, Baltoyannis P, Sze E: Protection of the rat lung from the harmful effects of laser smoke. Lasers Surg Med 8:248, 1988.
2. Baggish MS, ElBakry M: The effect of laser smoke on the lungs of rats. Am J Obstet Gynecol 156:1260, 1987
3. Batt RE, Naples JD: Microsurgery for endometriosis and infertility. In Hunt RB: Atlas of Female Infertility Surgery, pp 336–364. Chicago, Year Book Medical Publishers, 1986
4. Bellina JH, Hemmings R, Voros JI et al: Carbon dioxide laser in electrosurgical wound study with an animal model: Comparison of tissue damage and healing patterns in peritoneal tissue. Am J Obstet Gynecol 148:327, 1984
5. Bruhat M: Tubal surgery techniques. Presented at Applications of Carbon Dioxide Lasers in Reproductive Biology, New Orleans, Louisiana, 1981

6. Bruhat MA, Mage G, Manhes M: Use of the CO_2 laser by laparoscopy. In Kaplan I (ed): Proceedings of the Third International Congress for Laser Surgery, pp 274–276, Tel Aviv, Israel, Ot-Paz, 1979
7. Chatman DL: Pelvic peritoneal defects and endometriosis: Alan-Masters syndrome revisited. Fertil Steril 36:751, 1981
8. Daniell JF: Laparoscopic salpingostomy: Early clinical results. Lasers Surg Med 3:161, 1983
9. Daniell JF: Laparoscopic salpingostomy utilizing the CO_2 laser. Fertil Steril 41:558, 1983
10. Daniell JF: Laser laparoscopy. In Baggish MS (ed): Basic and Advanced Laser Laparoscopy in Gynecology, pp 343–356. Norwalk, Appleton-Century Crofts, 1985
11. Daniell JF, Feste JR: Laser laparoscopy. In Keye WR (ed): Laser Surgery in Gynecology and Obstetrics, pp 147–164. Boston, GK Hall Publishers, 1985
12. Daniell JF, Pittaway DE: Use of the CO_2 laser laparoscope in laparoscopic surgery: Initial experience with the second puncture technique. Infertility 5:15, 1982
13. Diamond MP, DeCherney AH: Pathogenesis of adhesion formation/reformation: Application to reproductive pelvic surgery. Microsurgery 8:103, 1987
14. Doyle JB: Paracervical uterine denervation by transection of the cervical plexus for the relief of dysmenorrhea. Am J Obstet Gynecol 70:1, 1955
15. Elkins TE, Stovall TG, Warren J et al: A histologic evaluation of peritoneal injury and repair: Implications for adhesion formation. Obstet Gynecol 70:225, 1987
16. Ellis H: The aetiology of post-operative abdominal adhesions: An experimental study. Br J Surg 50:10, 1962
17. Ellis H: Internal overhealing: The problem of intraperitoneal adhesions. World J Surg 4:303, 1980
18. Fayez Y: Assessment of the role of operative laparoscopy in tuboplasty. Fertil Steril 39:476, 1983
19. Feste JR: Laser laparoscopy: A new modality. Lasers Surg Med 3:170, 1983
20. Feste JR: Endoscopic laser surgery in gynecology. In Reproductive Surgery. Postgraduate Course Syllabus, pp 51–69. American Fertility Society, Chicago, Illinois 1985
21. Feste JR: Laser Laparoscopy, a new modality. J Reprod Med 30:413, 1985
22. Feste JR, Lloyd JM: A new valving system for removal of laser plume during pelvic CO_2 laser endoscopic procedures. Obstet Gynecol 69:669, 1987
23. Garden JM, O'Banion K, Shelnitz LS et al: Papilloma virus in the vapor of carbon dioxide laser-treated verrucae. JAMA 259:1199, 1988
24. Givens JR et al (eds): The Infertile Female, pp 272–292. Chicago, Year Book Medical Publishers, 1979
25. Gomel V: In Phillips JM (ed): Fertility Surgery in Laparoscopy, pp 212–218. Baltimore, Williams and Wilkins, 1977
26. Gomel V: Salpingostomy by laparoscopy. J Reprod Med 18:265, 1977
27. Jansen RPS, Russell P: Nonpigmented endometriosis: Clinical, laparoscopic, and pathologic definition. Am J Obstet Gynecol 155:1154, 1986
28. Joffe SN, Schroder T: Lasers in general surgery. Adv Surg 20:125, 1987
29. Levine RL: Economic impact of pelviscopic surgery. J Reprod Med 30:655, 1985
30. Lichten EM, Bombard J: Surgical treatment of primary dysmenorrhea with laparoscopic uterine nerve ablation. J Reprod Med 32:37, 1987
31. Martin DC: Laparoscopic and vaginal colpotomy for the excision of infiltrating cul-de-sac endometriosis. J Reprod Med 33:806, 1988
32. Martin DC, Diamond MP: Operative laparoscopy: Comparison of lasers with other techniques. Cur Probl Obstet Gynecol Fertil 9:563, 1986
33. Martin DC, Vander Zwaag R: Excisional techniques with the CO_2 laser laparoscope. J Reprod Med 32:753, 1987
34. McDonald MN, Elkins TE, Wortham GF et al: Adhesion formation and prevention following peritoneal injury and repair in the rabbit. J Reprod Med 33:436, 1988
35. McLaughlin DS: Evaluation of adhesion reformation by early second-look laparoscopy following microlaser wedge resection. Fertil Steril 42:531, 1984
36. Nezhat C, Winer WK, Nezhat F et al: Smoke from laser surgery: Is there a health hazard? Lasers Surg Med 7:376, 1987
37. Olive DL, Martin DC: Treatment of endometriosis-associated infertility with CO_2 laser laparoscopy: The use of one- and two-parameter exponential models. Fertil Steril 48:18, 1987
38. Semm K: Instruments and equipment for endoscopic abdominal surgery. In Semm K, Friedrich ER (eds): Operative Manual for Endoscopic Abdominal Surgery, p 94. Chicago, Year Book Medical Publishers, 1987
39. Semm K: Course of endoscopic abdominal surgery. In Semm K, Friedrich ER (eds): Operative Manual for Endoscopic Abdominal Surgery, pp 130–213. Chicago, Year Book Medical Publishers, 1987

40. Stripling MC, Martin DC, Chatman DL et al: Subtle appearance of pelvic endometriosis. Fertil Steril 49:427, 1988
41. Tadir Y, Kaplan I, Zuckerman Z et al: Actual effective CO_2 laser power on tissue in endoscopic surgery. Fertil Steril 45:492, 1986
42. Tadir Y, Ovadia J, Zuckerman Z et al: Laparoscopic applications of the CO_2 laser. In Atsumi K, Nimsakul N (eds): Proceedings of the Fourth Congress of the International Society for Laser Surgery, Vol 2, pp 25–26. Japanese Society for Laser Medicine, Tokyo, 1981
43. Taylor MV, Martin DC, Poston WM et al: Effect of power density and carbonization on residual tissue coagulation using the continuous wave carbon dioxide laser. Colpos Gynecol Laser Surg 2:169, 1986
44. Tomita Y, Michashi S, Nagata K et al: Mutagenicity of smoke condensates induced by CO_2 laser irradiation and electrocauterization. Mutat Res 189:145, 1981
45. Weed JC, Ray JE: Endometriosis of the bowel. Obstet Gynecol 69:727, 1987

14

Argon Laser Laparoscopy

William R. Keye, Jr.

During the past 10 years, lasers have become extremely popular in nearly every surgical discipline. To gynecologists, lasers offer the opportunity to dissect or ablate tissue with greater control and precision than ever before. However, the hope that this precision and control would lead to dramatically better clinical results has not yet been realized. As a result, skeptics and critics alike have labeled the laser as nothing more than a very expensive bovie. Indeed, lasers currently used in gynecology coagulate and cut tissue through the heating of tissue, much like electrocautery. Consequently, the results of laser surgery are not so much the result of any inherent properties of the laser but are dependent on the precision with which a surgeon directs the beam of laser light. It has even been claimed that a laser can make a good surgeon better and a bad surgeon worse.

However, the argon laser, the gold vapor laser, and the copper vapor laser, among others, are more than just tools for cutting, dependent on the photothermal effects of laser light. They have the ability to destroy pathologic tissue through photochemical or photothermal effect of laser light that depends on the color or chemical composition of tissue. As a result, they have the ability to destroy pathologic tissue selectively, thus decreasing the need for a surgeon to be precise in aiming the laser light.

Recognizing the principle of selective absorption of laser light by some tissues more than others, the author investigated the use of the argon laser in the treatment of endometriosis. Theoretically, the argon laser was an ideal laser for the treatment of this disease because the wavelengths of light generated by the argon laser (488 and 514.5 nm) are preferentially absorbed by red pigments such as hemoglobin and hemosiderin, both of which are present in abundant amounts in most endometriotic lesions. Fortunately, this has proved to be one of those rare situations in which the practical application has been as good as the theory.

INSTRUMENTATION

The argon laser currently approved for marketing by the Food and Drug Administration (FDA) for gynecological procedures is manufactured by HGM Medical Laser Products, Inc., in Salt Lake City, Utah. The laser is available with a maximum output of 5 watts (Model 8) or 16 watts (Model 20). Model 8 is 16 1/4 × 8 × 31.5 inches, weighs 120 pounds, is water cooled, and requires a 208-volt, 45-ampere, single-phase power source. Model 20 is larger (16 1/4 × 8 × 40 inches) and is also water cooled, requiring a 208-volt, 60-ampere, three-phase power source identical to that required by many Nd : YAG lasers. Model 20 is generally favored by most gynecologists because it is more powerful, making it possible to vaporize the uterosacral ligaments and lyse thick adhesions more quickly and therefore more safely than with the lower-powered model.

The energy of the argon laser is delivered through a flexible optical fiber either 300 or 600 micrometers in diameter. This fiber is extremely efficient and delivers to the tissue more than 85% of the output of power transferred by the laser tube. The fiber is composed of a central core of quartz surrounded by Teflon cladding. It is reusable and can be sterilized by gas or liquid agents. The fiber easily passes down the operating channel of any unmodified single-puncture operating laparoscope, an operative hysteroscope sheath, or any of several accessory suprapubic hollow probes. It may also be delivered through a directional single-puncture laser laparoscope (Figs. 14–1 through 14–4). The fiber is extremely durable and can be bent into a small circle without breaking.

Protective goggles or eye wear is essential when using the argon laser. The lens of the eye wear filters out 99% of the light within the visible spectrum from 488 to 514.5 nm. All medical personnel and the patient must wear protective goggles or glasses while the laser is in use, and all windows must be covered with blinds or

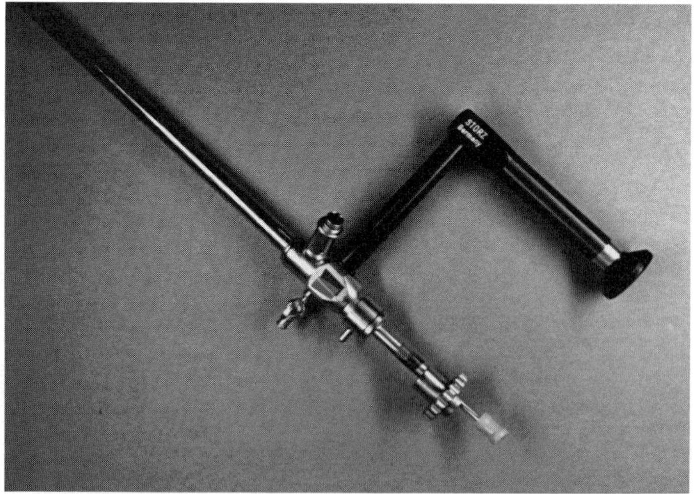

FIGURE 14–1. Storz single-puncture laser laparoscope with an argon fiber holder.

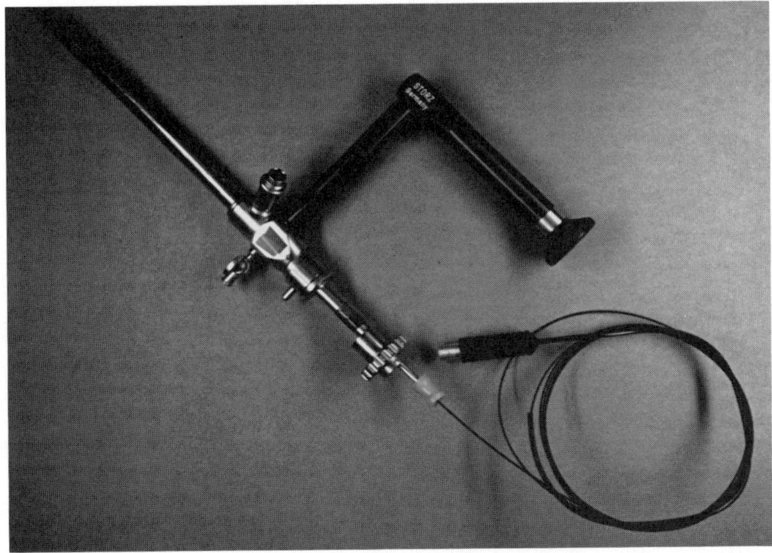

FIGURE 14–2. Argon laparoscope with 600-micrometer quartz fiber.

other opaque coverings. The operator may choose either to wear this protective eye wear or to cover the eyepiece of the laparoscope with a "Monoshutter." A Monoshutter is an electronically triggered device that interposes a protective filter between the operator and the laparoscope only when the laser is in use. The eyepiece of this Monoshutter is designed to fit most standard CCD endoscopic cameras, which permit video documentation.

The laser is triggered by a foot pedal with a protective covering that eliminates the accidental depression of the pedal by an assistant or by other operating room personnel.

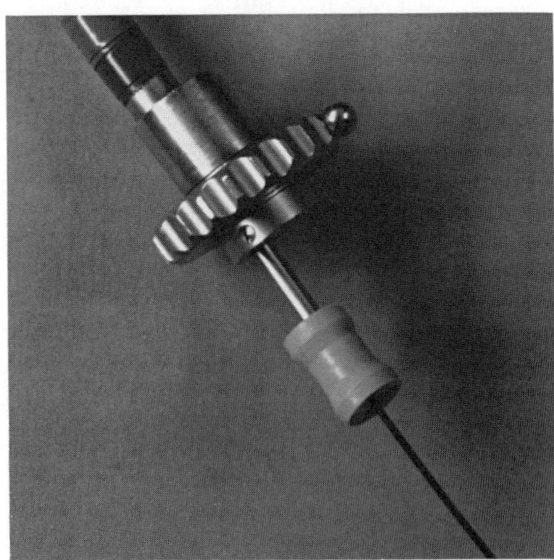

FIGURE 14–3. Adjustable hand piece to direct the laser fiber.

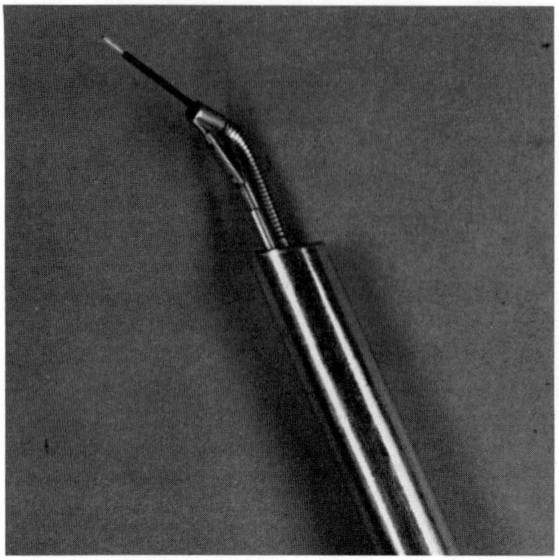

FIGURE 14–4. Tip of argon fiber as seen in a flexible laparoscope that can be used to deliver laser energy to relatively inaccessible areas.

RESULTS OF CLINICAL TRIALS

After a series of animal studies in which they demonstrated the efficacy and safety of the argon laser to treat experimental endometriosis, Keye and his colleagues[4] began clinical trials with the argon laser for the treatment of endometriosis in humans. Initially, five women received treatment for 31 superficial implants of endometriosis on the uterosacral ligaments, ovaries, fallopian tubes, bladder, and sigmoid; they experienced no complication.[2] Using Model 8, the researchers coagulated each implant with a no-touch technique. This technique involved advancing the fiber through the operating channel of the scope until it emerged into the abdomen and was within 1 to 5 mm from the implant. The aiming beam was directed at each implant, and the laser was set at 2 watts of power and fired until the implants were totally blanched and thus coagulated.

Two years later, in 1985, Keye and colleagues[5] reported performing adhesiolysis and excision of endometriosis or adhesions as well as vaporization or coagulation of endometriotic implants using a contact or touch technique in which the tip of the fiber actually contacted the tissue. They used 5.5 watts of energy and were able to prepare the pelvis for laparoscopic oocyte collection safely and effectively for *in vitro* fertilization. They reported their experience with 92 consecutive patients who were studied prospectively.[3] Each subject was observed for 6 to 36 months and evaluated for conception and reduction of pain. Sixty-seven percent had already failed to conceive after other therapies. All had additional infertility factors (average of 2.5) and had experienced long-standing infertility (average of 4.8 years). Nineteen of 56 (34%) of those with infertility became pregnant (average monthly fecundity rate of 2.5%). Nearly two thirds (64%) conceived within 6 months of therapy. Among a small group of women with infertility of less than 24 months, 63% conceived. These results compare favorably with life table analyses of other treatment modalities.

The most dramatic finding was the reduction of pain (dysmenorrhea, dyspareunia, and other pelvic pain) that occurred in 92% of the 50 women who had complained of preoperative pelvic pain. Similar results have now been achieved in nearly 600 patients treated between 1982 and 1988. Other investigators have reported similar findings.[1]

SURGICAL TECHNIQUES

Destruction of Superficial Implants

Implants overlying the uterus, fallopian tubes, ovaries, rectosigmoid, bladder, ureters, broad ligaments, and uterosacral ligaments can be safely treated with the argon laser. Individual implants can be coagulated or vaporized. For lesions overlying a hollow viscus or large vessel, coagulation is preferred. Experiments on animals have demonstrated that the pigment in the implant efficiently absorbs the energy of the argon laser and therefore "buffers" the underlying tissue from the thermal effect of the laser. In studies of rabbits in which concentrated hemoglobin was injected just below the serosa, the hemoglobin reduced the depth of thermal damage of normal tissues by approximately 50%. Thus, implants over the ureter, bladder, fallopian tube, rectosigmoid, and major vessels within the broad ligament can be completely coagulated without clinically significant damage to underlying structures. For this reason and the selective absorption of the argon laser light by the hemoglobin and hemosiderin within the implant, the argon laser is an extremely safe laser. The chance of acutely perforating a viscus is extremely low. In nearly 600 cases, Keye and his colleagues have not perforated a viscus with the argon laser.

To coagulate implants, the 600-micrometer fiber is delivered into the pelvic cavity through either the operating channel of a single-puncture laparoscope or the channel of any of a number of suprapubic probes used for smoke evacuation or irrigation. The fiber is advanced until it is within 2 to 5 mm of the lesion. Although the aiming beam aids in directing the fiber, the fact that the fiber is almost in contact with the lesion renders the use of the aiming beam unnecessary in the majority of cases. The laser power is set on 5 to 8 watts and in the continuous mode. Using a foot pedal, the laser is activated and the argon energy delivered to the implant until it either becomes extremely pale, as in the case of lightly pigmented lesions, or the hemoglobin turns black, resembling carbon. The operator turns the laser beam off by lifting his or her foot from the pedal and then moves on to the next implant.

In the case of implants of the uterosacral ligaments, nodules of endometriosis or non-pigmented endometriosis, vaporization of the implant is preferred. Vaporization is accomplished by touching the tip of the 600-micrometer fiber to the implant and adjusting the power setting to 5 to 12 watts in the continuous mode. The foot pedal is activated, and the implant is vaporized until it completely disappears and normal subserosal tissue is seen. The operator lifts his or her foot off the foot pedal and turns the laser beam off.

DESTRUCTION OF OVARIAN ENDOMETRIOMAS

The subject of treating ovarian endometriomas is very controversial. Some investigators believe there is no place for the laparoscopic drainage of any ovarian cyst other than small follicular cysts. They argue that a laparoscopist cannot always predict the histology of the cyst by its outward and gross appearance and that spilling the contents of mucinous cystadenomas, benign cystic teratomas, or cystic epithelial carcinomas is not only unwise but potentially fraught with long-term complications. Others believe that appropriate treatment requires only simple drainage of ovarian endometriomas. Yet others believe it is not only safe but effective to remove or destroy the cyst wall of an ovarian endometrioma.

Keye and colleagues follow a conservative approach by limiting the laparoscopic drainage of ovarian cysts to those no greater than 4 to 5 cm. All others are removed intact at laparotomy. When approaching an endometrioma laparoscopically, the goal is to drain the old blood, which often reduces pelvic pain, and to prevent its recurrence. Therefore, the quartz fiber is advanced until its tip touches the ovarian capsule overlying the thinnest part of the endometrioma. Using 10 to 15 watts of energy from the argon laser, a linear incision is made in the ovarian capsule and ovarian cyst wall. The bloody contents are then evacuated, and the cyst is irrigated with heparinized lactated Ringer's solution and biopsied or removed. By using one or two forceps introduced into the pelvis through suprapubic sites, the edges of small cysts are held open and the fiber directed into the cyst. Then, using 5 to 10 watts of argon laser energy, the inside of the cyst is coagulated or vaporized until it is completely destroyed. The cyst is then irrigated, and the debris is suctioned from the cyst and pelvic cavity. The cyst does not bleed when this technique is used and is left open to heal secondarily.

Brosens* recently described a new and novel technique with the argon laser and "ovarioscopy." Having identified an ovarian endometrioma, he passes the quartz fiber down through the operating channel of a single-puncture laparoscope. He then vaporizes a small defect in the ovarian capsule overlying the endometrioma but avoids incising the wall of the cyst. He then removes the fiber from the laparoscope and replaces it with a salpingoscope modified to include an operating channel. He punctures the cyst wall with the salpingoscope and irrigates the dark, old blood from within the cyst. The internal features of the cyst are then visualized by distending the endometrioma with normal saline or lactated Ringer's solution, and the quartz fiber is advanced into the cyst and through the operating channel of the salpingoscope. He then coagulates and vaporizes the cyst wall under direct vision and coagulates any small veins present at the base of the endometrioma. He then removes the salpingoscope from the endometrioma and is left with only a small puncture wound that is several millimeters in diameter. Long-term follow-up is not yet available to demonstrate the superiority of this technique over those just described. Nevertheless, it does have the theoretical advantage of a reduced rate of recurrence and fewer postoperative adhesions.

Adhesiolysis

The introduction of an argon laser capable of delivering between 14 and 16 watts of energy has facilitated adhesiolysis with this wavelength. In addition, the availability of a 300-micrometer fiber and 600 micrometer fibers with 100 micrometer tips has made it possible to obtain very small spot sizes and high power densities. Most

---

* *Personal communication.*

pelvic adhesions thus may be efficiently removed or incised with the argon laser. The advantage of this system over that of the carbon dioxide (CO_2) laser is the reduction in smoke created when vaporizing with the argon laser and a touch technique.

The principles of adhesiolysis are similar to those used with other modalities. The adhesion is isolated, placed under traction, and either incised or excised. The advantage of the argon laser flexible fiberoptic system over currently available CO_2 laser systems is the decreased need for a backstop behind the adhesion. The diverging beam of the argon laser loses its power density rapidly from the tip of the fiber, so that structures more than 1 to 2 cm past the fiber tip are generally spared from significant thermal damage.

The laser is activated just before or at the moment the fiber touches the adhesion, and the fiber is drawn across the adhesion while maintaining direct contact between the fiber tip and the adhesion. Once the adhesion is incised, the laser is turned off. If the laser is turned off while the fiber is still in contact with the tissue, the tissue often sticks to the tip and increases the chance that the fiber will burn out.

Neosalpingostomy

If the fallopian tube is freely mobile and the end of the tube easily visualized, the dilated terminal position of the tube can be incised and made patent with any of several lasers including the argon laser. With the increasing success of *in vitro* fertilization and the traditionally poor results of terminal salpingostomy, there is decreasing enthusiasm for subjecting patients to a laparotomy to perform this procedure. Thus, laparoscopic surgery for distal tubal disease has grown in popularity.

To perform a terminal salpingostomy, the tube is first distended with indigo carmine in normal saline and the scarred end of the tube identified. The tubal serosa overlying the ampulla is then grasped with a laparoscopic forceps introduced through a suprapubic site. The fiber is then introduced into the pelvis through the operating channel of a single-puncture laparoscope until it touches the end of the tube. Using a power setting of 10 to 12 watts and a 300-micrometer fiber or a 600 micrometer fiber with a 100 micrometer tip, the end of the tube is incised in a standard fashion with three or four radial incisions originating at the center of the scarred end of the tube. A second forceps may need to be introduced to grasp the flaps of the tube and facilitate incision once the initial opening is made into the tube and the tube collapses as the indigo carmine rushes out. No backstop is necessary because of the diverging beam.

Once the flaps are made, the power is turned down to 3 to 5 watts .Using a no-touch technique, the flaps are "flowered back" using the technique originally described by Bruhat.

Ectopic Pregnancy

The argon laser is ideally suited for the conservative management of an unruptured ampullary tubal pregnancy because of its ability to cut and coagulate simultaneously. The fiber can be delivered through either the operating channel of a single-puncture laparoscope or an accessory suprapubic port. After the base of the ectopic is injected with several milliliters of vasopressin in normal saline (10 units in 30 ml), the tip of the 600-micrometer fiber is placed on the antimesenteric edge of the tube, and with a power setting of 10 to 12 watts a linear incision is made. Generally, the incision is completely free of bleeding. The ectopic is then shelled out, and the tube is left to heal without suturing the edges together.

ADVANTAGES AND DISADVANTAGES

The argon laser laparoscopic system has several advantages over other laser systems (Table 14–1).

1. The flexible fiber delivery system is extremely easy to use. It can be introduced through either the operating channel of a single-puncture laparoscope or an accessory suprapubic port. The fiber is either in contact with the tissue or very close, so the tip of the fiber and the path of the laser beam are always in view. No special devices or couplers must be purchased, aligned, or maintained. If the fiber tip breaks (rare) or burns out (common), it can be easily and quickly repaired at the time of surgery.
2. The technique of using a flexible fiber is remarkably similar to those operative laparoscopic techniques already acquired by most laparoscopists. Therefore, the learning curve is short, and most laparoscopists feel comfortable using this system after performing only a few procedures.
3. Vaporization and coagulation can easily be performed, and the exact tissue effect can be controlled by the distance between the fiber tip and the tissue. Although the tissue effect can also be controlled by the size of the fiber and the power setting, most laparoscopists prefer to leave these constant during most of the operating time and instead to continuously change the distance between the fiber tip and tissue to achieve the desired effect.

TABLE 14–1
Advantages of Argon Laser Laparoscopy

1. Simple fiberoptic delivery
2. Easy to learn
3. Coagulation and vaporization
4. Color-selective absorption
5. No special equipment necessary
6. No need for backstop
7. No bulky articulating arm
8. No beam alignment necessary

TABLE 14–2
Disadvantages of Argon Laser

1. Tinted eye wear is required.
2. The system is water-cooled.
3. Three-phase electrical supply is needed.
4. Not approved for lower genital tract use.

4. There is no articulating arm to hinder motion of the laparoscope. In fact, the laser sits at the patient's feet and out of the way of the scrub technicians and the assistants. Only the fiber enters the operative field.
5. Less char and less smoke are created with the argon laser than with the CO_2 laser, often eliminating the need for a smoke evacuation system.
6. The argon laser is extremely dependable and requires little maintenance or upkeep. Keye and colleagues have used an argon laser for nearly 250 procedures without interruption for repairs. Only occasional minor adjustments were made between scheduled operating days to maintain optimal performance.

The major disadvantage of the argon laser is the need for tinted eye protection (Table 14–2). Goggles and glasses are cumbersome when performing endoscopy. In addition, they alter the color of the tissue and at times interfere with a surgeon's ability to identify subtle and lightly pigmented lesions. The electronically controlled Monoshutter that fits over the eyepiece of the laparoscope or hysteroscope largely eliminates this disadvantage. Until the laser is actually fired, the filter is not in place and does not distort the color of the tissue. By using pulses of 1 to 2 seconds, a surgeon can monitor the tissue effect almost continuously during the procedure. However, the monoshutter decreases the size of the field of vision, thus interfering slightly with the surgeon's comfort. However, this reduced field of vision is not obvious when a camera is attached to the eyepiece of the monoshutter and the surgeon works off the television monitor. A second-generation monoshutter that does not reduce the field of vision is currently being developed.

Another disadvantage of the argon laser is the need for running water to cool the machine and for a 220-volt three-phase electrical system identical to that used by many Nd:YAG lasers. These requirements limit the use of the argon laser to those sites supplying these water and power requirements.

CONCLUSIONS

During the past 5 years, the indications for the use of lasers in gynecology have expanded greatly. At least four different wavelengths are now used for gynecological endoscopy. Fortunately, gynecological pelvic surgeons do not need to purchase or to have access to each of these lasers, for new techniques and delivery systems have made it possible to perform most gynecological pelvic procedures with any of these wavelengths. Experience has demonstrated that the argon laser is extremely versatile, simple to use, effective, and safe.

REFERENCES

1. Diamond MP, Decherney AH, Polan ML: Laparoscopic use of the argon laser in nonendometriotic reproductive pelvic surgery. J Reprod Med 31:1011, 1986
2. Keye WR Jr, Dixon J: Photocoagulation of endometriosis by the argon laser through the laparoscope. Obstet Gynecol 62:383, 1983
3. Keye WR Jr, Hansen LW, Astin M et al: Argon laser therapy of endometriosis: A review of 92 consecutive patients. Fertil Steril 47:208, 1987
4. Keye WR Jr, Matson GA, Dixon J: The use of the argon laser in the treatment of experimental endometriosis. Fertil Steril 39:26, 1983
5. Keye WR Jr, Poulson AM, Worley RJ: Application of simplified laser laparoscopy in preparation of the pelvis for *in vitro* fertilization. J Reprod Med 30:418, 1985

15

Laser Laparoscopy Using the KTP Laser

James F. Daniell

The KTP laser is the newest laser to be evaluated clinically for laparoscopic surgery in North America. It is a visible light laser produced at a wavelength of 532 nm. The energy of the laser is generated from a neodymium:yttrium-aluminum-garnet (Nd:YAG) laser and is then passed through a crystal of potassium-titanyl-phosphate (KTP), producing a doubling of the frequency from 1064 to 532 nm. This laser has been referred to at various times as the frequency-doubled YAG laser, the KTP laser, the 532-nm laser, the Laserscope laser, and the Omniplus laser. For purposes of simplification, it will be referred to here as the KTP/532 laser.

PHYSICS OF THE KTP/532 LASER

The KTP/532 laser is a visible-light laser, in the green spectrum, which has characteristics similar to the argon laser. Its energy may be passed through fibers and fluids and penetrates tissue approximately 2 mm with some scatter. Although moderately color dependent, it is effective on all colored tissues. The laparoscopic delivery system consists of plastic-coated flexible fiberoptic quartz fibers. Fibers are available in two diameters: 400 and 600 micrometers. The major effect of this laser on tissue is vaporization when the fiber is touching the tissue and coagulation when the fiber is slightly off the tissue. It is necessary for the operator to use a protective eye filter because of the backscatter of the beam on impacting the tissue. A special filter that is provided fits over the eyepiece of the laparoscope. The filter only drops into place when the laser is activated, and the laser cannot be fired when the eye filter is removed. This laser requires external water cooling, so it is not as mobile as the carbon dioxide (CO_2) laser. However, this laser can be positioned in the corner of the operating room and the long fiber brought over to the operating field. Assistants thus have greater access to the operating room table for operative laparoscopy.

ANIMAL STUDIES

Animal investigations of this laser began in October, 1985, at West Side Hospital in Nashville, Tennessee.[1] Tissue effects both at open laparotomy and laparoscopy in rabbits were evaluated. The results of these studies revealed that effective vaporization, incision, and coagulation could be possible under laparoscopic control using the flexible fiber delivery system. Tissue studies did not demonstrate any penetration more than 2 mm from direct contact with the fiber tip to the bowel, bladder, or peritoneal surface in rabbits.

CLINICAL TRIALS

In November, 1985, after obtaining Food and Drug Administration (FDA) and hospital Institutional Review Board approval of the investigative protocol, laparoscopic use of the KTP laser was initiated by the author at West Side Hospital in Nashville, Tennessee. After the protocol was discussed with each patient, a signed informed consent allowing use of the experimental laser and videotaping for visual documentation was obtained. The initial investigative indications were for treatment of endometriosis, pelvic adhesions, distal tubal obstruction, polycystic ovarian disease, ectopic pregnancy, small subserosal uterine fibroids, and laparoscopic transection of uterosacral ligaments for dysmenorrhea.[2] Concomitantly, a clinical trial was also initiated to investigate the hysteroscopic use of the KTP laser for resection of uterine septi, vaporization of intrauterine adhesions, and small submucosal fibroids.[3]

Clinical results from early investigation of the KTP laser were excellent. There were no complications in the more than 100 patients studied. Clinical symptoms were evaluated in a retrospective questionnaire to determine the reduction of pelvic pain in patients presenting with pain and for the occurrence of pregnancy in patients whose primary indication was infertility. The results of these early studies were subsequently published.[1-3] Other investigators subsequently confirmed the initial findings.[4]

CLINICAL TECHNIQUES FOR LAPAROSCOPIC USE OF THE KTP LASER

More than 1000 laparoscopic operations using the KTP laser at West Side Hospital have been performed, and no complications have been reported. A fairly standardized technique has evolved that is effective, limits risk to the patient, and provides for rapid use of the KTP energy through the laparoscope. All patients are treated on an outpatient basis unless medical indications required early admission. Surgery is performed in the proliferative phase of the cycle in patients to avoid possible occult pregnancy and the necessity for dissecting around a corpus luteum of the ovary, which might bleed during laparoscopic manipulations. The laser is tested by the laser coordinator before the patient's arrival in the operating room. The laser remains stationary in the corner of the operating room, and after the patient is positioned, prepared, and draped, the laser fiber is brought over to the operating field. A straight catheter is temporarily inserted to drain the bladder, and a uterine manipulator is placed for dye injection and for positioning the uterus. All procedures are carried out under video control using the author's preference of a 90/10 beam splitter (Wolf Instrument Company, Rosewood, Ill.) attached to two video recorders. This setup allows for the making of videotapes for the patient as well as the author for teaching and medical/legal documentation. A microphone is available so that the surgeon may selectively talk to the patient during the procedure for her later review, which has great educational benefits for the patient. Two monitors are used so that the surgeon and assistant may easily view the endoscopic surgery simultaneously. A specially designed second-puncture dual-channel irrigation/suction probe (Gynescope, Willobough, Ohio) is used to allow for simultaneous suction and irrigation in the pelvis.

The fiber can be placed into the abdomen by various techniques (Table 15–1). It can be brought through the operating channel of an operating laparoscope, through the central portion of a 5-mm suction/irrigation probe (commonly used for CO_2 laser laparoscopy), or through a special 5-mm steerable probe that has been designed for ease of use in the pelvis (Gynescope, Willobough, Ohio). The fiber tip is cleaved and the plastic coating stripped off the distal 1 cm of the fiber. The fiber is cleaned by the circulating nurse by wiping it with an alcohol swab. If during the procedure the tip of the fiber melts back slightly, thereby reducing laser transmission, the fiber tip is grasped by the circulating nurse, who may cleave it, strip it, and recleanse it within 30 seconds. This process allows rapid recleaving of the fiber throughout the procedure. The fiber may be repeatedly used for several operations until it becomes too short. Operating room personnel should take care not to break the fiber by stepping on it and should avoid stepping on the eye filter cable. After the pelvis is laparoscopically evaluated for the location and type of pathology present, a decision is made about which of the three modes of entry for the laser fiber will be used. Because a 10-mm diagnostic laparoscope is used to enhance the picture quality for videotaping, the fiber is usually delivered through a 3- or 5-mm second-puncture

TABLE 15–1
Methods of Laparoscopic Delivery with the KTP Laser

Through the operating channel of the laparoscope
Through a 3-mm standard irrigation probe
Through the small central channel of a 5-mm irrigation/aspiration probe
Through special needle probes for fibers
Through a special steerable probe

device. Correct placement of the alternate probes vastly simplifies the procedure. Normally a 5-mm probe is placed in the midline suprapubically for use as the initial probe for manipulation. Then , if a third probe is to be inserted into the abdomen, it is usually positioned 3 or 4 cm lateral to the umbilicus on the side opposite from most of the disease. This lateral placement of the accessory third probe reduces the "clashing of swords" as the instruments are simultaneously manipulated. A final check of the laser's readiness is performed before beginning the application of the laser's energy. After the eye filter is attached to the eyepiece of the laparoscope, the power is usually set on 10 watts, and the laser is activated in the continuous mode. During the laser laparoscopy, the tissue effects are varied merely by adjusting the fiber to and from the tissue. The circulating nurse usually does not need to change the power setting during the procedures. If a combination of coagulation and vaporization is indicated for a particular disease process, the non-contact coagulation portions will be performed first to preserve the tip of the fiber, thus reducing the need for unnecessary recleaving. For instance, if the patient has implants of endometriosis over the bladder and adhesions to the lateral pelvic sidewall, the implants would first be photocoagulated by keeping the laser fiber 1/2 cm off the tissue and photocoagulating with a non-contact technique. Then the fiber tip would be touched to the adhesions, taking care to monitor what is beneath the adhesions, and then the adhesions would be vaporized by the contact technique.

It is important to remember that the laser fiber is never advanced more than 1 to 2 cm from the tip of the delivery probe. This is to reduce the likelihood of breaking the fiber and inadvertently losing it in the abdomen. If the probe through which the fiber is passed is being used for manipulation, which often is the case, the fiber should be retracted during the manipulation. Copious irrigation with heparinized lactated Ringer's solution is usually performed using a concentration of 5000 units of heparin in each liter of lactated Ringer's. The scrub nurse, standing at the patient's perineum, is responsible for smoke suction and irrigation, as well as for positioning the uterus during the procedure as she watches the monitor. She tries to keep her other hand free to hold and pass accessory instruments. In this way, the scrub nurse may become a valuable participant in the operative laparoscopy using the KTP/532 laser.

As the laser is fired, the eye filter drops in front of the eyepiece of the laparoscope, and the color of the view is changed slightly. The color change by the eye filter minimally distorts the view for the operator as well as for the video camera. Videotaping for the patient is usually done during selected portions of the operation and is controlled by a remote-control switch on the camera attached to the laparoscope. Normally the beginning and end of the procedure are videotaped along with certain portions of the surgery for the patient's edification (Table 15–2).

Smoke production with the KTP/532 laser is markedly less than with the CO_2 laser, but it still occurs. For this reason, a high-flow insufflator is used and smoke is vented off at the point of accumulation whenever possible. Smoke is vented from the suction probe into the disposable floor canisters, which have a biologic filter in line before entering the operating room's wall suction. Smoke production can be minimized by frequently irrigating the pelvis as well as by limiting the vaporizing effect of the laser. Normally a 600-micrometer fiber is used. It gives a larger spot size and can therefore be used to incise and ablate greater surface areas more rapidly.

TABLE 15–2
**Advantages of Video Use for
Gynecological Endoscopy**

Allows the assistant to really "help"
The resident is able to do more
Greater involvement by the operating room team
Improved teaching potential
Educational tapes can be produced
Enlightenment of patients
Increases referrals for surgery

However, when a hydrosalpinx is present or an ectopic pregnancy requiring a linear salpingostomy is encountered, the smaller-diameter 400-micrometer fiber is used to give a more powerful, narrower cut as a result of its smaller spot size. If it is noted during the procedure that there is decreased transmission of laser energy through the tip of the fiber, the fiber is removed, cleaved, stripped, and resterilized before continuing the operation.

Vaporization is accomplished by touching the tip of the fiber to the tissue (contact technique). Coagulation is accomplished by merely pulling the tip slightly back from the tissue (non-contact technique). Small vessels are usually prophylactically coagulated before cutting them by moving the fiber as needed (non-contact followed by contact techniques). After the surgery is completed, the pelvis is copiously irrigated with heparinized Ringer's solution, which is then completely removed by suction from the pelvis.

The patient is usually discharged the day of surgery unless she is too uncomfortable or lives too far away. Most patients have the standard postoperative discomfort after laparoscopy, and no different sensations have been observed in these patients following KTP/532 laser laparoscopy as opposed to other forms of operative laparoscopy involving other lasers or non-laser techniques. Operative times are approximately one-third less than with CO_2 laser laparoscopy. This is because less time is needed to set up for surgery, suctioning smoke, and reinsufflating the peritoneal cavity.

SPECIFIC CLINICAL PROCEDURES

Compared with other forms of laparoscopic laser surgery, the KTP/532 laser appears to be advantageous for procedures in which greater depth of penetration is needed or in which there is a potential for bleeding. For example, vaporization of polycystic ovaries with the KTP/532 fiber allows greater destruction of the ovarian stroma than can be obtained with the CO_2 laser, along with much less smoke production. Dense adhesions may be lysed with less risk of bleeding and smoke accumulation as well. Transection of the uterosacral ligaments may be rapidly accomplished with less risk of bleeding. Terminal neosalpingostomy, which can be done with the CO_2 laser, is easier to accomplish with a fiber tip. There is less risk of damage to the internal side of the occluded fallopian tube when using the KTP/532 fiber tip because of the tendency of the CO_2 laser to damage underlying tissue if a backstop is not used. The tendency for bleeding is also reduced with the KTP/532 laser, which provides superior coagulation over the CO_2 laser as tissue is transected. Tables 15–3 and 15–4 list some of the clinical results that have been obtained for specific diseases that have been treated by laparoscopic laser surgery using the KTP/532 laser.

ADVANTAGES OF THE KTP LASER FOR LAPAROSCOPIC SURGERY

As has already been stated, there are several advantages of using the KTP/532 laser for laparoscopic surgery instead of the CO_2 laser or non-laser techniques. The most important advantage is the ease of delivery of the system with the flexible fiber. A

TABLE 15–3
LUNA Results with KTP Laser
(6-Month Follow-Up)

	WORSE	SAME	IMPROVED
Endometriosis			
80 patients	3 (4%)	17 (21%)	60 (75%)
Primary Dysmenorrhea			
20 patients	2 (10%)	6 (30%)	12 (60%)
Totals			
100 patients	5 (5%)	23 (23%)	72 (72%)

LUNA, laparoscopic uterosacral nerve ablation.

TABLE 15–4
Results of Laparoscopic Neosalpingostomy with Lasers*
(1 Year Minimum Follow-Up)

TOTAL PATIENTS	OPEN TUBES AT 6 WEEKS HSG	ATTEMPTING PREGNANCY	PREGNANCY RESULTS		
			Intrauterine	Aborted	Ectopic
120	96 tested 80 open (83%)	101	22	10	15

* *Includes CO_2 laser use of well.*

surgeon does not have to have special couplers or delivery devices that are expensive or cumbersome to use or that require continued maintenance. All that is required is a simple probe or operating laparoscope through which the fiber may be passed. The green beam, generated by the KTP/532 and used for aiming as well as lasing, is much easier to visualize in the pelvis than the helium–neon aiming beam of the CO_2 laser. The KTP/532 laser's ability to lase through fluids allows a surgeon to use copious amounts of irrigating fluids, concomitantly reducing the accumulation of smoke, which is a major disadvantage of the CO_2 laser. Because the KTP/532 laser's energy is passed through the tip of its fiber without the benefits of a focusing lens, there is marked reduction of the power densities as the tip is retracted away from the tissue. Thus, a backstop is usually not necessary unless laser energy is applied within 1 cm of underlying vital structures.

The tissue effects of the KTP/532 laser are different from the CO_2 laser in that greater tissue coagulation is produced by the KTP/532 laser's energy. There is usually less bleeding when vascular structures are encountered during vaporization or incision with the KTP/532 laser. The ability to keep the laser stationary in the corner of the room away from the operating field is another major advantage. Access to the operating table is maximized, and none of the alignment problems with the CO_2 laser's articulating arm are encountered with the KTP/532 laser. (Mirror misalignment is a common sequela to repeated movement of the CO_2 laser.)

DISADVANTAGES OF THE KTP/532 LASER FOR OPERATIVE LAPAROSCOPY

Some disadvantages of the KTP/532 laser are apparent. The major disadvantage is the need for an eye filter, which reduces the diameter of the viewing field of vision slightly and requires the presence of another cord on the operating field. Although the present eye filter only slightly reduces visibility, it still can reduce the accuracy of visual control. The need for running water to externally cool the KTP/532 laser, along with special electrical hookups, limits the number of operating rooms that may be used with this laser. The mobile CO_2 laser, on the other hand, can be electrically connected in any operating room and does not need special plumbing. Another disadvantage of the KTP/532 laser is its cost, approximately $90,000, which is more than the initial cost of CO_2 laser laparoscopy. Although the KTP/532 fibers cost $100 each, if used carefully, they may be used for 30 or 40 procedures. This durability tremendously reduces the subsequent cost per case. The possibility exists that a piece of the fiber tip could break off in the abdomen and be lost during the procedure. This complication should not occur if proper precautions are taken never to introduce more than 1 cm of the fiber into the peritoneal cavity beyond the tip of the probe. The final dilemma for the KTP/532 laser is the lack of long-term follow-up of clinical results following this new technique of laparoscopic tissue destruction, because the KTP/532 laser has only been available for clinical use for a short time.

SAFETY PRECAUTIONS AND TRAINING IN USE OF THE KTP LASER

Because the KTP laser is a visible-light laser, the potential for it to cause eye damage, although certainly possible, is minimal. If the filter is not used or is short circuited accidentally, surgeons should immediately be aware of the bright lime-green beam and close their eyes. This same phenomenon occurs for other observers in the operating room, because the eyes immediately detect the bright lime color. The Nd:YAG laser, which is infrared and thus is invisible, is potentially much more dangerous to the eyes of surgeons and operating room personnel. The other potential danger of this laser is to the patient, in that the energy does penetrate more than the energy of the CO_2 laser. Theoretically, the risk of inadvertent damage to the bowel, ureter, or bladder is increased if the laser is applied too long in direct contact over these organs in the pelvis at laparoscopy. The safety of the KTP/532 laser appears to be greater than with the CO_2 laser because of the easier delivery system and the fact that the space interposed between the point at which the laser energy enters the abdomen and the tissue impact is minimized. With the CO_2 laser, unfortunately, there is a long open space in the peritoneal cavity through which the laser beam passes. Bowel or other vital structures may potentially enter this space and be inadvertently damaged with the CO_2 laser much more easily than with the KTP/532. Table 15–5 shows the safety record following the use of the KTP/532 at West Side Hospital.

Because of the short period of time that this laser has been clinically available, it is not widely available in residency programs. Therefore, interested gynecologists need to take special courses or participate in workshops to learn the safe applications of this laser and become familiar with its tissue effects. It is important to understand that just because a surgeon is experienced with the tissue effects of the CO_2 laser, it does not mean that he or she can immediately understand and use the KTP/532 laser safely. The KTP/532 laser uses a totally new and different wavelength and has different tissue effects.

The manufacturers of the KTP/532 laser have made a strong commitment to education and support courses for nurses and physicians interested in using this technology. These courses usually offer animal surgery experience and preceptor-

TABLE 15–5
Endoscopic Use of the KTP Laser in Gynecology at HCA West Side Hospital, Nashville, Tennessee

November, 1985–November, 1987	
Laparoscopic cases	380
Hysteroscopic cases	31
Totals	411
Complications	0

ships with physicians trained in laparoscopic use of the KTP/532 laser. Before using the KTP/532 laser laparoscopically, interested gynecologists should pursue one of the specific educational opportunities.

CONCLUSIONS

This is an exciting time in endoscopic gynecological surgery, with shifting trends in surgical care of patients. Many patients who previously underwent major operations are now being treated with outpatient or same-day surgery. The use of lasers has tremendously changed the author's patterns of gynecological surgery (Table 15–6). The list of applications includes the replacement of hysterectomy for menorrhagia with Nd : YAG laser ablation; laparoscopic treatment of ectopic pregnancies, hydrosalpinges, adhesions, and endometriosis; and laparoscopic removal of tubes and ovaries through operative laparoscopy (Table 15–7). All these advanced operative laparoscopic procedures tend to save patients time, money, and discomfort and are of benefit to all of us involved in health care today. All gynecologists interested in

TABLE 15–6
Changing Patterns of Gynecological Surgery with Lasers— Laparoscopy vs. Laparotomy

	ENDOMETRIOSIS	HYDROSALPINGX	ADHESIONS	ECTOPIC
1980	50/50	10/90	60/40	5/95
1987	80/20	90/10	90/10	95/5

Laparoscopy/laparotomy (major surgery)

TABLE 15–7
Shifting Trends in Gynecological Surgery

	OLD THERAPY	NEW THERAPY
Menorrhagia	Hysterectomy	YAG ablation
Severe endometriosis	Laparotomy	Laparoscopy
Ectopic gestation	Laparotomy	Laparoscopy
Uterine septum	Abdominal metroplasty	Hysteroscopic resection
Hydrosalpinx	Laparotomy	Laparoscopy
Cornual blockage	Cornual reanastomosis	Hysteroscopic probing and dilatation
Pelvic adhesions	Laparotomy	Laparoscopy
Ovarian pathology requiring removal	Laparotomy oophorectomy	Pelviscopy

operative endoscopy are encouraged to evaluate and investigate the use of lasers for gynecological procedures.

REFERENCES

1. Daniell JF: Initial evaluation of the use of potassium–titanyl–(IC9P/532) laser in gynecologic laparoscopy. Fertil Steril 46:373, 1986
2. Daniell JF, Meisels S, Miller W et al: Laparoscopic use of the KTP/532 laser in nonendometriotic pelvic surgery. Colpo Gynecol Laser Surg 2:107, 1986
3. Daniell JF, Osher S, Miller W: Hysteroscopic resection of uterine septa and visible light laser energy. Colpo Gynecol Laser Surg 3:217, 1987
4. Diamond MP, Boyers SP, Lavy G et al: Endoscopic use of the potassium–titanyl–phosphate 532 laser in gynecologic surgery. Colpo Gynecol Laser Surg 3:213, 1987

16

Laser Laparoscopy Using the Neodymium: Yttrium-Aluminum-Garnet Laser

Jack M. Lomano

Improved endoscopic techniques coupled with advances in laser technology have spurred an interest in using laser energy to treat gynecologic pathology. Laser therapy offers several advantages over other modalities, including its ability to produce precise tissue destruction, better hemostasis, and more rapid tissue healing. In addition, when combined with endoscopy, the laser increases accessibility to pelvic anatomy. Moreover, it achieves all of this at less expense and discomfort to the patient.

The neodymium: yttrium–aluminum–garnet (Nd:YAG) laser has been used in the United States and extensively in Europe for the control of gastrointestinal hemorrhage, destruction of bronchial tumors, and destruction of bladder tumors. Its use in gynecology has been overshadowed by the acceptance of the carbon dioxide (CO_2) laser in the treatment of lower tract and intra-abdominal pathology. At the present time, the CO_2, argon, KTP twin crystal, and Nd:YAG lasers all have application to gynecology in the treatment of intra-abdominal, lower tract, and intrauterine disease. Specifically, these lasers have been used to treat pelvic endometriosis, cervical dysplasia, condylomata acuminata, pelvic adhesive disease, and premalignant diseases of the vulva and vagina.

The Nd:YAG laser is a solid crystal made up of yttrium, aluminum, and garnet with surrounding neodymium. The Nd:YAG light is in the near infrared region and has a wavelength of 1064 nm. The beam is transmitted through clear liquids, thus allowing its optimal use in water-filled cavities, such as the eye, bladder, stomach, or uterus. Its absorption is not color specific like the argon laser, but

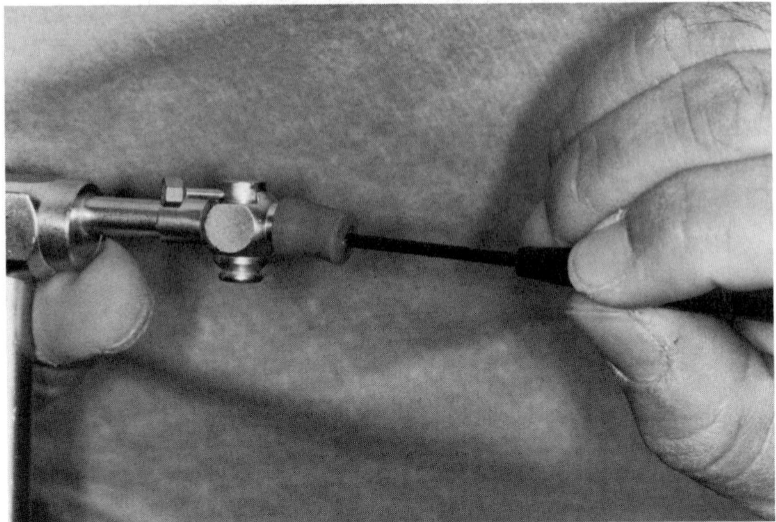

FIGURE 16–1. Nd : YAG laser fiber passed through the laparoscope.

the beam is selectively absorbed by any tissue of a dark color. The Nd : YAG laser has a characteristic physical property, in that it is scattered and penetrates on impact with tissue, resulting in a homogeneous zone of thermal coagulation that may extend from 1 to 5 mm beyond the site of impact. The Nd : YAG laser is an excellent tool for tissue coagulation and, like the argon and KTP/532 lasers, can be delivered through fiberoptic systems. By applying sapphire or diamond to the tip of the Nd : YAG laser fiber, one can concentrate the energy of the Nd : YAG laser, which then becomes a cutting tool with precision that is similar to that of the CO_2 laser.

The Nd : YAG laser can be passed through fiberoptic guides (Fig. 16–1), making it adaptable to the laparoscope. The flexible tip of the fiber allows an operator to reach difficult areas of the pelvis. The fibers can be bent with a steerable Albarran's system that resembles those used in cystoscopic work (Fig. 16–2). A newly developed sapphire crystal may be attached to the laser fiber, thus concentrating the energy and increasing the capacity of this laser to actually cut tissue (Fig. 16–3). The addition of the sapphire contact probes allows the YAG laser to vaporize and cut, as well as to coagulate.

SAFETY CONSIDERATIONS

The Nd : YAG laser carries a risk for operating physicians, as well as for patients. Eye injury from backscatter following tissue impact is a danger for surgeons. Use of special safety lenses is mandatory. For patients, the principal risk is occult damage to pelvic contents if the beam is inadvertently directed to an intra-abdominal organ that is not intended to be in the path of the laser energy. If a surgeon follows the principles of power density and laser safety that have been previously outlined in this

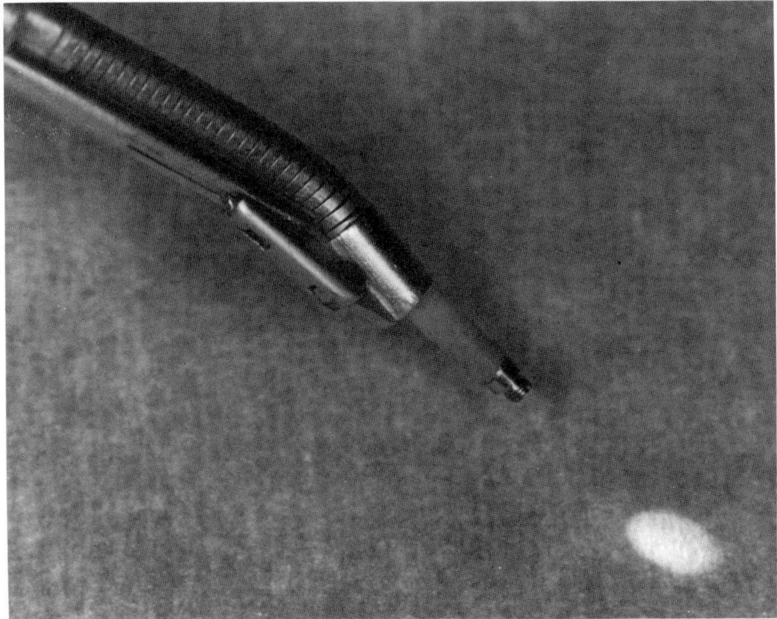

FIGURE 16–2. Laparoscopic Albarran's bridge allows deflection to the fiber.

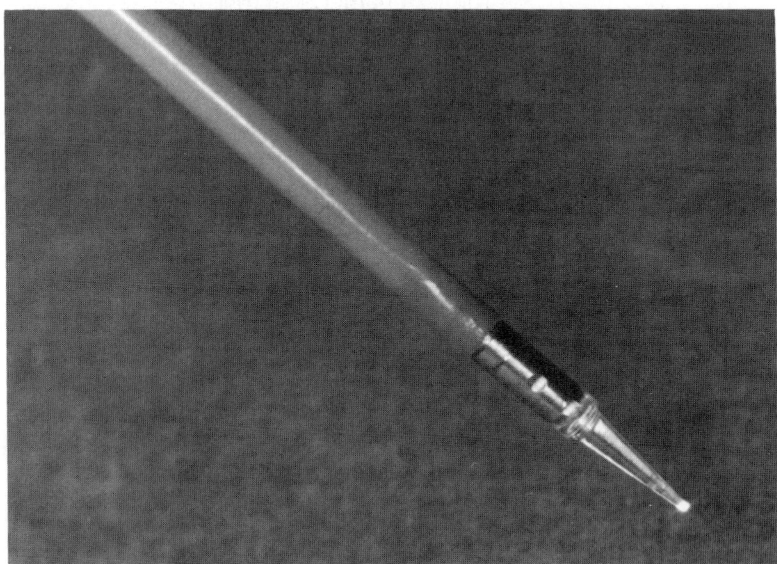

FIGURE 16–3. Close-up view of a sapphire contact probe.

textbook, this risk should be kept to a minimum. Nd:YAG laser light energy follows all of the physical principles of laser energy with regard to penetration. A more dramatic tissue effect is expected with increased power or decreased spot size. Penetration is also increased when the laser is left in place for a longer time. Nd:YAG laser energy may be applied to lesions overlying the ureters and bladder within the parameters that will be outlined in this chapter. Hofstetter has reported the use of the Nd:YAG laser in the bladder at power settings of 40 to 60 watts in order to treat bladder tumors.[8] There have been no reports of urinary tract fistulas despite the treatment of these tumors cystoscopically in the bladder, as well as in the ureters. The safety of the Nd:YAG laser in the treatment of lesions overlying bowel has not been established.

Although the safety record of laparoscopic Nd:YAG laser surgery has so far been good, more widespread use by inexperienced surgeons may increase the complication rate. Specific training in the use of the Nd:YAG laser, as previously discussed in this text, is mandatory.

LAPAROSCOPIC TREATMENT OF PELVIC ENDOMETRIOSIS

In 1936, Cattel and Swinton summarized the entire world's literature on endometriosis, which consisted of 20 cases.[2] Since then, the incidence of the disease has increased dramatically. This is particularly distressing because it is occurring at a time when many women in the United States are electively choosing to postpone childbearing to a later age. The association between endometriosis and an inability to conceive has been observed for years.[14] Premenstrual and menstrual pain caused by congestion of sclerosed ovaries and nodules in the uterosacral ligaments presents a significant disability annually to thousands of women. Because of the increasingly young age at initial diagnosis of endometriosis, hysterectomy and bilateral salpingo-oophorectomy are an unacceptable treatment. Conservative medical treatment with oral contraceptives, danazol (Danocrine), or gonadotropin agonists may have serious side-effects that may preclude their long-term use.[1,5,6,15] Conservative surgery has been reported to be effective in controlling the disease. However, sharp dissection of pelvic endometriosis is not only difficult, but often results in bleeding that may lead to adhesion formation, thus potentially further compromising fertility. Another option, electrocautery, although providing excellent hemostasis, can produce thermal necrosis and perforation of underlying bowel, bladder, or ureter.

Feste,[7] Martin,[13] Daniell and Pittaway,[3] and Kelly and Roberts[9] have reported using the CO_2 laser through the laparoscope to treat endometriosis. Keye and associates[10] have reported the laparoscopic treatment of endometriosis with the argon laser, and Daniell[4] has treated the disease with the KTP twin crystal laser. Photocoagulation of early pelvic endometriosis with the Nd:YAG laser was first reported by Lomano.[11] It is an excellent treatment modality because of its inherent ability to penetrate tissue without vaporization of the serosa, thus potentially having the advantage of fewer postoperative adhesions (Fig. 16–4). The Nd:YAG laser is capable of being delivered through an optical fiber, which is easily manipulated through the laparoscope. Because the Nd:YAG laser is a coagulating rather than a vaporizing

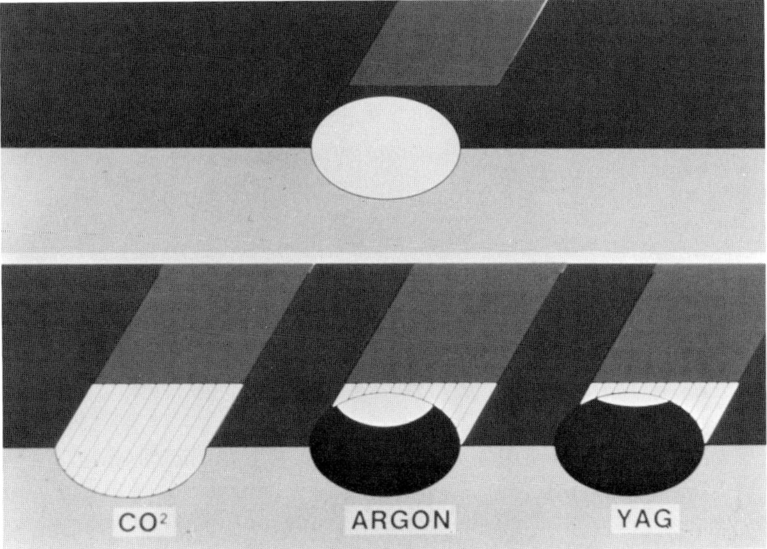

FIGURE 16–4. Comparison of tissue penetration with the CO_2 argon, and Nd : YAG wavelengths.

tool, a smoke evacuation system is not needed. The Nd : YAG laser also offers the advantage of color selectivity, because its particular wavelength is selectively absorbed by the dark colors of pelvic endometriosis. Patients eligible for this treatment may have shown signs and symptoms of early pelvic endometriosis, including pelvic pain, menstrual dysfunction, infertility, or nodularity found at pelvic examination. Patients who are discovered to have severe endometriosis are considered for open laparotomy, especially when the pelvic viscera are poorly visualized through the laparoscope.

Outpatient diagnostic laparoscopy is scheduled under general anesthesia. If early pelvic endometriosis is found, the Nd : YAG laser fiber is introduced through the operating channel of the laparoscope. A double-puncture technique is sometimes used so that additional instruments can be placed to facilitate the procedure. The fiber is placed approximately 2 to 5 mm from the observed lesion. A laparoscopic fiber deflector may be needed to direct the beam into relatively inaccessible areas of the pelvis. Photocoagulation is performed using 20 watts of power until a blanching effect is achieved 1 to 2 mm beyond the border of the lesion. Intermittent 1- to 3-second exposures with a spot size of 2 mm are recommended to avoid the buildup of heat and subsequent vaporization of the serosa.[15] The procedure can usually be completed in approximately 10 to 40 minutes.

Patients are discharged on the day of surgery and resume normal activity within 1 to 2 days after surgery. They are observed postoperatively at 3-month intervals. Adjunctive medical therapy may be used following treatment. This technique of photocoagulation of early pelvic endometriosis has been used at Grant Laser Center, Columbus, Ohio, during the past 5 years, and no serious complications have been encountered. A series of 61 patients with early pelvic endometriosis

TABLE 16–1
Results of Nd : YAG Laser Photocoagulation of Early Pelvic
Endometriosis* (61 Patients*; Average Follow-up 22 Months)

REPORT OF SYMPTOMS	NO. OF PATIENTS	PERCENT
Improved	45	74
Worsened	2	3
No change	12	20

** Results taken from 61 patients with an average follow-up of 22 months. Two patients were unavailable for follow-up.*

treated laparoscopically with the Nd : YAG laser has been reported by the author.[12] The patients were monitored for an average of 22 months. Symptoms improved after surgery in 45 patients (74%), worsened in two patients (3%), and did not change in 12 patients (20%). Two patients have been unavailable for follow-up (Table 16–1). Studies to establish the effectiveness of Nd : YAG laser photocoagulation of early pelvic endometriosis are now under way at multiple centers throughout the United States.

The early results indicate that the Nd : YAG laser is an apparently effective and safe modality in the treatment of early clinical endometriosis. Several characteristics of the Nd : YAG laser include its ability to penetrate tissue without vaporization of the serosa. Its ability to be delivered through an optical fiber and the fact that it is a coagulating, rather than a vaporizing tool, suggest that it may be an ideal system for treating early endometriosis through the laparoscope. Definitive evidence for the value of this therapy must await the results of long-term prospective comparative studies.

Nd : YAG LASER EXCISIONAL PROCEDURES

Peritubal and periovarian disease is a major cause of infertility in the United States. Diagnosis is most often made at the time of laparoscopy and can be corrected with the Nd : YAG laser at the time of diagnostic laparoscopy with the aid of a sapphire contact probe. Neosalpingostomy, fimbrioplasty, transection of the uterosacral ligaments, and lysis of adhesions all can be accomplished using the Nd : YAG laser contact probes.

Surgical Laser Technologies (SLT, Malvern, PA) has recently developed a sapphire tip for use with the Nd : YAG laser. The tip concentrates the laser energy into a small spot size and allows the laser to be used as a cutting modality rather than a coagulating one. Excisional procedures involving intraperitoneal disease can safely be performed with the sapphire tip attached to the Teflon cladding surrounding the quartz laser fiber. Because the tissue effect of the sapphire-tipped Nd : YAG laser is more hemostatic than that of the CO_2 laser, it has the potential benefit of less blood loss during excisional procedures. Excision with the sapphire tips results in a zone of thermal necrosis very similar to that of the focused CO_2 laser, thus making it suitable for treatment in delicate areas of the pelvis where precision is important

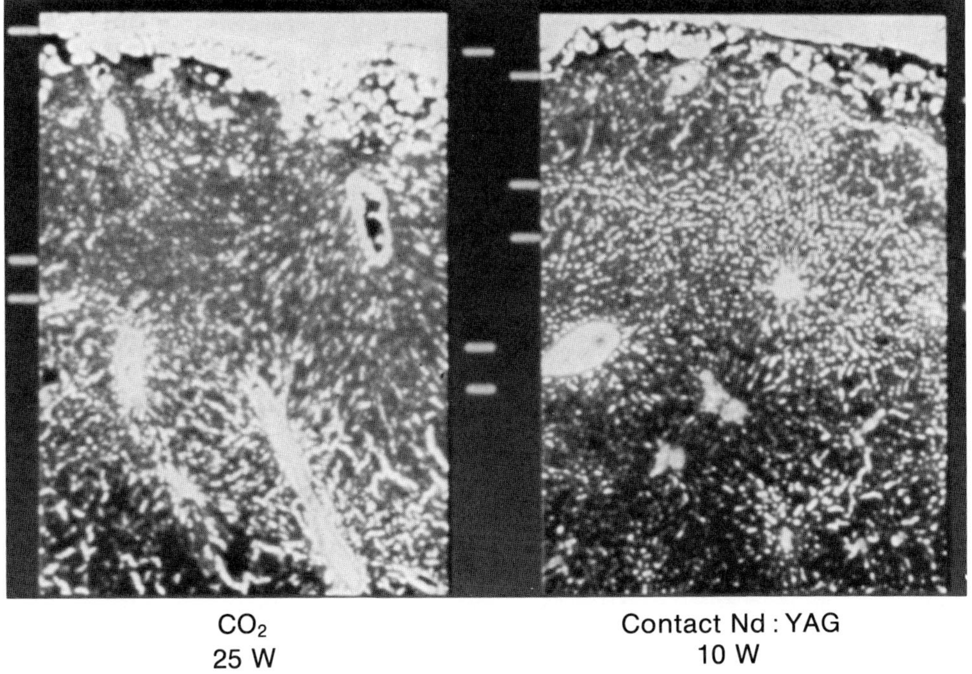

FIGURE 16–5. Comparison of thermal necrosis with the CO_2 laser and Nd : YAG sapphire contact probe.

(Fig. 16–5). The sapphire contact probes offer the distinct advantage of precise tissue removal with minimum damage to surrounding normal structures (see Chapter 20). In addition, these excisional procedures can be accomplished with less bleeding and less risk of damage to normal surrounding tissue.

INSTRUMENTATION FOR THE Nd : YAG LASER

As Nd : YAG laser energy is emitted from the lasing chamber, it can be collected and channeled through quartz fibers. These fibers vary between 100 and 600 μm in diameter. The fibers used for laparoscopy are usually 400 to 600 μm in diameter. As the Nd : YAG laser energy is discharged from the quartz fiber into a gas medium, such as air or CO_2, heat energy is generated. At power settings greater than 15 watts, this heat becomes significant and can result in the fracture of the fiber tip with subsequent loss of power density. By surrounding the quartz fiber with Teflon cladding, one can flow a gas coaxially over the tip of the fiber, thus cooling the fiber and avoiding fracture of the fiber tip. Nd : YAG laser manufacturers generally provide a two-step foot pedal. Initial pressure on the foot pedal begins the gas flow, and further pressure then releases the laser energy from the lasing chamber. Air, CO_2, or nitrous oxide can be used as a cooling gas. Because CO_2 is rapidly absorbed by the peritoneal cavity, it is the most ideal cooling gas for Nd : YAG laser laparoscopy.

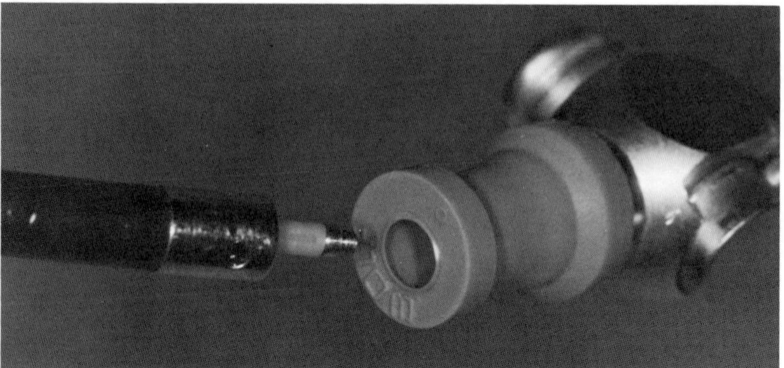

FIGURE 16–6. Close-up of a gas-cooled fiber.

Debris occasionally builds up on the end of the fiber, resulting in inadvertent concentration of heat at the fiber tip, melting the Teflon cladding and fracturing the quartz fiber. This problem is easily repaired by a laser technician, who can cleave the fiber along with its outer Teflon cladding, polish the end of the quartz fiber, and then reassemble. A small metal sleeve is inserted between the quartz fiber and the Teflon to allow the purging gas to flow around the entire circumference of the fiber (Fig. 16–6).

SUMMARY

Recent technical advances in laser surgery combined with improved laparoscopic techniques have provided a new horizon for laparoscopic laser surgery. The Nd:YAG laser has been used effectively in treating intra-abdominal pathology through a laparoscope. Photocoagulation of early pelvic endometriosis, excision of pelvic adhesions, neosalpingostomy, fimbrioplasty, and lysis of pelvic adhesions may be accomplished with a minimum of destruction to surrounding normal tissue. The Nd:YAG laser produces a simultaneous hemostatic tissue effect that has not been demonstrated with the CO_2 laser. The future of laser laparoscopy will be determined by the advances in laser biophysics as they are coupled to the needs of practicing physicians. This approach for laser laparoscopy offers advantages of simplicity and eventual lower cost. Physicians must become familiar with all wavelengths of laser energy as they are used through the laparoscope. The difficulties and potential benefits, as well as risks, must be understood by practicing physicians using these new modalities in an arena of rapidly changing technology.

REFERENCES

1. Biberoglu KO, Behrman SJ: Dosage aspects of danazol therapy in endometriosis: Short-term and long-term effectiveness. Am J Obstet Gynecol 139:645, 1981
2. Cattel RB, Swinton NW: Endometriosis with reference to conservative treatment. N Engl J Med 214:341, 1936

3. Daniell JF, Pittaway DE: Use of the CO_2 laser in laparoscopic laser surgery: Initial experience with the second puncture technique. Infertility 5:15, 1982
4. Daniell JF, Miller JF, Tosh R: Initial evaluation of the use of the potassium-tithanyl-phosphate (KTP-532) laser in gynecologic laparoscopy. Fertil Steril 46:373–377, 1986
5. Dmowski WP, Cohen MR: Treatment of endometriosis with an antigonadotropin, danazol: A laparoscopic and histologic evaluation. Obstet Gynecol 46:147, 1975
6. Dmowski WP, Cohen MR: Antigonadotropin (danazol) in the treatment of endometriosis. Evaluation of post-treatment fertility and three-year follow-up data. Am J Obstet Gynecol 130:41, 1978
7. Feste JR: CO_2 laser neurectomy for dysmenorrhea. Lasers Surg Med 3:27, 1984
8. Hofstetter A: Lasers in urology. Lasers Surg Med 6:412–414, 1986
9. Kelly RW, Roberts DK: CO_2 laser laparoscopy: A potential alternative to danazol in the treatment of Stage I and II endometriosis. J Reprod Med 28:638–640, 1983
10. Keye WR, Matson GA, Dixon J: The use of the argon laser in the treatment of experimental endometriosis. Fertil Steril 39:26–29, 1983
11. Lomano JM: Photocoagulation of early pelvic endometriosis with the Nd:YAG laser through the laparoscope. J Reprod Med 30:77–81, 1985
12. Lomano J: Nd:YAG laser ablation of early pelvic endometriosis: A report of 61 cases. Lasers Surg Med 7:56–60, 1987
13. Martin DC: CO_2 laser laparoscopy for the treatment of endometriosis associated with infertility. J Reprod Med 30:409–412, 1985
14. Naples JD, Batt RE, Sadigh H: Spontaneous abortion rate in patients with endometriosis. Obstet Gynecol 57:409, 1981
15. Seibel MM, Berger MJ, Weinstein F et al: The effectiveness of danazol on subsequent fertility in minimal endometriosis. Fertil Steril (Suppl) 37:310, 1982.

17

Laser Hysteroscopy

William M. Jamieson
Milton H. Goldrath

Hysterectomy is now the most commonly performed major surgical procedure in the United States. During the past decade, 500,000 to 700,000 hysterectomies have been performed annually. Nearly 40% of the hysterectomies performed have been for abnormal uterine bleeding. Almost two billion dollars is spent annually in the United States for hysterectomies and resulting complications. This figure does not include the dollars lost for disability, which affects both the patients and their employers. It is significant that one fourth to one half of the hysterectomies performed are followed by some type of surgical morbidity; more than 600 patients die each year as a direct result of hysterectomies and their complications.[25] These statistics plus the reluctance of many women to have their uterus removed have led many women to seek surgical alternatives to remedy the problem of persistent abnormal menstrual bleeding.

In the not too distant past, it was stated that the hysteroscope was an instrument waiting for an indication. During the past 15 years, hysteroscopy has slowly evolved into a vital diagnostic procedure and has also played a major role in advancing the surgical specialty of gynecology. Like its abdominal counterpart, the laparoscope, the hysteroscope has replaced many procedures that formerly required a major abdominal incision. The advent of surgical laser systems incorporating fiberoptics that could readily be passed through the hysteroscope's operating channel greatly enhanced the quality and expanded the number of surgical procedures that could be performed transcervically in an outpatient surgical setting. In 1981, the first published report, by Goldrath,[12] described the successful use of the neodymium : yttrium-aluminum-garnet laser (Nd : YAG) for ablating the endometrium in women who had intractable menorrhagia. Since that time, numerous investigators have published data demonstrating the value of this technique as an alternative to hysterectomy for selected patients.[6,15,16,20] The effectiveness of the Nd : YAG laser is based on its optical wavelength, 1064 nm, which produces a coagulation tissue effect. This results from nonspecific beam absorption with marked forward scatter on impact. This scattering spreads the beam energy over a much larger tissue area than occurs with other lasers. The result is coagulation, rather than vaporization, which is both uniform and predictable. This effect differs from the temperature isotherms seen with high-frequency electrocautery, which tend to follow paths of least tissue resistance (*e.g.,* nerve fibers and blood vessels).

The safe and predictable effects of the Nd : YAG laser were originally described by two Norwegian urologists, Hofstetter and Frank. In their initial studies performed on bladders, they determined that the temperatures created on the front and back wall of a hollow organ differ depending on the type of laser used. Although the front wall temperatures are roughly the same with the Nd : YAG and the carbon dioxide (CO_2) lasers, the back wall temperatures following the Nd : YAG laser are much higher. Despite the higher powers used with the Nd : YAG laser (40 to 55 watts) as opposed to the CO_2 laser (5 to 10 watts), only a fraction of laser energy is absorbed in the bladder tissue. Most of the energy diffuses backward (30% to 40%) and forward (25% to 30%) as it scatters. The net effect is tissue destruction with minimal risk of hollow viscus perforation. This safe penetration depends on the characteristic scattering of the Nd : YAG beam. As necrosis proceeds, the incident radiation is automatically more strongly rejected by the tissue, and the absorption becomes minimized at the time of mechanical injury of the surface. These characteristics of the Nd : YAG laser thus allow deep tissue necrosis with minimal risk of perforation.

The safe application of the Nd : YAG laser in the human uterus was initially described by Goldrath in his original article.[12] Thermocouples 1 cm below the endometrial surface of an extirpated uterus were placed, and a maximum temperature of 49.9°C was recorded after using a power setting of 55 watts for 5 seconds. Tissue destruction usually does not occur until 55°C, the thinnest portion of the human uterus is 1.5 cm, and circulation in the intact uterus should carry some heat away, resulting in less tissue penetration. The thermal effects and safety of the Nd : YAG laser were further substantiated by Mosely et al, who demonstrated minimal conduction of heat to the serosal surface of the uterus.[19] Thus, uterine perforation or damage to surrounding pelvic structures should be remote following Nd : YAG laser endometrial ablation. Since 1986, the Nd : YAG laser has been approved by the Food and Drug Administration (FDA) for this indication.

PATIENT SELECTION FOR ENDOMETRIAL ABLATION

It is important to select and evaluate patients carefully, as well as to anticipate any technical difficulties. The clinical evaluation of a patient with abnormal uterine bleeding should include a thorough history and pelvic examination followed by endometrial sampling and hysteroscopy examination. Patients should be rejected for Nd : YAG laser endometrial ablation if advanced endometrial hyperplasia or malignancy, acute pelvic inflammatory disease, or large submucous myomas are encountered. Uterine size *per se* should not be a contraindication if the endometrial lining is

TABLE 17–1
Patient Selection for Nd : YAG Laser Endometrial Ablation

1. Debilitating uterine bleeding that is unable to be controlled by nonsurgical means and a desire to retain the uterus
2. A benign endometrial sampling within 1 year of the procedure
3. Does not demand total amenorrhea
4. Does not want to remain fertile
5. Medically or surgically poor candidate for hysterectomy

completely accessible. Candidates for laser ablation should have a history of abnormal menstrual bleeding that is unable to be controlled by more conservative nonsurgical methods. These patients have frequently undergone multiple dilatation and curettages and are either unable or unwilling to control their bleeding hormonally. In the past, these patients could opt for a hysterectomy or live with debilitating bleeding. The Nd : YAG laser now offers these patients a third alternative. It should be strongly emphasized that this procedure should be carried out only for those patients who are candidates for hysterectomy. For a patient who merely wants to stop menstruating, endometrial ablation is not advised. This procedure should not be performed "cosmetically," but it should be offered to those women who for personal or psychological reasons wish to retain the uterus *in situ*.

Patients undergoing endometrial ablation should understand that not all women achieve total amenorrhea. If a patient is unwilling to accept normal or less than normal menstruation (two to four pads per day for 4 days), then she is probably not a good candidate for the procedure. Although patients with pure menorrhagia (more than 30 pads per menses) are probably the best candidates for the procedure, patients with menometrorrhagia may also be treated. It is imperative that patients undergoing endometrial ablation not desire any future childbearing. Although the Nd : YAG laser ablation procedure is not considered a means of sterilization *per se,* it will most likely render patients infertile as a result of scarring. There is one known case of pregnancy following an ablation procedure that rendered the patient totally amenorrheic for 9 months.★

A large number of candidates for the Nd : YAG laser ablation are those patients who are medically or surgically poor candidates for hysterectomy and have debilitating or life-threatening menorrhagia. Patients who have cardiac disease and are taking coumadin, patients with renal disease, and patients who have either blood dyscrasis or clotting disorders would likely benefit from endometrial ablation as opposed to hysterectomy. Massive obesity is not a contraindication to endometrial ablation (Table 17–1).

★ *Shirk G: Personal communication. 1988.*

THE PROCEDURE

The technical concept of endometrial ablation using the Nd:YAG laser is simple. The Nd:YAG laser fiber is passed through the operative channel of a hysteroscope, and the entire endometrium is destroyed under direct vision. However, achieving optimal results can present several technical problems. For 4 to 6 weeks before the endometrial ablation, the endometrium should be suppressed (to less than 1 mm in thickness) using danazol (Danocrine), intranasal synarel (Nafarelin), or leuprolide (Lupron). The procedure may be performed using general anesthesia, regional block, or, in medically compromised patients, paracervical block with light intravenous sedation. If general anesthesia is used, narcotics and nitrous oxide are preferred as opposed to inhalation anesthetics such as enflurane or isoflurane, as these cause uterine relaxation and vasodilation, which could result in fluid overload and pulmonary edema. The anesthesiologist should not preload the patient with intravenous fluids before the procedure, as is often done in routine surgical procedures. The anesthesiologist should particularly note the patient's pulmonary status and periodically auscultate the lungs as well. Proper draping of the patient before the procedure is important in order to account for all the fluid used to distend the uterus (Fig. 17–1). If the draping and fluid retrieval system are inadequate, there is no accurate way to determine the exact amount of fluid absorbed by the patient. The distending medium used may be any balanced salt solution (*e.g.,* lactated Ringer's solution, normal saline) that can be delivered under pressure. These solutions offer excellent visibility, are inexpensive, and are easier to deliver through the hysteroscope than the very viscous dextran 70 (Hyskon). Hyskon may be used, but the total volume infused should be restricted to less than 300 ml to eliminate the possible fluid compli-

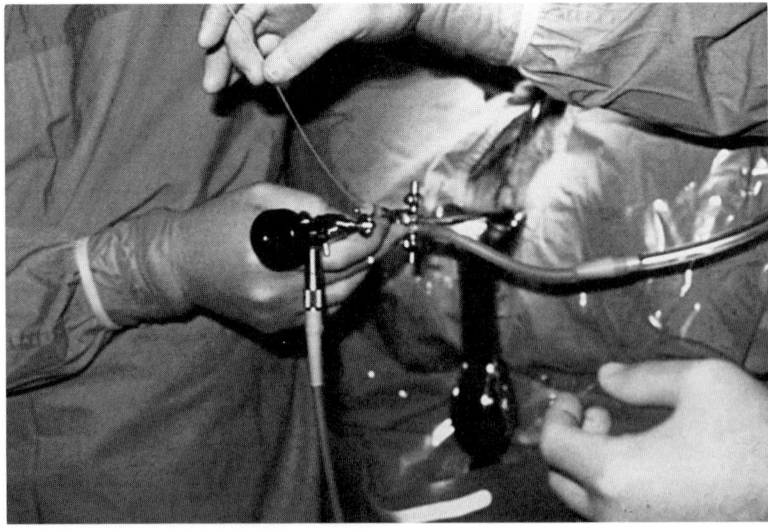

FIGURE 17–1. Proper draping technique is demonstrated, along with the use of the protective eyepiece filter.

cations from dextran overdose. The hypertonicity of dextran 70 enables each milliliter to retain about 3 to 4 ml of body fluid.[18] Fatal anaphalactoid reactions also have been reported with the use of dextran 70. *Under no circumstances should carbon dioxide ever be used as the distending medium during laser hysteroscopy, as fatal air embolism has occurred.*[17]

The procedure may require large volumes of distending medium when using lactated Ringer's or normal saline. This often presents technical problems for maintaining a high-flow system at a constant pressure (75 to 150 mm Hg). Transfusion pump systems or low-pressure nitrogen-powered pneumatic insufflators may be used to pressurize the infusion medium directly and deliver a uniform high-pressure flow.

When actually performing the procedure, the cervix should be grasped with a tenaculum and gently dilated to 9 mm. If perforation of the uterine cavity occurs during cervical dilation or with insertion of the hysteroscope, the procedure should be terminated. Perforation will decrease uterine pressure, and the subsequent lack of uterine distinction will result in poor visibility as well as an increase in peritoneal fluid accumulation. Although the intact thick myometrium is an excellent physical barrier during endometrial ablation, if it is damaged by perforation, possible bowel or bladder injury could result. A perforation should be healed within a week, and the procedure may be rescheduled later.

Using a dual-channel hysteroscope (Fig. 17–2) especially designed for endometrial ablation allows the irrigating fluid to flow freely into and out of the uterus through the hysteroscope while still maintaining adequate uterine distention. After inspection of the atrophic endometrial cavity, a 0.6-mm quartz fiber clad in a 1.1-

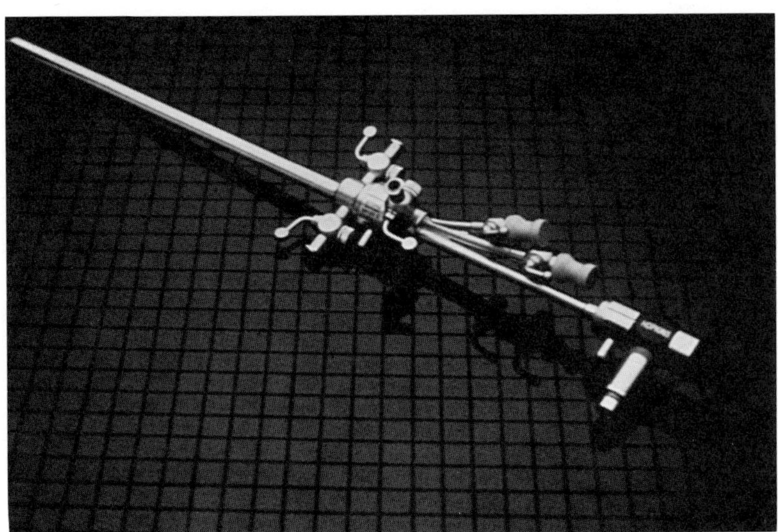

FIGURE 17–2. A dual-channel laser hysteroscope is used to allow adequate circulation inside the uterus to facilitate visualization as the procedure progresses.

mm Teflon sheath is passed through the operating channel of the hysteroscope into the uterus. The distal 5 mm of the Teflon coating should be cleaved before insertion to adequately expose the bare quartz fiber. The protective eyepiece filter should then be placed over the hysteroscope to protect the surgeon's retina from possible Nd:YAG laser backscatter (see Fig. 17–1). Even if the operator prefers to perform the procedure indirectly by means of a video monitor, protective eye wear should be worn in the event of inadvertent breakage of the quartz fiber outside the hysteroscope. Laser power should be set between 40 and 75 watts, depending on the operator's experience. Depth of tissue photocoagulation by the laser depends on wattage and exposure time to that tissue. It is recommended that less-experienced surgeons use lower wattage and that the fiber be dragged across the endometrium more slowly in order to retain adequate control. Beginning at the tubal ostia, the endometrial tissue is systematically destroyed to the juncture of the lower uterine segment and the internal cervical os. Take care to avoid ablating the internal cervical os, which may result in scarring and subsequent hematometra.

Whether to use the contact technique, in which the bare fiber tip actually touches the endometrial surface, or the non-contact technique, in which the fiber is kept 1 to 3 mm away from the surface, is controversial. Many investigators prefer the contact technique, which offers a better rate of amenorrhea and facilitates visualization of tissue destroyed. The white endometrial blanching that occurs with the non-contact technique is very difficult to distinguish from the already white atrophic endometrium following pretreatment administration of hypoestrogenic agents. In contrast, the contact technique displays a predictable charring effect that allows the operator to readily distinguish between the treated and untreated endometrial tissue (Fig. 17–3). The main disadvantage of the contact technique, particularly for patients with compromised cardiac or renal function, is that by opening venous sinusoids directly, there is a greater likelihood of absorption of the distending medium, which may result in fluid overload and pulmonary edema. In a study of 30 patients who underwent Nd:YAG laser endometrial ablation using contact technique, however, Jamieson and Chamberlain found that the average fluid absorbed was 735 cc.[15] In practice, most gynecologists combine both the contact and non-contact techniques. Whenever a patient's intraoperative fluid absorption reaches 2000 ml, the procedure should be terminated and 20 mg of furosemide (Lasix) should be given intravenously. If a patient has normal renal function, this fluid overload is usually self-limiting. Procedure time is directly proportional to the amount of fluid absorption because of an increasing number of venous sinusoids that are opened as the procedure continues. An experienced operator is usually able to complete the Nd:YAG laser endometrial ablation within 30 to 45 minutes, depending on the size of the endometrial cavity. The key is to be aware of the patient's fluid absorption at all times by using a proper draping and fluid retrieval system.

The entire endometrial cavity should be photocoagulated in a systematic fashion until all the surface is charred from the laser carbonization. It is important that the laser be fired *only* when the helium–neon beam is seen and *only* when the fiber is being dragged toward the cervix. It is unsafe to use the Nd:YAG laser if the small 0.6-mm fiber has perforated the uterine wall inadvertently could be laser energy as fired into the peritoneal cavity.

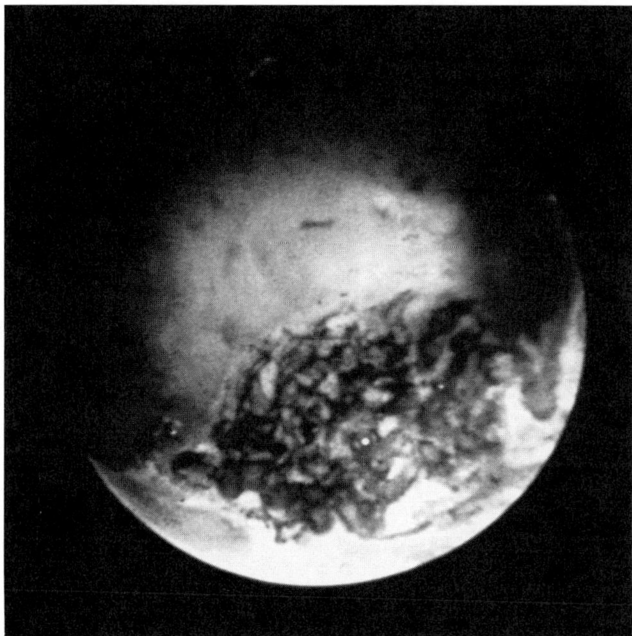

FIGURE 17–3. Endometrial charring is seen on the posterior uterine wall after application of the Nd : YAG laser's energy using the contact technique. The desired atrophic endometrial appearance on the anterior uterine wall is seen after appropriate pretreatment with hypoestrogenic agents.

Results

Total amenorrhea or scant monthly bleeding (fewer than three pads per menses) should be considered excellent results. Flow that requires fewer than 12 pads per menses, although not ideal, should be considered acceptable, if indeed the patient had debilitating menorrhagia. Patients who return to their preoperative bleeding patterns are considered treatment failures. Large series from several investigators show an overall combined success rate of approximately 95% (Table 17–2). At least 80% of treated patients have had excellent results. If poor results follow initial therapy, repeat treatment offers 75% of these patients an eventually excellent result.[10] Most treatment failures are either due to operator error (incomplete ablation of the uterine cavity) or severe adenomyosis, in which the endometrial glands are beyond the penetration of the laser beam. Experience and proper selection of patients should minimize treatment failures. Preoperatively, patients should be informed that the final results of the procedure will not be known for at least 4 months, as Goldrath described continued endometrial scarring for 4 to 12 months after the procedure.[11] In their study of 30 patients, Jamieson and Chamberlain found that 80% of their patients were very satisfied with their results at 6 months.[15]

TABLE 17–2
Percentage of Amenorrhea After Endometrial Ablation Using the Nd : YAG Laser—Summary of Reported Data

REPORT	NO. OF PATIENTS	EXCELLENT	GOOD	POOR	REPEAT
Lomano[17]	10	8 (80%)	2 (20%)	0	0
Daniell et al[6]	18	7 (39%)	7 (39%)	4 (22%)	0
Loffer[16]	33	24 (73%)	7 (21%)	2 (6%)	2
Shirk et al[22]	48	29 (61%)	17 (35%)	2 (4%)	6
Goldrath[12]	216	206 (96%)	3 (1%)	7 (3%)	4
Gimpelson[10]	23	16 (70%)	7 (30%)	0	1
Jamieson[15]	30	24 (80%)	6 (20%)	0	0

Complications

Postoperatively, some patients may experience severe menstrual cramps (Table 17–3), possibly because of the large amounts of prostaglandins released during destruction of the endometrium. Nonsteroidal anti-inflammatory agents usually help control this type of postoperative pain. The majority of patients return home the same day of surgery and return to work within 48 to 72 hours. Patients usually experience a serosanguineous discharge, which at times may be frankly bloody for up to 6 weeks postoperatively. This discharge appears to be secondary to the loss of cellular integrity at the burn site. Some patients may actually have a heavy "menstrual flow" during the immediate postoperative period; it may represent shedding of the original eschar in the uterine cavity. These patients should be reassured that this may not significantly affect the final outcome. Patients should be seen 3 and 12 weeks postoperatively. At those visits, the cervical canal should be probed to ensure cervical patency in order to avoid cervical stenosis, which could result in a later hematome-

TABLE 17–3
Complications of Endometrial Ablation Using the Nd : YAG Laser

1. Severe postoperative cramping
2. Postoperative hemorrhage (immediate or delayed) that may require hysterectomy
3. Hematometra
4. Endometritis or acute pelvic inflammatory disease
5. Delay in diagnosing a future carcinoma of the uterus
6. Thermal injury to bowel or bladder

tra. Even if the patient reports "bloody drainage," it is imperative to dilate the cervix to ensure adequate patency. To date there have been no reported cases of endometritis or acute pelvic inflammatory disease following endometrial ablation, but this complication is certainly possible. Prophylactic antibiotics are usually not employed at the present time.

The Nd:YAG laser ablation procedure has been criticized for possibly masking a future underlying carcinoma of the endometrium. Theoretically, if the resultant scarring were to block off a portion of still functioning endometrium, which could become malignant at a later time, the abnormal egress of blood would be delayed. This could result in a more advanced stage of carcinoma at the time of detection. There has never been a suggestion that the laser light *per se* causes cancer, however.

For the past 10 years during which this procedure has been performed, there have been no reported cases of carcinoma of the endometrium following Nd:YAG laser endometrial ablation. Uterine biopsy specimens have uniformly shown necrotic myometrium up to 4 months postoperatively. The tissue shows little inflammatory reaction other than foreign body giant cells surrounding carbon particles. After 5 months, only minute normal endometrial fragments are seen in occasional patients.

Pathological examination of uteri following hysterectomy in women who had previously undergone endometrial ablation has shown a single layer of cuboidal epithelium with ciliated and brush borders. Cytogenic stroma was sparse, and only rare endometrial glands were present. The epithelium contained only minimal hemosiderin and virtually no evidence of functioning endometrium.[11] Additionally, scarring following endometrial ablation occurs from outside in, usually resulting in a patent channel for egress of blood and endometrial debris. A patient who has undergone an endometrial ablation may eventually develop endometrial cancer. By virtue of the very types of patients who are referred for the procedure (obese, hypertensive, anovulatory women), this patient population is statistically at even greater risk than the general population.

Accidental thermal injury to bowel or bladder following Nd:YAG endometrial ablation has been reported, with at least one fatality encountered.[17] With proper training, technique, and observation of common safeguards, this severe complication should not occur.

Conclusion

Hysteroscopic Nd:YAG laser endometrial ablation has become a safe, cost-effective alternative to hysterectomy (Table 17–4). It behooves gynecologists to realize that today's modern women, who often have many career and family responsibilities, cannot afford the disability associated with a hysterectomy. If a simpler procedure may be used to accomplish the same results but with less morbidity, then it should be made available to the patients who are appropriate candidates. Contemporary gynecologists should become increasingly more aware that many women wish to avoid hysterectomy for a multitude of reasons and yet attain relief from debilitating menorrhagia. Endometrial ablation using the Nd:YAG laser offers these women a reasonable option.

TABLE 17–4
**Advantages of Nd : YAG Laser
Endometrial Ablation Versus
Hysterectomy**

1. Same-day surgery
2. Patient returns to work in 48 to 72 hours
3. Shorter surgical operating time
4. Less bleeding
5. Less postoperative infection
6. Lower cost
7. Patient retains her uterus

HYSTEROSCOPIC METROPLASTY

The uterus, cervix, and upper third of the vagina in the embryo develop from fusion of two lateral müllerian ducts. In the majority of women, the medial aspects of these ducts are absorbed and a single uterine cavity, cervix, and upper third of the vagina result. However, lack of medial absorption accounts for a persistent septum, which occurs in approximately 1% to 3.5% of women. Although its actual incidence is unknown, this anomaly is probably even higher secondary to the large number of female offspring exposed to diethylstilbestrol (DES). From the late 1940s until 1971, an estimated 2 to 3 million women received DES during their pregnancies, exposing 1 to 1.5 million female progeny to the drug *in utero*.[1] Although many other congenital reproductive anomalies are described in the gynecological literature, the persistent uterine septum is the most interesting because of its known association with increased spontaneous abortion, premature labor, and fetal malpresentation.

The first reported excision of a uterine septum was performed in 1882 by Ruge; the patient, who had had two previous miscarriages, subsequently delivered at term. Strassmann in 1907 perfected the reunification procedure that today bears his name.[21] The first transcervical incision of a uterine septum was reported in 1919, when Hirsh removed a large uterine septum by dilating the cervix to 4 cm and manually cut the septum with scissors. The patient subsequently delivered a term infant. Luikart, in 1936, also reported a similar successful procedure performed vaginally. Despite these early successes, the abdominal removal of these septa remained popular for the next four decades.[21] Both the Jones procedure of resecting the septum and the Tompkins procedure of incisional metroplasty have been uniformly successful. Because of the potential morbidity of the transabdominal approach, there has been a renewed interest in the transcervical approach to treat this disorder. In 1974, Edstrom[9] first reported incising a septum using a hysteroscope; other investigators, using scissors or electrocautery, also reported successful outcomes with less surgical morbidity than with the abdominal approach.[2,4,5,8,14,16,23]

Transcervical metroplasty had its own inherent set of problems. Resecting with scissors either with or without injected vasopressin (Pitressin) was often bloody, and visualization was often impaired. When electrocautery was used, hemostasis was maintained, but the degree of thermal damage was both unpredictable and potentially hazardous. For these reasons, Goldrath[11] first reported the use of the Nd:YAG laser to remove a uterine septum hysteroscopically. Because the laser coagulated as it cut, a virtually bloodless field was maintained.

Patient Selection

Patients who are known to have a uterine septum and a history of repeated spontaneous abortions or premature labor are candidates for this procedure. Patients with a history of recurrent abortion should have a thorough evaluation to rule out other known causes of habitual abortion before surgical intervention. Removal of an asymptomatic uterine septum in a nulliparous woman at this time is probably unwarranted except for unique or exceptional circumstances, which will be discussed later.

Hysteroscopic procedures should be scheduled either in the very early proliferative phase of the menstrual cycle or after pretreatment with danazol or a gonadotropin agonist. Minimal endometrial buildup and maximal hysteroscopic visibility are thus ensured.

The Procedure

Laser hysteroscopic metroplasties should be performed in coordination with direct laparoscopic vision to ensure that the uterine anomaly is not a bicornuate uterus. Direct vision also helps control the uniform depth of the laser's incision of the septum at the uterine fundus. As the laser light passes transversely across the uterine fundus, the light of the helium–neon beam can easily be seen. The uniform transmission of hysteroscopic laser light ensures the proper depth of incision into the uterine fundus, facilitating more complete resection of even a very broad-based septum, which is very difficult to complete with scissors.

To initiate the procedure, the hysteroscope is passed through the cervix into the uterine cavity and the distention medium is infused. The laser fiber is passed through the operative channel of the hysteroscope. The entire uterine cavity should be visualized in both cornua, as both tubal ostia should be clearly and definitely seen before starting the laser metroplasty. Avoidance of these ostia with the laser energy is critical, because these patients wish to preserve their fertility. The septum should be delineated in its entirety. The procedure is best begun at the proximal tip of the septum. When using the argon or KTP laser, the wattage should be set at 10 watts, and when using the Nd:YAG laser, it should be set at 40 watts. If using the Nd:YAG laser with contact tips, the wattage should be lowered to 15 watts. It is important to incise the septum in its midline throughout the procedure. This plane is virtually bloodless when using the laser, and damage to the surrounding myometrium is avoided. The operator must keep the uterine orientation (anteverted, retroverted) in mind at all times in order to maintain this midline incision of the septum. As the septum is divided in this transverse manner, the uterine walls progressively distend and the wider cavity helps maintain proper orientation. The incision is carried to within 1 cm of each tubal ostium. Should bleeding occur, it is usually a

TABLE 17–5
**Results of Hysteroscopic Laser
Vaporization of Uterine Septa***

Patients treated	18
Attempting to conceive	14
Conceived	11
Delivered	10
Aborted	1

** San Filippo J: Gynecologic endoscopy and pelviscopic surgery and laser laparoscopy. Personal communication, 1988*

sign that the base of the septum has been reached, and further resection is unneeded. At this point, the laparoscopic observer should see a uniform light source as the laser is moved transversely from the uterine cornu to cornu. The hysteroscopic surgeon also should see both tubal ostia in one panoramic view when the hysteroscope is positioned at the level of the internal cervical os. The procedure should be terminated at this point. The operation usually takes about 15 minutes to perform. The placement of an intrauterine device and postoperative antibiotics are not needed. These patients should be placed on cyclic high-dose estrogen and progestin therapy for 2 months postoperatively. Conception should be delayed at least 3 months to allow for endometrial regeneration.

Results

Hysteroscopic metroplasty results published by Daly and colleagues[3] using excisional laser techniques with a 6-year follow-up, showed a term pregnancy rate of 92% and normal fecundity consistent with the normal fertile population. They also found an overall cost savings of 45% with hysteroscopic metroplasty, taking into account the cost of the initial procedure as well as the cost savings of a subsequent vaginal delivery. San Filippo reported equally good results (Table 17–5).*

Conclusion

Hysteroscopic metroplasty has become the preferred method for removing a uterine septum. The advantages are numerous (Table 17–6). The minimal morbidity along with the cost-effectiveness of this procedure might indicate its future use as a prophylactic procedure to minimize the risk and cost of early pregnancy loss and premature delivery. Of particular interest would be those infertile patients who are known to have a uterine septum and who are candidates for *in vitro* fertilization or gamete intrafallopian transfer. It could be strongly argued that these patients should

---

* *San Filippo J: Gynecologic endoscopy and pelviscopic surgery and laser laparoscopy. Personal communication, 1988.*

TABLE 17–6
**Advantages of Hysteroscopic Metroplasty
versus Abdominal Metroplasty Procedures**

1. Outpatient procedure
2. Less surgical morbidity
3. Less adhesion formation
4. Less cost to patient and third-party payers
5. Less blood loss (<30 ml vs. >400 ml)
6. Less operating time (about 30 minutes vs. >1 hour)
7. Less disability and time away from work (2 days vs. 4–6 weeks)
8. No need for cesarean section with subsequent pregnancies

undergo hysteroscopic metroplasty to avoid possible miscarriage or premature birth. It remains controversial whether the procedure increases pregnancy rates in unexplained infertility. Within the past 10 years, hysteroscopic metroplasty has become the procedure of choice for treating uterine and cervical septa. It is hoped that as laser and endoscopic technology becomes more sophisticated, gynecologists will be further stimulated to use hysteroscopic laser metroplasty to treat more effectively their patients who have a uterine septum.

HYSTEROSCOPIC RESECTION OF SUBMUCOSAL LEIOMYOMAS AND ENDOMETRIAL ABLATION USING ELECTROCAUTERY

A major disadvantage of the hysteroscopic use of the Nd:YAG laser is the presence of large submucosal myomas that obstruct the endometrial cavity. Small, pedunculated myomas may often be removed hysteroscopically with the laser. The larger, broad-based myomas are very difficult to excise with the laser, however, as their physical size makes it impossible for the laser fiber to make contact with the entire endometrial surface. Because the tissue effect of the laser's energy is so precise, it is virtually impossible to destroy or coagulate the entire obstructing myoma. Therefore, large submucosal fibroids are a relative contraindication to using the Nd:YAG laser for endometrial ablation. However, using electrocautery and a resectoscope, these submucosal myomas may be removed simply and safely. If the patient does not wish to remain fertile, endometrial ablation may also be performed simultaneously.

In 1927, von Mikuliez–Radecki and Freund performed the first intrauterine electrocoagulation,[24] but the electric cutting loop was not used until 1957, by Norment and colleagues.[19] In 1976, Neuwirth first described hysteroscopic resection of submucosal leiomyomata, and 7 years later, he reported 28 patients who were treated in this manner.[18]

Patient Selection

The surgical candidate should have a history of persistent menorrhagia, recurrent pregnancy loss, or infertility and should obviously desire to retain her uterus. The first criterion for hysteroscopic resection of myoma is confirmation of a submucosal myoma by direct hysteroscopic observation. Hysterosalpingograms most often result in false-positive filling defects and should not be used alone to establish the diagnosis of submucosal myoma. As many gynecologists know, a blind dilatation and curettage often misses a large myoma because the curette can easily glide over the myoma on its pedunculated stalk. Diagnostic accuracy is greatly increased by direct visualization through a hysteroscope.

Contraindications to the procedure include endometrial hyperplasia, gynecologic malignancy, or acute pelvic inflammatory disease. The patient should accept the fact that if complications should occur, a hysterectomy may be required. As with the Nd : YAG laser ablation procedure, uterine size is only a relative contraindication to the resection procedure. It seems appropriate to consider hysteroscopic myoma resection because of its lower morbidity than to perform a hysterectomy in a medically compromised patient. For healthy patients who also have other pelvic pathology in addition to submucous myoma, hysterectomy may be more appropriate.

Instruments and Equipment

Hysteroscopic equipment used for resection of intrauterine myoma is similar to the standard operative hysteroscope, but there are also marked differences. The continuous-irrigation hysteroscope is made of four integrated working components. First, the innermost working element is the zero-degree telescope. This differs optically from the 30-degree scope that most hysteroscopists use when performing their operative or laser surgery through the hysteroscope. This "direct-vision" scope changes an operator's orientation from the familiar intrauterine view and requires some additional practice to master. The next outer sheath is the retractable electric loop system, which is the main working element of the instrument. Pushing the hand-held thumb loop forward extends the electric wire into the uterine cavity while allowing the hysteroscope itself to remain stationary. Releasing the thumb apparatus retracts the curved wire loop and allows cutting of the myomatous tissue. Outside of this component is the first sheath for the inflow of liquid, and finally a second concentric sheath for the fluid outflow (Fig. 17–4).

It is preferred to use a high-pressure insufflation pump to keep the uterine cavity distended during the procedure. The high pressure provides a tamponading effect that reduces intraoperative bleeding, and the constant closed-irrigation system provides excellent visibility during the resection.

The fluids used are most often isotonic sterile glycine (1.5%) and sorbitol. Dextran 70 may be used, but its potential complications when used under pressure must be kept in mind. Under no circumstances should any balanced salt solution (lactated Ringer's solution, normal saline) be used with electrocautery. The cautery

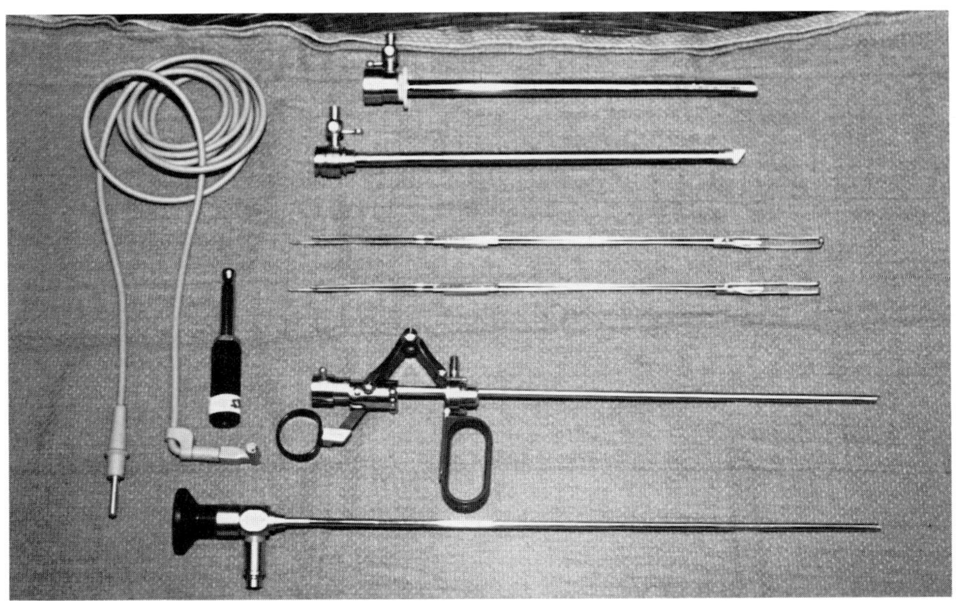

FIGURE 17–4. Components of a hysteroscopic resectoscope.

will not work correctly, and these solutions could cause potentially severe electrical shock or burns to the patient and operating room personnel. Again, the patient should be draped in a manner that allows retrieval of all irrigating fluid. It is important to know the amount of fluid that the patient has absorbed during the procedure in order to avoid complications from fluid overload. The unipolar cautery used should have a blend mode in addition to the cut and coagulate modes. As always, patients should be grounded before using unipolar cautery.

Procedure

For the best results, the procedure should be scheduled in the early proliferative phase or the patient should be pretreated with danazol or a gonadotropin agonist for 4 weeks. Either general or regional anesthesia may be used. If a patient is a poor surgical risk, paracervical block may be advisable. The endocervical canal is dilated to 10 mm, and the hysteroscope is passed gently into the endometrial cavity. There should be some egress of fluid flow around the outer sheath of the scope, but not so much as to decrease the distention of the uterine cavity. Inspection of the endometrial cavity should delineate the extent of the myoma. Further inspection should reveal any large vessels, which often envelope a solitary myoma; selective coagulation of these vessels should be performed in order to decrease the bleeding that may be encountered during the actual resection. Finally, methodic electroresection is performed either during direct vision or indirectly by the television monitor by moving the mobile electric cutting loop back and forth in order to remove the entire myoma "chip by chip." Forty to 120 watts of electric current has been used. If the myoma is attached by a narrow, pedunculated stalk, take care to leave it on the stalk until the end of the procedure. If the myoma is prematurely excised from its base before adequate resection is accomplished, the procedure is complicated by the lack of a stable base from which to shave off the remaining myoma. An operator must then "bob for apples" while trying to stabilize the myoma in the fluid-filled uterus and resect it at the same time. As the chips accumulate, the hysteroscope should be withdrawn and the uterine cavity explored with ovum forceps to remove them. Once the cavity is cleared of the myomatous debris, the scope is reinserted into the uterus and the procedure is continued until the cavity is emptied. It is not imperative to remove the entire myomatous base if it extends deeply into the uterine musculature. Submucosal fibroids cause bleeding because the endometrial stroma is lost and the mucosal epithelium lies stretched over the myoma. After the myoma is removed to the plane of the uterine cavity, the mucosa should regenerate over the site, and normal menstrual function often returns.[18]

Operating times vary with the size of the myoma, but most surgeons need less than 1 hour. If patient desires normal menstrual function or fertility, cyclic estrogen and progesterone should be prescribed for 2 months postoperatively to facilitate endometrial regeneration over the resection site. If a patient does not wish normal menstruation or is beyond her reproductive years, then electrocoagulative ablation of the remaining endometrial cavity should be discussed preoperatively.

Potential Complications

As with the Nd : YAG endometrial ablation, fluid overload may be encountered if one is not careful. Draping of the patient must be meticulous in order to retrieve fluid and accurately measure the amount. The anesthesiologist must be able to recognize signs of impending pulmonary edema if dextran 70 is used, and signs of hyponatremia if an isotonic solution such as glycine or sorbitol is used. The anesthesiologist may prefer regional anesthesia when glycine is being used so that early signs of water intoxication may be observed (Table 17–7). Electrolytes should be checked if more than 500 ml are absorbed.

Hemorrhage is a potential complication but most often may be controlled by using further electrocoagulation or by tamponading the endometrium with a 30-ml

TABLE 17–7
Progressive Signs of Water Intoxication

1. Hypertension
2. Bradycardia
3. Restlessness
4. Confusion
5. Pulmonary congestion
6. Vascular collapse
7. Seizures
8. Hyponatremia or hypokalemia

Foley bulb inserted into the endometrial cavity. If bleeding cannot be controlled by these conservative measures, hysterectomy may be required.

Inadvertent cauterization of pelvic viscera is a potentially devastating complication following this procedure. Although the cutting current's depth of destruction is limited, the use of the coagulation current presents a different dilemma. No studies to date have shown what depth of electrical burn is seen with the various wattages used during hysteroscopic electrocautery surgery. For this reason, great care must be used with this instrument. Concomitant use of the laparoscope would be of little value in avoiding a bowel burn with delayed necrosis. Pneumoperitoneum or flooding of the pelvis with cool liquid may possibly prevent this potential complication. Until studies of extirpated uteri are carried out to show the depth of cauterization following the use of various wattages and time exposures, great care must be taken when performing a hysteroscopic myoma resection. This procedure should be abandoned if a uterine perforation is encountered. The foot pedal should not be depressed if visibility is poor or if the loop cannot be completely visualized. Prophylactic antibiotics are not needed after the procedure because endometritis and postoperative pelvic inflammatory disease have yet to be reported.

Results

Most investigators have consistently found this procedure to be safe and to have predictable results. In 1983, Neuwirth published results of 28 patients: 17 returned to normal menstruation, and 8 conceived.[18] Hallez and colleagues[13] reported normal menses in 30 of 32 patients. Secondary dysmenorrhea disappeared in 6 of 7 women, and 7 of 11 patients conceived with no evidence of placenta accreta. Most patients are discharged from the outpatient facility the same day and may return to work in 48 hours. Menstruation usually returns to normal.

Hysteroscopic Endometrial Electroablation

In 1987, DeCherney and associates[7] first reported the use of electrocautery delivered through the hysteroscope for ablation of the endometrium. All the patients were medically compromised, and excellent results showing total amenorrhea in 6 months for 18 of 19 patients were described. Their technique involved using the same electrical loop selected for resecting myoma and ablating the entire endometrial surface using 30 watts of coagulation current. The average operating time was 15 to 30 minutes.

Other investigators[22,26] have modified this technique using the "roller-ball cautery." The difference between this and the electrical loop is a wider zone of coagulation and easier passage of the loop over the endometrial cavity (see Fig. 7–8). The technique of roller-ball ablation is similar to that using the loop electrocautery for submucosal myoma resection. The hysteroscope is passed to a stationary point in the uterine cavity. The roller-ball apparatus is controlled by the operator's thumb into all areas of the endometrial cavity, beginning first with each tubal ostium. Thirty to 120 watts has been used; some investigators use a blend mode, and others have used pure coagulation. Vancaillie is recommended using a maximum of 80 watts at a rollerball speed of 1 cm/second. The visual effect of cauterization is not as readily apparent as that seen with the Nd : YAG laser; therefore, more than one pass is often made on the endometrial surface. The internal cervical os should not be cauterized. Fluid absorption should be accurately measured at all times during the procedure because of the risk of fluid overload. Townsend[22] has reported complete amenorrhea in 67% of his treated patients.

This procedure has become popular as another alternative to using the Nd : YAG laser for ablating the endometrium. The main advantage for considering electrocautery over the Nd : YAG laser is cost. Very few smaller hospitals are willing to spend $100,000 for a piece of laser equipment that may only be occasionally used. The cost of the hysteroscopic electrocautery unit is indeed much less. Another advantage of the roller-ball electroablation is that its wider coagulating base allows surgeons to ablate larger uterine cavities in shorter periods of time. Although safety and predictable penetration for the Nd : YAG laser have been well established, such safety has not been conclusively demonstrated for hysteroscopic electrocautery. Until such safety standards are met and appropriate laboratory and clinical safety trials are undertaken, caution should be exercised by any gynecologist who may use this device. Additionally, when using isotonic solutions for uterine distention, hyponatremia and water intoxication have been reported.[18] This potential fatal complication is not nearly as recognizable and treatable as pulmonary edema, which may be encountered with Nd : YAG laser ablation. Finally, from a technical standpoint, the wider base of the roller-ball apparatus sometimes makes it difficult to ablate the cornual areas of the uterus adequately.

The future of the ablation procedure and the possibility of 100% amenorrhea in nearly all treated patients may lie in combining the Nd : YAG laser and the roller-ball cautery techniques. The Nd : YAG laser could be used for the more inaccessible areas and the roller ball for more general "cleanup" of the entire cavity. This combined technique would markedly reduce the exposure time of the roller-ball cautery on the endometrial surface, thereby possibly improving its safety. At the same time, it would readily coagulate small areas of the endometrium that may have been missed by the small fiber of the Nd : YAG laser. Perhaps the two techniques—roller ball and Nd : YAG laser—can be melded in much the same way that pelviscopy and laparoscopic laser surgery have been. Both technologies have advantages, and it may be time to use the advantages of each to treat patients more safely and effectively.

REFERENCES

1. Buttrum VC, Reiter RC: Surgical Treatment of the Infertile Female, 1st ed, p 153. Baltimore, Williams & Wilkins, 1985
2. Chervenak FA, Neuwirth RS: Hysteroscopic resection of uterine septum. Am J Obstet Gynecol 141:351, 1981
3. Daly DC, Maier D, Soto-Albors C: Hysteroscopic metroplasty: Six years' experience. Am J Obstet Gynecol 73:201, 1989
4. Daly DC, Tohan N, Walters CA et al: Hysteroscopic resection of the uterine septum in the presence of a septate cervix. Fertil Steril 39:560, 1983
5. Daly C, Walters CA, Soto-Albors CE et al: Hysteroscopic metroplasty: Surgical techniques and obstetric outcome. Fertil Steril 39:623, 1983
6. Daniell J, Tosh R, Meisels S: Photodynamic ablation of the endometrium with the Nd : YAG laser hysteroscopically as a treatment of menorrhagia. Colpo Gynecol Laser Surg 2:43, 1988

7. DeCherney A, Diamond M, Lavy G et al: Endometrial ablation for intractable uterine bleeding: hysteroscopic resection. Obstet Gynecol 70:668, 1987
8. DeCherney A, Polan ML: Hysteroscopic management of intrauterine lesions and intractable uterine bleeding. Obstet Gynecol 61:392, 1983
9. Edstrom KG: Intrauterine surgical procedures during hysteroscopy. Endoscopy 6:175, 1974
10. Gimpelson RJ: Hysteroscopic Nd:YAG laser ablation endometrium. J Reprod Med 33:872, 1988
11. Goldrath MH: Hysteroscopic laser surgery. In Baggish MS (ed): Basic and Advanced Laser Surgery in Gynecology, ed 1, p 357. Norwalk, Appleton-Century-Crofts, 1985
12. Goldrath MH, Fuller T, Segal S: Laser photovaporization of endometrium for the treatment of menorrhagia. Am J Obstet Gynecol 140:14, 1981
13. Hallez JP, Netter A, Cartier R: Methodical intrauterine resection. Am J Obstet Gynecol 156:1080, 1987
14. Israel R, March CM: Hysteroscopic treatment of the septate uterus. Am J Obstet Gynecol 67:253, 1986
15. Jamieson WM, Chamberlain JA: Patient response to endometrial ablation with the Nd:YAG laser. Las Surg Med 7:37–42, 1989
16. Loffer RD: Hysteroscopic endometrial ablation with the Nd:YAG laser using a non-touch technique. Obstet Gynecol 69:679, 1987
17. Lomano JM: Photocoagulation of the endometrium with the Nd:YAG laser for the treatment of menorrhagia: A report of ten cases. J Reprod Med 31:148, 1986
18. McLaughlin DS: Complications of laser endoscopy. In Baggish MS (ed): Laser Endoscopy, ed 1. New York, Elsevier-Dutton, 1990
19. Mosely H, Morris JD, McLeod PW et al: Thermal effects of intrauterine Nd:YAG laser endometrial ablation. Lasers Med Sci 2:77–82, 1987
20. Neuwirth RS: Hysteroscopic management of symptomatic submucous fibroids. Obstet Gynecol 62:509, 1983
21. Norment WB, Sikes CH, Berry FX et al: Hysteroscopy. Surg Clin North Am 37:1377, 1957
22. Shirk GD, Ostergard D, Everett R et al: A multicenter investigation of hysteroscopic endometrial ablation using the Nd:YAG laser. Presented at the Third World Congress on Hysteroscopy, Miami, Florida, 1987
23. Te Linde RW, Mattingly RF: Operative Gynecology, 4th ed, pp 281–282. Philadelphia, JB Lippincott, 1970
24. Townsend DE: A new technique for ablating the endometrium. Contemp Obstet Gynecol 34:90, 1989
25. Valle RF, Sciarra JJ: Hysteroscopic treatment of the septate uterus. Am J Obstet Gynecol 61:392, 1983
26. Vancaillie TG: Electrocoagulation of the endometrium with the ball-end resectoscope. Obstet Gynecol 74:425, 1989
27. Van Mikulicz-Radecki F, Freund A: Ein neues hysteroskop und seine praktische anwendung in der gynakologi. Z Geburtshilfe Gynaekol 92:13, 1927
28. Wingo PA, Huezo CH, Rubin GL: The mortality risk associated with hysterectomy. Am J Obstet Gynecol 152:803, 1985

Part Four

CURRENT CONTROVERSIES

18

Photodynamic Therapy

Rocco V. Lobraico
Leonard I. Grossweiner

Photodynamic therapy (PDT) is an experimental cancer treatment based on the combined action of light and a drug that localizes selectively in tumor tissue. The evolution of PDT can be traced to its beginnings early in this century, when biologic reactions in the presence of oxygen were induced by adding a dye and illuminating with visible light.[24] This process was termed *photodynamic action.*[28] Early efforts to treat tumors with topical dyes and sunlight were unsuccessful because of inadequate dye uptake and insufficient illumination.

In the 1920s, researchers noted that tumor cells emit a reddish fluorescence when exposed to near-ultraviolet or "black light." This light emission was identified with the presence of endogeneous porphyrins.[23] Later studies demonstrated that fluorescent tumors are susceptible to destruction by light.[2]

Hematoporphyrin derivative (HPD) was the first effective PDT drug. The drug[6] is a reaction product of crude bovine hematoporphyrin. A chromatographic analysis of HPD showed that it is a mixture of metal-free porphyrins, one constituent of which is responsible for its useful properties.[29] The tumor-localizing affinity of HPD after intravenous injection was first demonstrated by Lipson in 1961.[17] Photosensitization of tumor destruction by HPD was first reported in human subjects in 1978.[7]

A more refined product of HPD is dihematoporphyrin ether (DHE). This component has been tentatively identified as a covalent dimer or small oligomer of porphyrin units. The exact composition of DHE has yet to be unambiguously established. It tends to bind to plasma lipoprotein with a distribution *in vivo* consistent with a low-density lipoprotein.[14] Recent trials have shown that other synthetic porphyrins such as phthalocyanins, naphthalocyanins, chlorins, and purpurines are tumor localizing and photosensitizing.[11,33] Only Photofrin II★ (DHE) is approved in the United States by the Food and Drug Administration.

The putative mechanism in PDT involves a photodynamic action that leads to the formation of singlet molecular oxygen by efficient energy transfer from the optically generated DHE triplet state. Singlet oxygen is an unstable species that oxidizes biomembranes and is toxic to cells.[26] The specific PDT targets have been tentatively identified as mitochondrial membranes of cancer cells,[12] fibroblasts, elastic fibers, and the endothelial cells lining the tumor microvasculature.[5,22] Although a low concentration of DHE accumulates in endothelial cells, they exhibit a high degree of photosensitivity. The action mechanism in PDT differs from x-ray and cobalt-60 gamma ray therapy in which damage to chromosomal DNA inhibits tumor cell growth. This may explain why PDT is repeatable and does not interfere with radiation therapy.

METHODS OF USE

PDT has been used effectively for recurrent squamous cell carcinoma of the oral cavity,[15] skin metastasis from breast cancer,[30] basal cell carcinoma of the skin,[31] transitional cell carcinoma of the bladder,[16] and recurrent superficial gynecologic cancer.[18] It is palliative by destroying obstructive lesions in clinically advanced malignant lesions of the esophagus[21] and bronchus.[3] It has recently been found to be effective when used to treat carcinoma *in situ* or early invasion.

The affinity of porphyrins and metalloporphyrins for neoplastic, embryonic, and traumatized tissue enables treatment to be concentrated at the tumor site.[9] Red light at 630 nm is used to optimize tissue penetration and light absorption by DHE in order to initiate the photochemical reaction (Fig. 18–1). A tunable argon–pumped dye laser is the usual light source, although other light sources are practical, including arc lamps, projection lamps, copper vapor laser, and a pulsed gold vapor laser at 628 nm.[27]

The light dose depends on the geometry of the tumor and the methods of light delivery. A quartz optical fiber with a microlens at its tip delivers a uniform beam in a conical shape. For front-surface illumination, the fiber tip is suspended above the vulvar perineal and perianal regions (Fig. 18–2). To enable the conical beam to conform to the size of the treatment area, the fiber tip is moved nearer to or farther away from the tissue surface. Deeper lesions are treated by inserting an interstitial optical fiber with its cladding removed 5 to 20 mm from the termination (Fig. 18–3). Intracavitary tumors can be reached by extending the optical fiber through an endoscope or a transparent glass tube for vaginal PDT (Figs. 18–4 and 18–5). The quartz optical fiber used in endoscopy is prepared in the same way as the interstitial fiber to give a cylindrical diffusion of light. It is essential that every part of the tumor receive at least the threshold light dose required for tumor eradication.[13]

★ *Product of Quadra Logic Technology, Vancouver, British Columbia, Canada.*

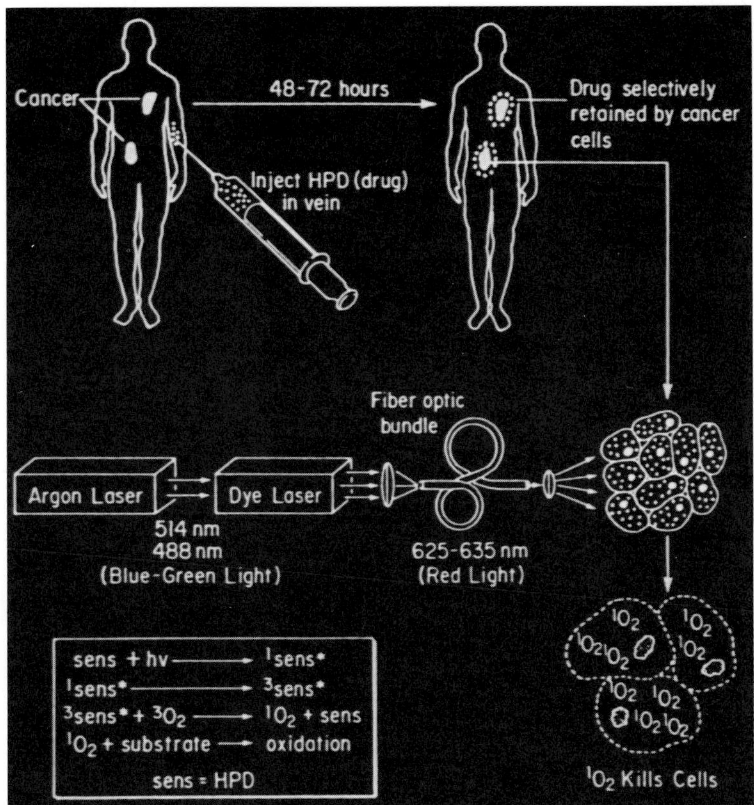

FIGURE 18–1. Schematic representation of PDT procedure. The putative action mechanism involves the generation of singlet molecular oxygen ($^1O_2$) by the combined action of light and HPD or DHE localized in the tumor and its attack on tumor tissue membranes. The molecular reactions are indicated in the box at the lower left. Likely targets of $^1O_2$ include the plasma membranes, the mitochondrial membranes of cancer cells, and the endothelial cells lining the tumor tissue microvasculature.

TREATMENT

Prerequisites for PDT require ruling out renal or hepatic impairment because DHE is metabolized by the liver and excreted by the kidneys. Other factors to be excluded are evidence of bone marrow depression, known hypersensitivity to porphyrins, and pregnancy.

After patient selection complies to protocol, an intravenous injection of 2.0 to 2.5 mg/kg of body weight of DHE is administered. A few hours later, the lesion is illuminated with a bank of black–light fluorescent lamps. A salmon-colored fluorescence appears, revealing the entire extent of the lesion. Visualization of the fluorescence requires accommodation to a darkened room and is enhanced by wearing amber goggles. Careful examination of these fluorescent areas before light treatment

(text continued on page 270)

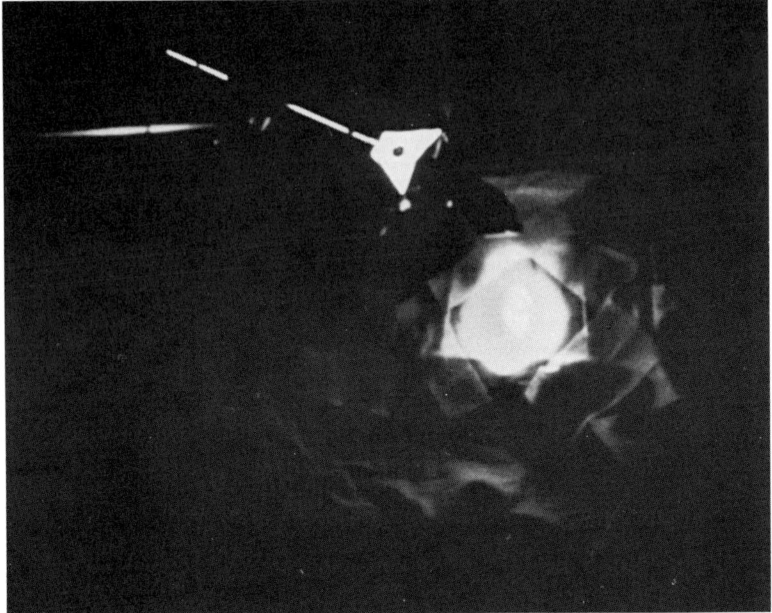

FIGURE 18–2. Delivery of PDT light to the vulva with a microlens fiber. The treatment area is defined by the distance from the fiber tip to the tumor surface and masking.

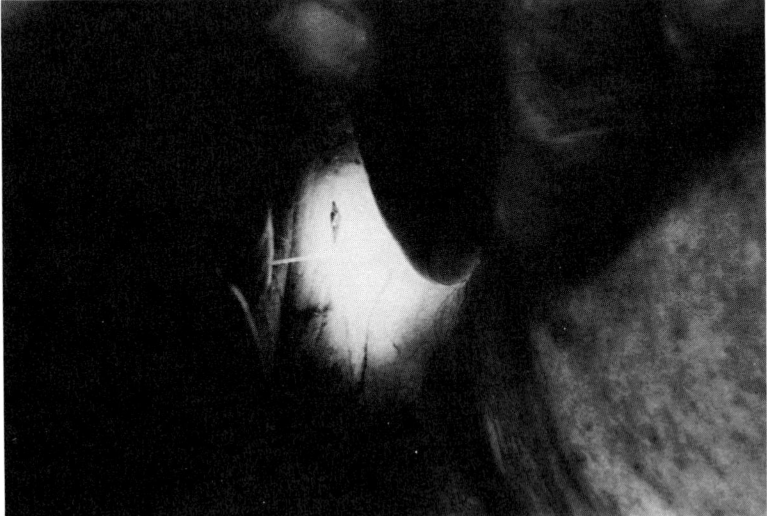

FIGURE 18–3. Treatment of a tumor extending into the perianal region with a cylindrical tip interstitial fiber. The effective treatment field is determined by the tip length and the extension of light from the tip into the tumor tissue. Several insertions may be required for large tumor masses. Interstitial delivery may be preceded by front surface delivery with a microlens fiber.

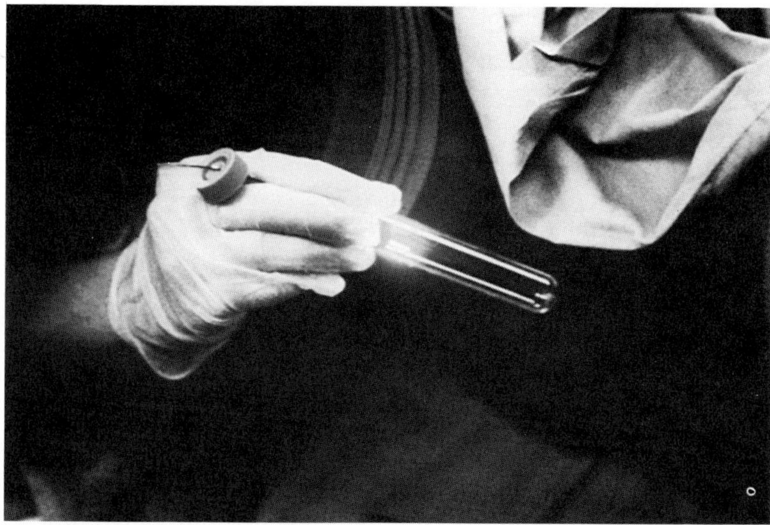

FIGURE 18–4. Carcinoma *in situ* of the vaginal epithelium is treated with a cylindrical tip fiber centered in a glass tube.

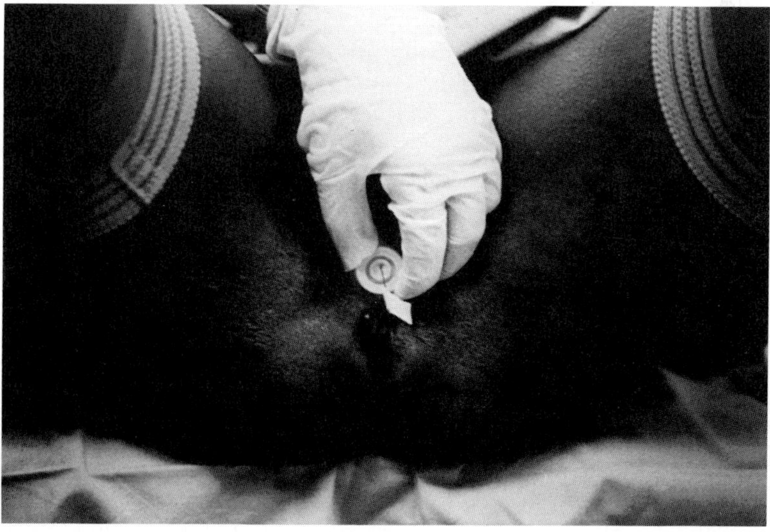

FIGURE 18–5. PDT of the vagina after insertion of the glass tube fiber holder.

aids in the delineation or measure of irregular tumor margins. A delay of 24 to 72 hours after the injection of DHE allows time for absorption in the tumor cells, while at the same time, a partial release of porphyrins occurs from benign tissue.[10] The treatment light is delivered by an argon-pumped dye laser.[4] The optimum wavelength of 630 nm is obtained by adjustment of a birefringent filter and is measured by a spectrometer provided with the laser system.

The output of the delivery fiber is measured with a calibrated power meter. The beam diameter at the tumor site is measured and the area calculated. Knowing the laser beam area and the power of the laser as it emerges from the fiber tip, the surface intensity is calculated in mW/cm^2. The exposure time is determined from a published dose chart. A masking shield with a measured aperture is placed over the tumor site, permitting 1 to 2 cm of exposure beyond the determined margins of the lesion.

The typical treatment time varies from 10 to 30 minutes. Patients occasionally experience a warm sensation at the tumor site during treatment. If the power density is too high for a patient's tolerance, the power must be reduced, and in order to attain the calculated light dose, the exposure time must be extended.

Diffuse ecchymosis may occur either during the light treatment or soon after because of the destruction of the elastic fibers and endothelial cells disrupting the capillary vascular walls. Induration of tissue with tumor necrosis and eschar formation appears within 24 to 36 hours after the photochemical reaction initiated by the laser beam. The associated process is often painful. This discomfort may persist for 24 to 48 hours and will subside with cold compresses. Analgesics must be given for support. The duration of pain and healing is directly proportional to the amount of tissue exposed to the incident beam and the extent of necrosis.

SKIN PHOTOSENSITIVITY

A transient side effect of PDT is photosensitivity of the skin to sunlight or unusually bright illumination such as a dental lamp. It begins when the porphyrin is given intravenously and may persist from 30 to 60 days. Any area of the skin exposed to the sun or bright light may respond. The tissue appearance in all exposed cases is rated from one to five in degrees of minimal, moderate, and severe erythematous and edematous reactions. Severe reactions show fiery erythema with edema and blistering. Moist desquamation or necrosis may occur.

To minimize these reactions in the surrounding normal tissue, an opaque masking is applied during light exposure as previously described. Some light may leak under the masking, extending the area of sensitization reaction. To avoid this, the masking must be tightly applied.

The face, neck, shoulders, hands, and feet are the sites most commonly affected with edema if not properly covered. Instructions should be given to wear sunscreen cream (SPF 15), sun glasses, wide-brim hats, high-neck sweaters, gloves, slacks, covered shoes, and stockings. Avoid or delay treatment of patients who have taken doxorubicin (Adriamycin) or have had x-ray therapy within the previous 3 months.

DISCUSSION

The effectiveness of PDT is determined 3 months after treatment. A complete response requires a negative gross and histologic finding. A partial response requires more than 50% of the lesion destroyed, and no response when more than 50% of the lesion remains or the lesion is progressive.[8]

Because light is attenuated by passing through tissue, blood and melanin pigment in the skin limit light penetration of deep tumors, requiring an increase in the incident light dose. The effective light dose also depends on the local concentration of DHE because only the light absorbed by DHE can initiate tumor eradication. The effective reaction of PDT in a thick tumor can be viewed as the formation of a necrotic band that migrates from the irradiated surface through the tumor as the treatment proceeds. Benign tissue adjacent to the tumor is also damaged to an extent determined by the light exposure and the residual DHE concentration. This factor places an upper limit on the light dose that can be used for PDT. Accurate PDT dosimetry can improve the therapeutic ratio between the probability of effecting tumor eradication and the probability of inducing unacceptable normal tissue damage.

The factors that determine the uptake and retention of a photosensitizing agent have not been identified. High uptake creates a dilemma because skin photosensitivity may become extreme. However, the sensitizing effect of porphyrins leaves no residuals and does not have the usual dark toxic effects associated with cancer therapeutic agents. A program should be continued to investigate other agents that could be eliminated more rapidly from the body or to identify a vehicle that could be introduced to stimulate clearance of the photosensitizing agent from the body. Topical application with local absorption might be the solution because it would eliminate the prolonged systemic involvement.[25]

Tumor margins should be addressed by allowing an adequate region at the periphery of the tumor to be illuminated with an effective light dose.

Data gathered from studies of tumors in animals suggest that hyperthermia may enhance the action of PDT.[19,32] Therapeutic planning requires considerable development to optimize a complete response.

CONCLUSION

PDT is an economical procedure that seldom requires hospitalization, reduces costs, and does not incapacitate patients, except for their need to avoid direct sunlight. The treatment is repeatable. It does not interfere with chemotherapy or ionizing radiation therapy and is non-carcinogenic. PDT can be used as an adjunctive therapy for advanced invasive lesions without interfering with or hindering the use of other therapeutic measures.

PDT has a promising future in attacking early invasive cancer, either as a primary or adjunctive approach. It may serve as the treatment of choice for severe dysplasia or carcinoma *in situ*. Superficial lesions are amendable to a uniform incident laser beam. PDT may prove useful in treating endometriosis as well.[20]

The techniques and instrumentation involved in PDT are rapidly being improved to include new light sources, other potential photosensitizing porphyrins, and improved dosimetry.

The use of fluorescence as a diagnostic and therapeutic guide for treatment must be accepted with reservation.[1] In neoplastic areas, DHE fluorescence was appreciable in ulcerative tissue. It was weak or sometimes not observed in non-ulcerated tissue. The fluorescent intensity cannot be related to the relative drug concentration because of the different photophysical properties of this compound in its monomeric and aggregated forms. In fact, some cases had highly positive responses to treatment although no fluorescence could be observed. Therefore, the visual examination of the tumors, when positive, must be accepted as informative and for the present serves as our only guide for determining the extent of a lesion.

REFERENCES

1. Andreoni A, Cubeddu RJ: Fluorescence Properties of HPD and Its components. Porphyrins in Tumor Photo Therapy. Proceedings of an International Symposium held in Bruzzano, Milano, Italy, May 16–28, 1983. New York, Plenum Press, 1984
2. Auler H, Banzer G: Untersuchungen uber die Rolle der Porphyrins bei geschwul stkranken menschen und tieren. Z Krebsforsch 53:65, 1942
3. Balchum OJ, Doiron DR: Photoradiation therapy of endobronchial cancer. Clin Chest Med 6:255, 1985
4. Castro DJ, Saxton RE, Fetterman HR et al: Rhodamine-123 as a new photochemosensitizing agent with the argon laser: Non thermal and thermal effects on human squamous carcinoma cells *in vitro*. Laryngoscope 7:554, 1987
5. Coleridge-Smith PD, Brown SG, Tralau CJ et al: Is tumor destruction by laser photodynamic therapy mediated by vascular effects (abstr). Br J Surg 74:547, 1986
6. Dougherty TJ, Grindey G, Field R et al: Photoradiation therapy II cure of animal tumors with hematoporphyrin and light. J Natl Cancer Inst 55:115, 1975
7. Dougherty TJ, Kaufman JE, Goldfarb A et al: Photoradiation therapy for the treatment of malignant tumors. Cancer Res 38:2628, 1978
8. Epstein JH: Adverse cutaneous reactions to the sun. In Malkinson FD, Pearson RW (eds): Yearbook of Dermatology, pp 5–43. Chicago, Year Book Medical Publishers, 1981.
9. Figge FHJ, Weilarid GS, Manganiello LL: Cancer detection and therapy. Affinity of neoplastic, embryonic, and traumatized regenerating tissue for porphyrins and metalloporphyrins. Proc Soc Exp Biol Med 68:640, 1948
10. Fingar VH, Potter WR, Henderson BW: Drug and light dose dependence of photodynamic therapy: A study of tumor cell clonogenicity and histological changes. Photochem Photobiol 45:643, 1987
11. Firey PA, Rogers MAJ: Photo-properties of a silicon naphthalocyanine: A potential photosensitizer for photodynamic therapy. Photochem Photobiol 45:535, 1987
12. Grossweiner LI: Membrane photosensitization by hematoporphyrin and porphyrin derivative. In Doiron D, Gomer C (eds): Porphyrin Localization and Treatment of Tumors, pp 391–404. New York, Alan R. Liss, 1984
13. Grossweiner LI: Optical dosimetry in photodynamic therapy. Lasers Surg Med 46:911, 1987
14. Grossweiner LI, Goyal GC: Photosensitization of liposomes by porphyrins. J Photochem 25:253, 1984
15. Grossweiner LI, Hill JH, Lobraico RV: Photodynamic therapy of head and neck squamous cell carcinoma. Optical dosimetry and clinical trial. Photochem Photobiol 46:911, 1987
16. Kelly JF, Snell ME: Hematoporphyrin derivative: A possible aid in the diagnosis and therapy for carcinoma of the bladder. J Urol 115:150, 1976
17. Lipson RL, Baldes ES, Olsen AM: The use of a derivative of hematoporphyrin in tumor detection. J Natl Cancer Inst 26:1, 1961
18. Lobraico RV, Waldow SM, Harris DM et al: Photodynamic therapy for severe dysplasia and carcinoma *in situ* of the lower female genital tract. Lasers Surg Med 6:208, 1986
19. Mang TS, Kemme T, Chapman ID: Combination studies in hyperthermic induced by Nd:YAG as an adjuvant to photodynamic therapy (abstr). Lasers Surg Med 7:105, 1987

20. Manyak MJ, Nelson LM, Solomon D et al: Photodynamic therapy of rabbit endometrial transplants: A model for treatment of endometriosis. Fert Steril 52:140, 1989
21. McCaughan JS Jr, Hicks W, Laufman L et al: Palliation of esophageal malignancy with photoradiation therapy. Cancer 54:2905, 1984
22. Musser DA, Wagner JM, Weber FG et al: The binding of tumor localizing porphyrins to a fibrin matrix and their effects following photoradiation. Res Commun Chem Pathol Pharmacol 28:505, 1980
23. Policard A: Etudes sur Les aspects offerts par des tumerurs experimentales examine'es a La Luminere de Woods. Compt Rend Soc Biol 91:1423, 1924
24. Raab O: Uber die Werkung Fluorescierendes Staffe and Infusorien. Z Biol 39:524, 1900
25. Rettenmaier MA, Berman ML, Di Saia RJ et al: Gynecologic Uses of Photoradiation Therapy, Porphyrin Localization and Treatment of Tumors, pp 767–775. New York, Alan R. Liss, 1984
26. Straight RC, Spikes JD: Photosensitized Oxidation of Biological Molecules. In Frimer A (ed): Singlet O_z, IV pp 91–143. Boca Raton, CRC Press, 1985
27. Straight RC, Waner M, Lawrence IC et al: Laser photodynamic therapy of experimental tumors comparing the effectiveness of pulsed gold vapor, copper vapor, flashlamp-dye and continuous wave argon-dye lasers (abstr). Lasers Surg Med 7:74, 1987
28. Tappeiner HU, Joblbauer A: Die Sensibilisierend Wirkung Fluorescieren der substanzen. In Fogel FCW (ed): Gesammelte Undersuchungen uber die Photodynamische Erscheinung, Leipzig, 1907
29. Tsutau M, Carrano C, Tsutsu EA: Tumor localizers porphyrins and related compounds (unusual metalloporphyrins XXIII. In Alder AD (ed): The Biological Role of Porphyrins and Related Structures, pp 674–684. New York, New York Academy of Sciences, 1975
30. Waldow SM, Lobraico RV, Harris DM et al: Clinical trials utilizing photodynamic therapy for cancer. Lasers Surg Med 6:277, 1986
31. Waldow SM, Lobraico RV, Kohler IM et al: Photodynamic therapy for treatment of malignant cutaneous lesions. Lasers Surg Med 7:451, 1987
32. Waldow SM, Morrison PR, Grossweiner LI: Nd:YAG laser-induced hyperthermia in a mouse tumor model. Lasers Surg Med (in press)
33. Zanelli GD, Kaelin AC: Synthetic porphyrins as tumor localizing agents. Br J Radiol 54:403, 1981

19

Laser Surgery for Invasive Malignancies

Helmut F. Schellhas

HUMAN PAPILLOMAVIRUS INFECTION AND MALIGNANT LESIONS

Laser surgery is widely applied for preinvasive neoplastic genital lesions in gynecology and therefore plays mostly a preventive role in oncology. The convenient technique of tissue vaporization, however, may easily mask the presence of an invasive lesion that would require more aggressive treatment. Therefore, the adherence to detailed diagnostic criteria before laser vaporization, as outlined in other chapters in this book, is very important. The laser should be used as a tool for excision of genital preinvasive lesions rather than for vaporization. A slightly wider margin of excision than required for steel scalpel surgery should be obtained to provide for the small zone of marginal tissue coagulation that may impair optimal pathology evaluation of the tissue specimen.

Laser surgeons must be informed about the biologic behavior and the oncogenic potential of human papillomavirus (HPV) infections (Table 19–1). HPV causes characteristic benign proliferations of epidermal and mucosal surfaces but is also detected by the use of HPV-DNA probes in the majority of premalignant and primary malignant lesions of the female lower genital tract including distant metastatic sites. The malignant potential of the HPV infection can be determined by hybridization methods that have an acceptable sensitivity level. HPV types 6/11 have usually been associated with low-risk lesions and morphological characteristics such as diploidy and polyploidy of the cellular DNA, koilocytosis, and nuclear atypia. These lesions show frequent regression. High-risk lesions are generally associated with HPV types 16, 18, 31, 33, and 35 and are found to have aneuploidy, koilocytosis, nuclear atypia, atypical mitosis, and atypical vascularity. These lesions

TABLE 19–1
Morphological Characteristics of Condylomatous Lesions of the Vulva and Cervix Uteri

	LOW-RISK LESIONS	HIGH-RISK LESIONS
HPV type	6, 11	16, 18, 31, 33, 35
DNA	Diploid, polyploid	Aneuploid
Histology	Koilocytosis, nuclear atypia	Koilocytosis, nuclear atypia, atypical mitoses, atypical vascularity
Clinical behavior	Frequent regression	Oncogenic potential

have a high risk of progression to malignant lesions, and regular clinical follow-up is mandatory (see Table 19–1). These findings apply mostly to lesions of the cervix and vulva. Kurman and associates[9] found type 16 involved with cervical carcinoma *in situ* in 37% and with invasive carcinoma in 41%. Type 18 was found associated with carcinoma *in situ* in 3% and invasive carcinoma in 22%. They suspect a rapid transit time through the intraepithelial neoplastic stage for type 18, requiring close clinical surveillance. Barnes and associates[2] reported more poorly differentiated tumors and more frequent lymph node metastasis for type 18 as compared with type 16. Squamous cell carcinoma arising in condylomata acuminata of the vulva requires clinical recognition as described by Downey and associates.[6] These lesions are mostly found in elderly patients. In women over the age of 40, recurrent condylomata acuminata may be associated with immunosuppression and malignant disease.[10] Buscema and associates[5] identified HPV type 16 in four and type 6/11 in one squamous carcinoma of the vulva. Sutton and associates,[21] however, found HPV type 6/11 in 78% of 24 patients with squamous carcinomas of the vulva but found HPV type 16 or 18 in only 33% of malignancies. Viral typing alone is not diagnostic, although latent high-risk HPV infections can be found in women with negative Pap smears.[12] Viral typing has become commercially available and should be used in the management of patients found to have condylomata and benign and malignant epithelial neoplastic lesions.

Screening for HPV infection contributes to the recognition of the natural history of genital and neoplastic lesions. In an immunohistological study of vulvar intraepithelial neoplasia (VIN) by Rueda-Leverone and colleagues,[14] the presence of HPV infection was associated with multicentric lesions in 50% of patients and associated with cervical intraepithelial neoplasia (CIN) or cervical invasive carcinoma in 30%. In patients without evidence of HPV infection, multicentric VIN was found in only 10% of patients, and no cervical neoplasia.[14] Comprehensive diagnostic evaluation of the entire lower genital tract is required before any vaporizing laser surgical procedure is performed, otherwise malignant lesions will be masked. For the detection of HPV infection, hybridization tests are more sensitive than colposcopy, cytology, or histopathological sections, which often do not reveal the typical morphological characteristics of HPV infection (Table 19–2).[20]

TABLE 19–2
Sensitivity of Methods for the Detection of HPV Infection of the Female Lower Genital Tract in Human Papillomavirus-Positive Patients*

	%
1. Hybridization tests	100
2. Colposcopy of cervix	70
3. Colposcopy of vagina	59
4. Cytology of cervix	15
5. Cytology of vagina	7

* *Tested for HPV types 6/11 and 16/18*
(From Schneider A, Sterzik K, Buck G et al: Colposcopy is superior to cytology for the detection of early genital papillomavirus infection. Obstet Gynecol 71:236, 1988

Vulva

Carbon Dioxide Laser Surgery

Premalignant and invasive vulvar lesions should be excised and not vaporized with the carbon dioxide (CO_2) laser. The peripheral margins need to be slightly more extended than with scalpel surgery to allow for the thermal defect and shrinkage of tissue. The advantage of CO_2 laser surgery is decreased use of instrumentation, decreased blood loss, probable sealing of lymphatics, minimal touch technique, and bloodless development of surgical planes.

Indications. Standard vulvectomies and groin dissection are best performed with the steel scalpel because the procedure can be performed much quicker than with the CO_2 laser. Blood loss can be kept low with good standard surgical technique. CO_2 laser excision is advantageous in radical vulvectomy in the following instances:

1. Tumors extending into adjacent areas such as the ischiorectal fossa or pubic bone (Figure 19–1).
2. Groin dissection when groin nodes are clinically positive.
3. Recurrent tumors, especially in close approximation to the urethra and rectum (Fig. 19–2).
4. Preinvasive lesions extending into the vagina or anal canal.
5. Skinning vulvectomy for preinvasive lesions.

Technique. The articulated arm is preferred for vulvar surgery, and power densities between 50 and 100 kW/cm^2 are used with the beam focused on the tissue. Good tension is important for the tissue to be incised. Compression of blood vessels lateral to the incisional line using moist laps and finger pressure improves hemostasis. Dryness of the surgical field is important for adequate absorption

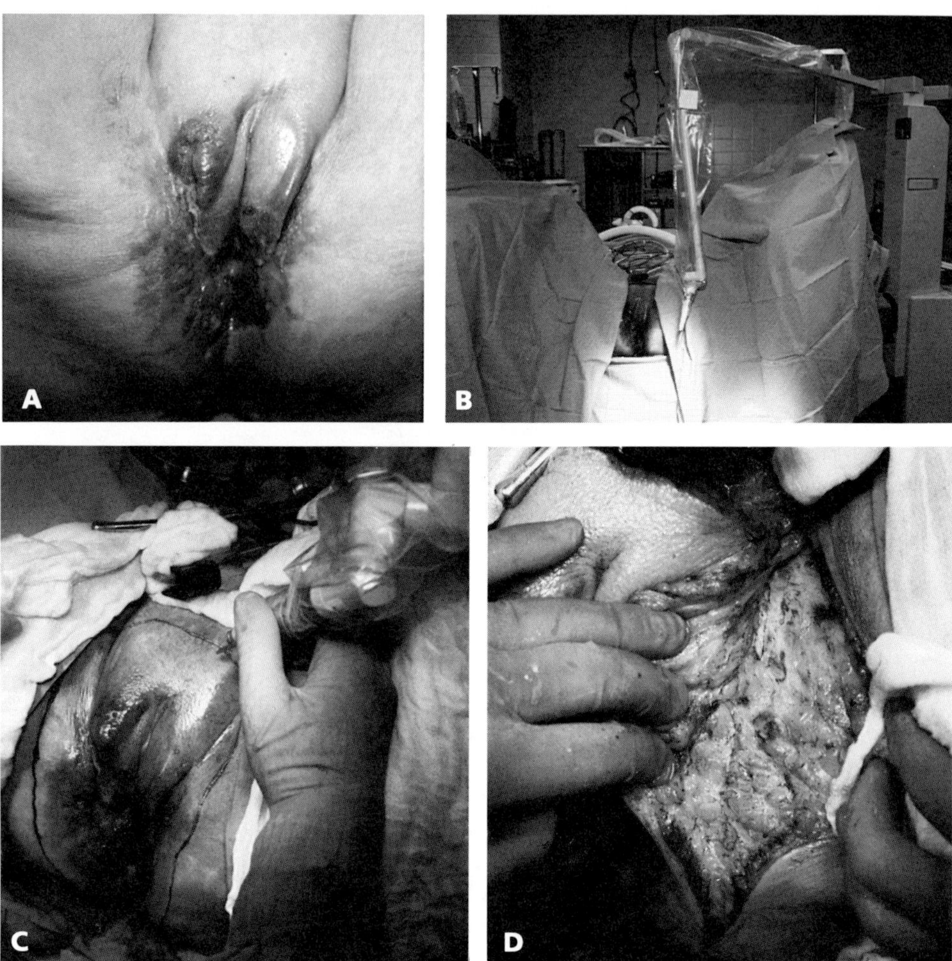

FIGURE 19–1. (*A*) Clinical data: Recurrent squamous carcinoma of anus previously treated by a Miles operation, radiation therapy, and chemotherapy in a 69-year-old woman. The tumor extension involves the perineum, vulva, and lower third of vagina. Parametria and groin nodes are clinically positive. The surgical procedure is performed for palliative purposes. (*B*) Positioning of the CO_2 laser. A powerful CO_2 laser is positioned cephalad. The articulated arm swings in from over the abdomen, providing optimal access to the operative field. A suction device and an electrosurgical scalpel are positioned above the surgical field. (*C*) The line of resection is marked with the surgical hand piece using low power. Moist gauze laps cover the periphery of the surgical field to absorb stray beams. The suction device is positioned over the pubis. (*D*) The plane of dissection has been developed. A focused beam with 50-watt power superpulse is used. Bleeding points are coagulated with electrosurgical cautery.

(*continued*)

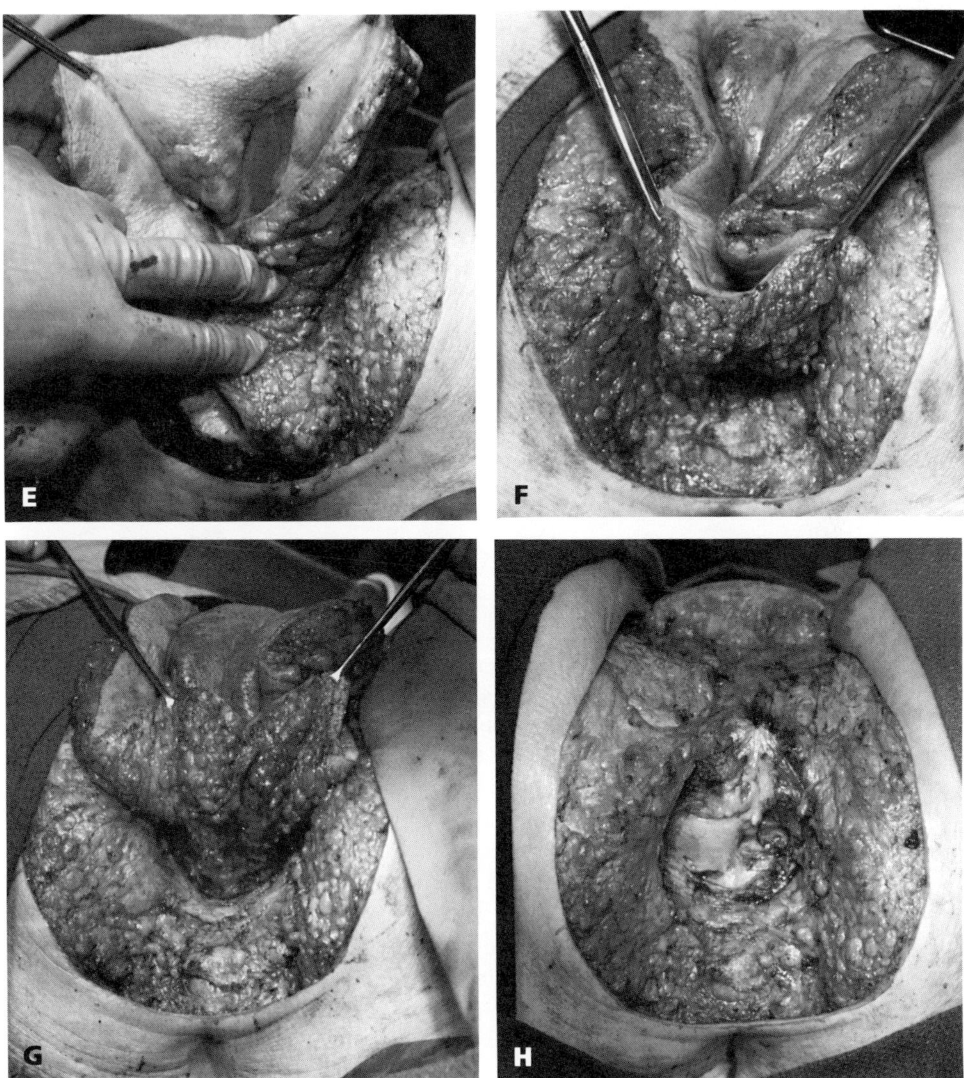

FIGURE 19–1. (Continued)
(*E*) The anterior and lateral parts of the vulva have been dissected with very little blood loss. (*F*) A plane of dissection has been developed over the sacrum. (*G*) Most of the posterior vagina has been dissected. (*H*) The surgical wound after resection is being left open for healing by secondary intention. The total blood loss was 350 ml.

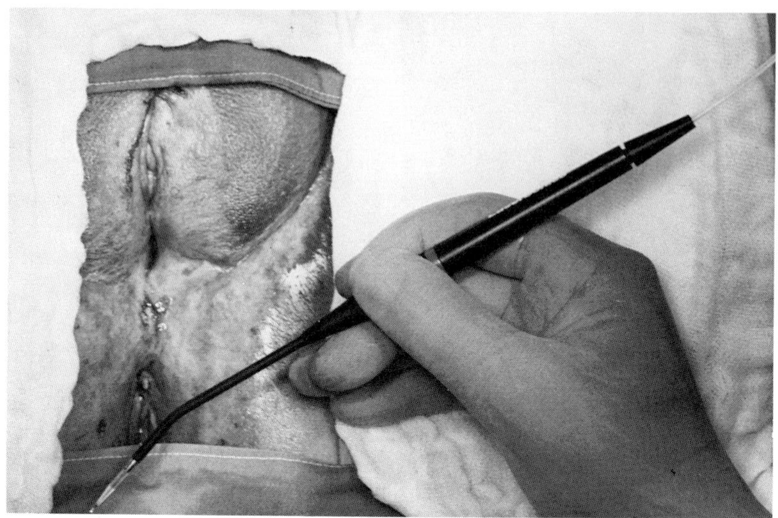

FIGURE 19–2. Recurrent squamous carcinoma of the vulva.

of the beam. Bleeding vessels are best cauterized with the electrosurgical knife, which is more effective than CO_2 laser coagulation. In groin dissection with the CO_2 laser, skin flaps are dissected with a power density of 2500 watts/cm². Flaps take well when developed with the CO_2 laser. Along the femoral vessels, tissue is gently dissected with a power density of 600 watts/cm².

Contact Neodymium : YAG Laser Surgery

Contact cutting probes combine the coagulation properties of the neodymium : YAG (Nd : YAG) laser with the incisional capabilities of the CO_2 laser scalpel (see Chapter 20).[7] Contact Nd : YAG laser surgery is applicable in surgery of the lower genital tract.

The contact probe for Nd : YAG laser surgery is made from a synthetic sapphire crystal and allows the delivery of a very small spot size with high power density. Various tip forms have been devised to be used for cutting, coagulation, or vaporization. The tips are attached to a hand piece for open surgery. Tip diameters of 0.2, 0.6, and 0.8 mm are available for surgical scalpels. They are available in non-frosted and frosted versions. The frosted end tip radiates both forward and laterally to increase coagulation in parenchymal organs. An increase of scalpel diameter results in a decrease in power density and a lengthening of the incision time. On the other hand, a decrease in the contact diameter results in a proportionate decrease of hemostasis. At a power of 25 watts, the 0.2-mm scalpel delivers a power density of 70,000 watts/cm² at the tip of the non-frosted contact probe (Table 19–3).[7] The crystal melts with higher powers used. There is little or no backscatter. Compared with the steel scalpel, the tensile strength of Nd : YAG 0.2-mm probe incision scars in rat skin was similar.[19] Contact laser liver resection produces minimal laser plume. Special protective goggles are required for the eyes.

TABLE 19–3
**Power Density at Tip of Contact Probes
(Watts/cm^2)**

POWER	LASER SCALPEL (TIP DIAMETER IN MM)			
(WATTS)	0.2	0.4	0.6	0.8
25	70,000	18,000	7,800	4,400
20	56,000	14,000	6,200	3,500
15	42,000	11,000	4,700	2,600
10	28,000	7,000	3,100	1,800
5	14,000	3,500	1,600	880
1	2,800	700	310	180

(From Joffe SN, Schroder T: Lasers in general surgery. In Mannick JA [Ed]: Advances in Surgery 20, pp 125–154. Chicago, Year Book Medical Publishers, 1987

Vagina

The standard treatment for the rare primary carcinoma of the vagina is radiation therapy, radical surgery, or a combination of radiation therapy and surgery in which one or the other method has to be reduced in extent to avoid major complications. Radiation therapy or chemotherapy is the first choice in the treatment of metastatic tumors to the vagina, such as from a primary endometrial or ovarian carcinoma. Following failure of standard cancer treatment methods, laser technology offers excellent means for palliative treatment and, in regard to small-volume tumors, possibly also for cure.

Carbon Dioxide Laser

For the treatment of vascular tumors, a low power density has a better hemostatic effect than a higher power density. A high power density beam cuts through tissue, whereas a lower power density beam seals capillaries and small vessels up to a diameter of 0.5 mm. A large capillary hemangioma of the cervix, for instance, was successfully treated with a power density range of 100 to 150 watts/cm^2.[3] On the other hand, high power density vaporizes a larger tissue volume. A focused laser beam should be used rather than a defocused beam. The latter will cause more thermal tissue damage and carbonization of the tissue, which then requires frequent débridement. The speed of beam movement is also important because the longer the beam remains directed against one spot, the deeper is the marginal damage of tissue dehydration and carbonization.

Combination of Carbon Dioxide Laser Surgery and Cryosurgery

The CO_2 laser beam is quickly absorbed by a thin layer of blood and is ineffective for the vaporization of tumor tissue. For this reason, we have frozen bleeding tumor tissues with a liquid nitrogen spray before commencing tissue vaporization with the CO_2 laser.[16] The ischemic frozen tissue absorbs the focused laser beam and can then be vaporized. The frozen tumor layer is continuously vaporized until intact vessels below the frozen zone are reached; refreezing is then required. Clinically, the combination of cryosurgery and CO_2 laser technique was applied in patients with hemorrhaging metastatic carcinoma of the cervix to the vagina and vulva and to the intra-abdominal treatment of cervical carcinoma metastatic to the pelvic bone. An extraperitoneal approach was used to gain access to the tumor site.[15]

Neodymium : YAG Laser

The Nd : YAG laser is very effective in the destruction of vascular or bleeding tumors. The beam emits at 1060 nm in the near-infrared portion of the electromagnetic spectrum and has the deepest tissue penetration of all surgical lasers. The Nd : YAG laser is basically a tissue coagulator, because the beam scatters within the tissue and produces a high volume absorption. The thermal effect depends on the power of the beam and the forward and backscatter of the beam in specific tissues. Necrotic tissue favors Nd : YAG laser beam absorption because it causes less backscatter than healthy tissue.[4] Low radiation energy causes tissue heating, whereas high laser energies result in tissue coagulation and necrosis. Tissue vaporization can be achieved by further heat generation of the coagulated and desiccated tissue with high energy densities and an added time factor. Large non-contact incisions with extensive marginal necrotic tissue zones can be made with absolute hemostasis using high power. Necrotic tissue can either slough off or cause tissue inflammation that results in fibrosis. The tissue changes following Nd : YAG laser radiation are not immediately recognizable to surgeons because the depth of the necrosis is deep and develops over several days. In CO_2 laser surgery, on the other hand, the tissue effects can be appreciated immediately. Adjacent organs such as the bladder, rectum, and also small bowel loops, especially when they are fixed in the cul-de-sac as a result of previous surgery and radiation therapy, can easily be perforated. The author has used the Nd : YAG laser in the palliative treatment of patients with hemorrhaging tumors of the cervix and ovary metastatic to the vagina.[18] The laser beam was delivered by means of a hand piece. A power of 40 to 100 watts was used continuously. The total energy used ranged between 630 and 12,100 watt-seconds. It is advisable to reduce the air or gas flow used to purge the end of the manipulator to avoid gas or air embolism, especially in vascular tumors. We also have used the fiberoptic Nd : YAG laser light guide through an endoscope, such as a hysteroscope or gastroscope, to vaporize tumors in narrow vaginas. The gastroscope was used repeatedly to control postoperative or late pelvic bleeding following pelvic exenteration.

Hematoporphyrin Derivative Photoradiation Therapy

Photoradiation therapy uses the cytotoxic property of a hematoporphyrin derivative (HPD), which is activated by photoradiation (see Chapter 18). Malignant cells are selectively destroyed after exposure to photosensitizing light. Because the tissue penetration of photosensitizing light is limited to depths approaching 1 cm, mostly superficial tumors are selected for treatment. For large-volume tumors, various illumination techniques have been developed, such as direct, single, or multiple fiber insertion into the tumor. Multiple treatment applications after a single injection of HPD can be applied and are usually performed at 48-hour intervals. A cylindrical fiber is used for diffuse vaginal lesions. In order to keep an equal distance between the light source and tissue lesions, the light guide fiber can be placed in the axis of a cylindrical laboratory glass tube. For vaginal treatment, therapeutic light doses have to be carefully calculated. Tissue inflammation adjacent to the necrotic tumor develops because normal tissue also retains a small amount of HPD and can be damaged. In addition, the heat energy of the light source can directly burn tissue irrespective of photosensitivity. Damage to the bladder or rectum may therefore occur.

We have used Photofrin I, 3 mg/kg intravenously.[17] Dosages of 76 to 720 joules/cm^2 were given for surface radiation and 1300 joules/cm^2 interstitially. Photoradiation was given 2 days and 5 days after injection. Rettenmaier and associates[13] used Photofrin I, 3 mg/kg, and used radiation power of 800 mW with exposure times ranging from 280 to 480 seconds. A newer, more purified substance, Photofrin II, is now available.* Cell necrosis is instant. Adjacent tissue inflammation develops. Transient spiking fever for several days after radiation is sometimes observed. All patients are hypersensitive to direct sunlight or intense artificial light for periods of 3 to 8 weeks after HPD therapy because of the presence of residual HPD in normal tissue. For this period, patients should avoid bright lights both indoors and outdoors.

Cervical Carcinoma

Laser surgery has found no application in the treatment of primary carcinoma of the cervix. Radical surgery or radiation therapy or a combination of surgery and radiation therapy with reduction of the extent of one of the treatment modalities is standard treatment. A primary tumor could conceivably be vaporized or coagulated with a laser system as a preliminary measure in a pregnant patient, for instance, who may refuse immediate treatment. Destruction of a primary cervical tumor by laser surgery before a radical hysterectomy to avoid wound implantation of viable tumor cells is still an untried application. Systemic chemotherapy, however, has been used as an adjuvant treatment method before radical surgery or with radiation therapy to decrease the volume of cervical cancer.

Endometrial Carcinoma

Endometrial ablation through a hysteroscope by means of the Nd-YAG laser is an established endoscopic procedure for the destruction of benign endometrium or submucous leiomyomas in patients with abnormal bleeding (see Chapter 17). The destruction of premalignant or malignant endometrial lesions in high-risk patients who are not candidates for hysterectomy is not an approved indication for endometrial ablation. Intracavitary cesium insertion is a treatment option for both premalignant and malignant lesions. Postradiation bleeding, however, might call for laser coagulation of the uterine cavity. McCaughan and colleagues[11] treated a patient with

---

* *QuadraLogic Technologies, Inc., 520 West 6th Avenue, Vancouver, British Columbia, Canada V5Z 4H5*

uncontrolled uterine bleeding caused by a primary carcinoma of the breast metastatic to the endometrium and cervix. They used HPD photoradiation through a hysteroscope.[11]

Disseminated Intra-Abdominal Carcinoma

No surgical laser system is now of great help in controlling disseminated intraperitoneal carcinomatosis typically found with primary ovarian carcinoma. The CO_2 and Nd:YAG laser systems are too difficult to use for safe application on bowel surfaces. Photoradiation therapy might be applicable in the future if the proper beam wavelength can be effectively delivered over large tissue surfaces. In the future, this might be accomplished with a beam scanner or a strobe flash with high light intensity. Jolles and associates[8] observed decreased systemic immunoresponsiveness induced by peritoneal photodynamic therapy in a murine model.

The Cooper Ultrasonic Surgical Aspirator (CUSA) is a very useful instrument for the removal of intraperitoneal metastatic disease and is superior to any available surgical laser system.[1]

REFERENCES

1. Adelson MD, Baggish MS, Seiter DB et al: Cytoreduction of ovarian cancer with cavitron ultrasonic surgical aspirator. Obstet Gynecol 72:140, 1988
2. Barnes W, Delgado G, Kurman RJ et al: Possible prognostic significance of human papillomavirus type in cervical cancer. Gynecol Oncol 29:267, 1988
3. Bellina JH, Gyer DR, Voros JI et al: Capillary hemangioma managed by the CO_2 laser. In Bellina JH (ed): Gynecologic Laser Surgery. New York, Plenum Publishing, 1981
4. Bucholz J, Haverkamt K, Meyer HJ et al: Scattering effects in laser surgery. In Kaplan I (ed): Laser Surgery II, Jerusalem, Jerusalem Academic Press, 1978
5. Buscema J, Naghashfar Z, Sawada E et al: The predominance of human papillomavirus Type 16 in vulvar neoplasia. Obstet Gynecol 71:601, 1988
6. Downey GO, Okagaki T, Ostrow RS et al: Condylomatous carcinoma of the vulva with special reference to human papillomavirus DNA. Obstet Gynecol 72:68, 1988
7. Joffe SN, Schroder T: Lasers in general surgery. In Mannick JA (ed): Advances in Surgery 20, pp 125–154. Chicago, Year Book Medical Publishers, 1987.
8. Jolles CJ, Ott MJ, Straight RC et al: Systemic immunosuppression induced by peritoneal photodynamic therapy. Am J Obstet Gynecol 158:1446, 1988
9. Kurman RJ, Schiffman MH, Lancaster WD et al: Analysis of individual human papillomavirus types in cervical neoplasia: A possible role for type 18 in rapid progression. Am J Obstet Gynecol 159:293, 1988
10. Marshburn PB, Trofatter KF: Recurrent condyloma acuminatum in women over age 40: Association with immunosuppression and malignant disease. Am J Obstet Gynecol 159:429, 1988
11. McCaughan JS Jr, Schellhas HF, Lomano J et al: Photodynamic therapy of gynecologic neoplasms after presensitization with hematoporphyrin derivative. Lasers Surg Med 5:491, 1988
12. Parkkinen S, Syrjanen S, Syrjanen K et al: Screening of premalignant cervical lesions for HPV 16 DNA by sandwich and *in situ* hybridization techniques. Gynecol Oncol 30:251, 1988
13. Rettenmaier MA, Berman ML, DiSaia PJ et al: Photoradiation therapy of gynecologic malignancies. Gynecol Oncol 17:200, 1984
14. Rueda-Leverone G, Di Paola GR, Meiss RP et al: Association of human papillomavirus infection and vulvar intraepithelial neoplasia: A morphological immunohistochemical study of 30 cases. Gynecol Oncol 26:331, 1987
15. Schellhas HF: Laser surgery in gynecology. Surg Clin North Am 58:151, 1978
16. Schellhas HF: Cryogens and carbon dioxide laser in cyclic combination for volume reduction of vascular tumors. In Kaplan I (ed): Laser Surgery III, Part I, Tel Aviv, OT-PAS, 1979

17. Schellhas HF, Schneider DF: Hematoporphyrin derivative photoradiation therapy applied in gynecology. Colpo Gynecol Laser Surg 2:53, 1986
18. Schellhas HF, Weppelmann B: The neodymium-YAG laser in the treatment of gynecologic malignancies. Lasers Surg Med 3:225, 1983
19. Schneider D, Fidler J, Schroder T et al: Comparison of wound healing between the superpulse CO_2 laser, electrosurgical knife and steel knife incision (abstr) Lasers Surg Med 6:1986
20. Schneider A, Sterzik K, Buck G et al: Colposcopy is superior to cytology for the detection of early genital human papillomavirus infection. Obstet Gynecol 71:236, 1988
21. Sutton GP, Stehman FB, Ehrlich CE et al: Human papillomavirus deoxyribonucleic acid in lesions of the female genital tract: Evidence for Type 6/11 in squamous carcinoma of the vulva. Obstet Gynecol 70:564, 1987

20

Use of the Nd : YAG Laser
With Sapphire Scalpels

Gerald J. Shirk

The search for the perfect surgical laser has led researchers to explore many wavelengths and delivery systems. The ideal thermal laser should have a fiberoptic delivery system to provide simple delivery and the ability to channel the laser to any area of the body with minimal damage to healthy tissue surrounding the lesion being treated. It should cause minimal lateral thermal damage to the surrounding healthy tissue but should still be able to create an incisional tissue effect or a coagulative tissue effect as needed. It should have maximal hemostatic abilities. It should have a precisely controllable focal point. It should create a minimal number of technical problems. Certainly no single laser wavelength can meet these criteria. The other way to achieve the ideal is to create a delivery system that has the capability of altering a specific laser's tissue effect.

One of the earliest lasers explored for medical use was the Nd : YAG laser. It was found to be an excellent coagulator of tissue. This laser has a wavelength of 1.064 nm, which is in the near infrared region of the light spectrum. This wavelength can be transmitted through a fiberoptic cable and is generally delivered to the surgical site using this type of a delivery system. Adding sapphire contact scalpels to the delivery system minimizes lateral thermal damage and achieves the power densities necessary to create incisional and coagulative tissue effects.

SAPPHIRE CONTACT LASER SCALPELS

Most medical lasers today are used for their thermal effect. This effect is dependent on the specific way the laser light energy is transferred to thermal energy in the tissue. This transferral to thermal energy depends on four factors: (1) laser wavelength, (2) power density, (3) tissue color, and (4) tissue vascularity. The property of the far infrared laser wavelength is to compact its light energy in a very small volume of tissue. Because the carbon dioxide (CO_2) laser's wavelength is in the far infrared spectrum, its light is opaque to cellular water. It is totally absorbed by water and rapidly converted to thermal energy in a very short distance.

Lasers that are used for gynecological surgery have a fiberoptic cable delivery system and are either in the visible or near visible light spectrum. These lasers can therefore be transmitted through water for long distances with little energy loss. The conversion of light energy to heat in tissue must be the result of light absorption by the proteinaceous structure of tissue. This conversion creates two obvious results. First, a much larger volume of tissue is involved in the laser thermal effect. Second, coagulation is the initial effect, with vaporization occurring only after protein is heated to greater than 100°C. Some lasers depend on absorption by colored cellular elements, but the Nd : YAG laser's light absorption is nonspecific and has a thermal depth of penetration of approximately 4 mm. This coagulative effect has been used successfully in gynecology to achieve endometrial photocoagulation using a hysteroscopic delivery system.

The use of this tissue effect for advanced operative laparoscopic procedures has only limited value. The same disadvantages occur with other lasers in the visible light spectrum.

The tissue effect of any laser is determined by power density, which is generally introduced as a concept associated with the CO_2 laser (watts/cm²). Its limited light scatter in tissue and its limited tissue penetration allow the calculation to be treated as two-dimensional. However, laser wavelengths in the visible or near visible range penetrate a significant distance into the tissue. The energy calculation therefore involves a volume factor (watts/cm³). The highest power density is created at the center of the tissue mass, with decreasing energy levels laterally. If these lasers are to achieve tissue effects similar to the incisional ability of the CO_2 laser with limited lateral damage, the delivery system must establish marked limitations on the light scatter properties of these lasers in tissue.

Fiberoptic delivery of laser light energy is generally through flexible quartz fibers, which are easy to use and relatively inexpensive. These fibers are capable of transmitting laser light through very small diameters (typically less than 1 mm), and they can be threaded to almost any part of the body, causing little or no damage to surrounding normal tissue. This delivery system is ideal for use with endoscopy. However, these light transmission systems are non–contact systems. If they come in contact with tissue or blood, the fiber is significantly damaged. This damage results in distortion and disruption of laser light transmitted from the fiber, the major disadvantage. The other disadvantage is the loss of the coherent property of the laser light during transmission through the cable. This loss of coherent property does not allow the laser to be focused below the diameter of the optical cable by an optical lens.[5]

Contact between the fiberoptic cable and tissue produces a marked change in the tissue effect. The depth of penetration of the laser light is significantly reduced. Most of this effect is secondary to significant blockage of light transmission from the optical cable. This blockage results in conversion of the light energy to heat at the contact point and heats the cable contact point to very high temperatures. These temperatures destroy the optical quartz cable. The variable surrounding tissue effect is the result of imperfect and variable transmission of light into the tissue and thermal damage from the hot fiber.

This effect, although it has an unpredictable tissue damage pattern, has been used for many surgical purposes. The contact stripping technique for endometrial ablation, initially described by Goldrath and colleagues,[7] uses this effect. The incisional technique produced by contacting the fiberoptic cable of the argon or potassium-titanyl-phosphate (KTP) lasers uses the same effect.

Destruction of the quartz fiber with disruption of its light-transmitting ability does not constitute an ideal surgical system. In 1985, Daikuzono and Joffe[3] described the use of a sapphire rod that allowed contact with tissue to take advantage of this altered tissue response without destruction of the sapphire optical fiber. The thermal tissue effect was predictable and depended on the geometry of the sapphire rod. The use of longer rods was described for open surgical use. Microlaser tips were described for endoscopic incisions and photocoagulation. Daikuzono and Joffe noted the following advantages: (1) easy control for incision by changing tip diameters and power; (2) a more homogeneous photocoagulation zone around the incised tissue and less tissue coagulation in the vertical direction; and (3) high thermal efficiency and use of laser light energy.

Considerable controversy still exists about the exact biophysical mechanisms of the sapphire contact rods. The central issue is whether there is really an altered absorption of laser light energy in the tissue affected or whether the thermal conversion is totally inside the sapphire rod. This is a key issue, because the answer determines whether or not the sapphire contact probes are expensive heater probes or actually have a specific laser reaction.

Current data support a combination effect. There is no question that a significant amount of laser energy is trapped in the sapphire probe. The probe is rapidly heated to more than 800°C at the contact surface. This is greater than the 600°C required for tissue disruption, so that the contact thermal effect plays a significant role. The conversion of light energy to thermal energy is caused by carbonization of tissue at the contact point, resulting in blockage of significant transmission of laser light into the surrounding tissue. This contact state has to be initiated at the beginning of each use; the probe has to be "burned in." The initial starting effect is tissue coagulation with a thermal injury zone wider than desired. This effect is followed by a gradual, then more rapid, vaporization effect until maximal function is achieved with minimal lateral thermal damage. Some laser light energy (20%) is still transmitted to the lateral tissue. This transmission can be demonstrated by observing the difference in lateral thermal effect on light-colored tissue such as chicken breast muscle and dark tissue such as liver.

Studies involving live animals have demonstrated the ability of the contact scalpels. Joffe and colleagues[8] reported on the use of the Nd:YAG laser for hepatic resections in rats. The resections were accomplished by using both a non-contact technique and the sapphire contact scalpels. Joffe was able to show that the contact scalpels could be used effectively for this procedure to provide not only excellent incising ability, but also hemostasis. The non-contact technique resulted in later thermal damage of 1 to 4.4 mm. The immediate lateral tissue damage from the contact scalpels was noted to be 0.6 to 0.8 mm. Late follow-up at 15 days demonstrated rapid healing, with a minimal margin of healed lateral damage. In the same study, Joffe reported on a series using the laser contact blade for hepatic resections in humans. Corson and associates[2] also described the extent of thermal injury and healing in the rabbit ovary and uterine wall. He measured the depth of injury to be from 0.3 to 0.6 mm. The residual thermal laser effect was 0.051 mm, measured at 14 days. The healing was complete at 21 days. Doty and Auth[4] developed a laser scalpel that they called a photocoagulating dielectric waveguide. They used an argon laser for their experiments, but their data could be applied to the use of the Nd:YAG laser. They used it to create a burn wound model in pigs. They demonstrated that this unit could be used to excise burn sites and to apply a skin graft with the same or better efficiency than the standard RF electrosurgical units. Joffe and Schroder[9] have done extensive studies on tissue effect and range of transmission of laser light energy into the tissue by different probe geometries. Their studies demonstrated the ability of the laser scalpels to create various thermal tissue effects.

Special Treatment of Tip Surfaces

The index of refraction can be changed significantly by altering the smooth air–sapphire interface. The easiest alteration is simply to frost or roughly etch the surface. This etching creates loss of light laterally with drastic changes in the amount of energy delivered to the tip of the sapphire scalpel. These scalpels are used for photoirradiation of tissue masses. The scalpels used most frequently are "precarbonized" (Fig. 20–1). This term is a misnomer because the tips are actually coated by vapor spraying heavy metals on the area to be used as the contact surface. The area is then covered with a ceramic coating to hold the process and provide a smooth surface. This process is used to achieve rapid heating of the sapphire tips at the contact point, because there is greater use of energy at the interface. Precarbonization presets the effect created by the initial "burning in" phase. These scalpels start immediately. The difference in incisional speed muscle in tissue is graphically illustrated in Figure 20–2.

Contact Tip Configurations

The main advantage of the contact tips is their ability to create various tissue thermal effects by changing their geometric conformation. Four major conformations used

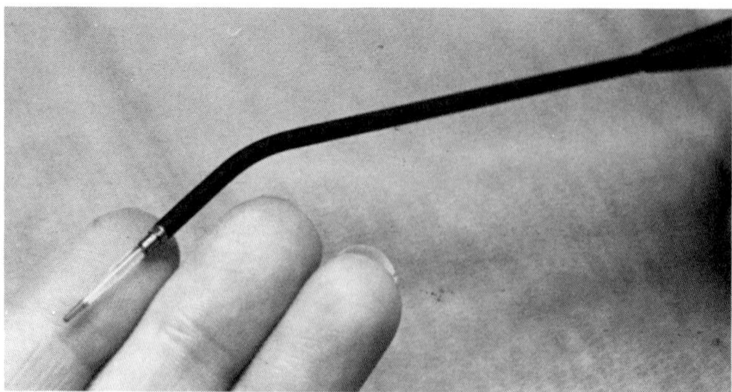

FIGURE 20–1. Precarbonized sapphire contact blade.

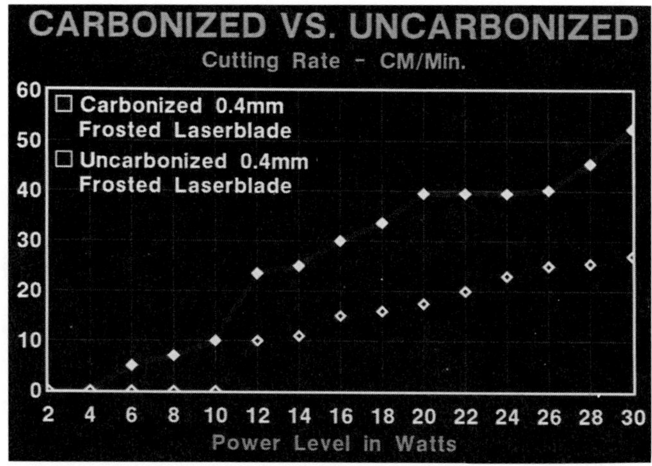

FIGURE 20–2. Incisional speed. (Data from LaserSonic's study)

are the cone or cylinder, the hemisphere, the flat, and the wedge. Other designs for special effects are available. Their thermal distribution patterns are demonstrated in Figure 20–3.

The cone scalpels and endoscopic tips are used to create power densities for incisional vaporization. This configuration concentrates the laser light energy in a very small volume of tissue. This compaction of the Nd:YAG laser energy creates power densities needed for tissue vaporization. The lateral tissue damage is limited to less than 0.5 mm (Fig. 20–4). The amount of energy compaction is related to the tip diameter, as demonstrated in Figure 20–5. This scalpel configuration is the major

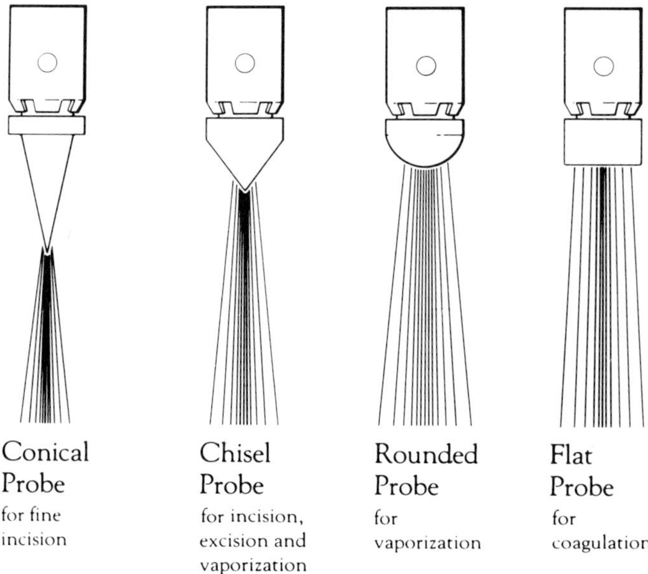

FIGURE 20–3. Contact scalpel geometries. (Courtesy of SLT)

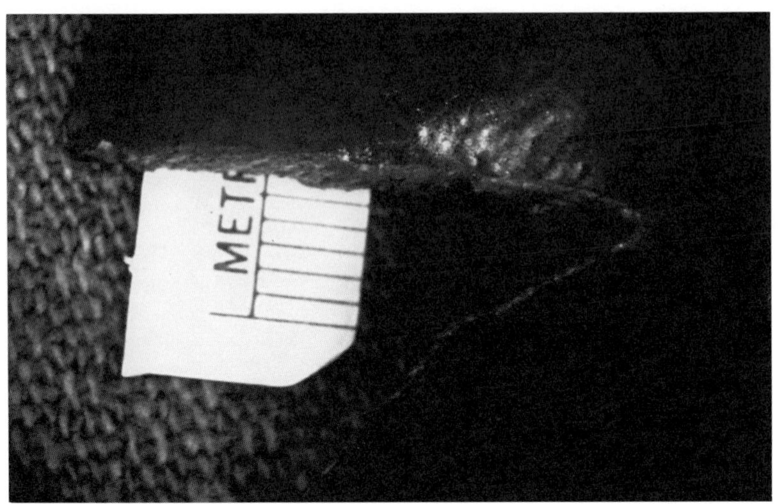

FIGURE 20–4. Lateral thermal effect in the liver. (Courtesy of J. Brumsted, University of Vermont)

(watts/cm2)

Tip Dia.	Area (cm2)	Power Levels					
		1.5	2.0	2.5	3.0	3.5	Watts
.2 mm	.0006283	2,387	3,183	3,979	4,775	5,571	w/cm2

Tip Dia.	Area (cm2)	Power Levels					
		5	10	20	30	40	Watts
.4 mm	.0025133	1,989	3,978	7,957	--	--	
.6 mm	.0056549	884	1,768	3,536	5,305	7,073	
.8 mm	.0100531	497	994	1,989	2,984	3,978	
1.0 mm	.015708	318	637	1,273	1,920	2,546	
1.2 mm	.0226195	221	442	844	1,326	1,768	

*Note: Calculations and formulas used are based on hemispherically-shaped blade tip.

FIGURE 20–5. Operating power density of laser blades.

way to change the diameter of the fiberoptic cable. It serves as a lens, because an optical lens cannot focus the laser light to a diameter less than the diameter of the fiberoptic cable. The 0.4-mm or 0.2-mm contact tips are most commonly used for laparoscopic procedures. The 0.4-mm to 0.8-mm blades are used with the hand-held probe, at 4 to 12 watts of continuous-wave Nd:YAG laser energy.

The hemisphere scalpel acts like a convex lens. It creates a central area of high power density, resulting in tissue vaporization. The lateral heating and leak of laser light energy, however, create a zone of lateral tissue coagulation. The final result is central vaporization with a small zone of lateral tissue coagulation. This configuration is used to vaporize large tissue masses. The central area of vaporization has an extended depth of tissue effect of 0.5 to 0.7 mm. This tip is especially useful for treating highly vascular tissue because of its excellent hemostatic ability. The longer bullet blade is used for hand-held procedures. The laparoscopic tip is shorter, and the energy settings for use of this tip are 12 to 20 watts of continuous-wave energy.

The flat tip has the effect of spreading the energy over a large contact zone, causing tissue coagulation. The laser penetration is limited but deeper than with the other tips used. This tip is used mainly for photocoagulation and hemostasis. It has a 1-mm depth of penetration[18] and is used at 16 to 25 watts of continuous-wave energy.

The wedge-shaped scalpel has a combination of effects. It is mainly a flat tip with a variable surface area. The surgical effect can be altered from coagulation, when using the flat sides, to vaporization, when using the blade edge. This altered position creates various depths of tissue damage according to the surface area used. This tip is used from 12 to 25 watts of continuous-wave energy.

Technical Variances

The largest technical problem that exists with the use of a sapphire contact scalpel is cooling. The scalpel operates at approximately 800°C. The time required to cool the sapphire from operating temperature to 60°C with a gas coolant is 8 seconds (Laser-Sonic's data). The tip is secured in a metal retainer, which also becomes hot during use and has a significant cool-down time. The major hazard from the sapphire scalpel is inadvertent contact with normal or vital tissue immediately after use.

Heating of the metal connecting device during lasing prohibits the use of this scalpel while it is secured only to the coaxial fiberoptic cable. The heated connector can melt the plastic catheter securing the metal connection. The risk is dropping the superhot laser scalpel onto the surgical site; therefore, this arrangement is unacceptable. The attachment of the contact scalpel should be to a secure foundation. Laser blades are easily secured in hand-held probes. Laparoscopic probes have also been developed to provide an excellent delivery system for the tips. These probes provide an efficient joining of the coaxial fiberoptic cable and the sapphire scalpels. The mechanism for changing scalpel configurations is simple.

The laparoscopic probe that was developed by the author provides the ability to change tips simply and rapidly to use different configurations. On the probe are the female threads, and on the tip are the male threads of the metal connector. This configuration allows the metal connection to be protected by a lateral shroud that serves as a thermal shield. Lateral tissues are therefore protected from inadvertent thermal damage. The risk of the tip becoming a hot free body in the abdomen is negated by the use of this probe (Fig. 20–6).

A prospective study of the efficiency and safety of the probe in 32 laparoscopic procedures was carried out.[1] The delivery system proved to be safe and provided easy access to all areas of pelvic pathology. The potential advantages over the CO_2 laser include improved hemostasis, decreased plume formation, the ability to incise adhesions safely without a backstop, and effective transmission of the laser energy through fluids.

The cooling medium can be either air or water. The sapphire has an index of refraction in air that provides complete transmission of laser light energy to the contact point. The blades are always cooled by air. Water cannot be used to cool the blades, because the heat gradients that are created fracture the sapphire. The cooling process with gas after use, however, is slow. The operator has to be careful not to contact tissue during this cool-down phase. Water can be used to cool the much smaller endoscopic tips.

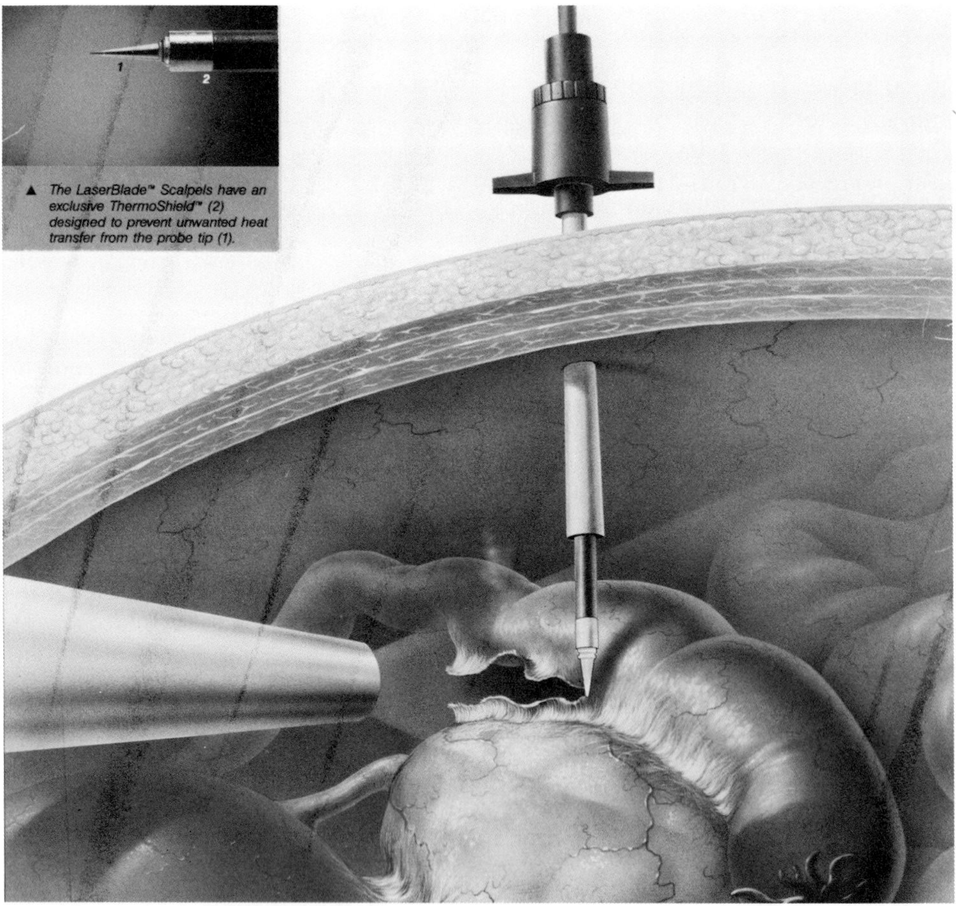

FIGURE 20–6. Laparoscopic probe.

Cooling with water has the benefit of speed but creates some major technical problems with tip function. Sapphire tips are designed to be used in air. The index of refraction for an air-sapphire interface is 1 and ensures that 97% of the laser light energy is transmitted through the tip. The index of refraction with water is 1.4. This difference creates a problem with the loss of light laterally from the sapphire tip and dispersion of the laser light energy, rather than transmission of maximal energy to the contact point. The tips are rapidly cooled after use, but this cooling effect severely affects the tip while functioning. LaserSonic's studies show a marked change in the performance energy curve (Fig. 20–7). Fortunately, this problem is not a major factor with all geometric configurations. The function of the fine conical tips can be altered significantly. The shroud on the probe allows the flow of water coolant to remain concentrated around the proximal tip. Unless the saline flow rate is high or the probe is placed in a vertical position during use, the distal tip remains in a gas and functions on the air interface curve.

The alternative, using CO_2 as a gas coolant, requires the operator to be extremely careful to avoid contacting the heated tip and metal retainer to vital tissue. The procedure with this technique requires immediate retraction of the tip into the operating sheath at the termination of use, while the operator compulsively watches the tip until the retraction is complete. The tips have a superior function when used with this type of cooling. Any procedure requiring extremely fine thermal tolerances should be done with gas cooling to provide maximal function of the tip.

Tissue sticking is a minor problem that occurs when the scalpel is allowed to cool while in contact with coagulated tissue. This problem is not unique to the contact scalpel; it can happen with electrocautery probes, fiberoptic cables using any laser wavelength, and other thermal probes. Tissue sticking is avoided by rapidly removing the scalpel from the tissue at the termination of use.

Fracturing of the sapphire crystal lattice from thermal stress is unlikely if the blades are used correctly. The main factor that could create a fracture is allowing a large buildup of coagulated tissue to occur on the surface of the blades. The large

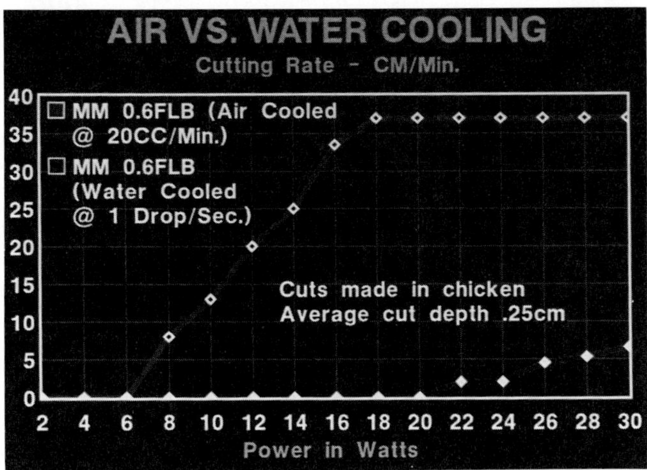

FIGURE 20–7. Water cooling. (Data from LaserSonics study)

carbon residual can be heated to above 2000°C. This temperature exceeds the thermal stress limits of the sapphire. The buildup of residual coagulated tissue on the blades requires immediate termination of use. The residual should be cleaned from the blades before resuming operative function.

CLINICAL USES OF THE SAPPHIRE CONTACT TECHNOLOGY

Treatment of Lower Genital Disease

The treatment of disease involving the lower genital tract has traditionally been the realm of the CO_2 laser. The Nd:YAG laser equipped with a contact scalpel can be used effectively to treat most lesions, with similar effects and results. The benign vulvar diseases that can be treated include condyloma venereum, carcinoma *in situ,* lichen sclerosis et atrophicus, and Bartholin's gland abscess. The contact scalpels are especially effective with large verrucous condyloma. The large masses can be excised hemostatically and then the base photocoagulated to the lower epidermal or upper dermal layers. The hemostasis provided makes the procedure faster and technically easier than similar therapy with the CO_2 laser.

In addition, use of the contact blades for excisional cone biopsy of the cervix provides an excellent result. Use of the contact blades for conization was reported in a group of 41 cases of cervical intraepithelial neoplasia in which preoperatively there was extension into the endocervical canal, inability to visualize the entire squamocolumnar junction, abnormal endocervical curettage, or disagreement between the colposcopic findings and the Pap smear.[6] All cones were successfully performed, with minimal thermal damage to the margins. The average blood loss was 9 ml without the use of vasopressin or other hemostatic measures. Delayed postoperative bleeding was a problem in only one patient. Healing was similar to that with the CO_2 laser. This technique has also been used by other investigators, who reported similar results.[17] The Nd:YAG laser can easily be used to perform incisional cone biopsy of the cervix. It is superior to the CO_2 laser in hemostasis and when working in a moist field. The procedure is a simpler surgical technique. The healed treated cervix cannot be differentiated from a cervix treated by the CO_2 laser.

Hysteroscopic Use of the Contact Tips

Endoscopic contact tips can be used for the treatment of intrauterine disease, but they have not been shown to be more effective or even as effective as contact with the bare urologic fiber. A study by Zumwalt and colleagues[18] on the use of the sapphire contact tips for photoablation of the endometrium suggested that the contact tips created too limited a depth of penetration and a variable tissue effect. This effect would prevent adequate destruction of the entire thickness of the basal endometrium. The problem with the contact tips is secondary to the liquid distention media required for operative hysteroscopy. Liquid media cool the tips and create significant energy loss. Further alterations of contact tip configurations may overcome this in the future.

The techniques used for endometrial ablation are varied. The contact technique for stripping the endometrium from the myometrium has been shown to be capable of creating total amenorrhea. The tissue effect created by contacting the bare fiber has been previously described. The added lateral tissue damage is beneficial. Limiting the lateral thermal effect further by a sapphire contact tip whose function is significantly altered by placing it in a fluid medium would serve no particular advantage. The future use may be to increase the size of the thermal "paintbrush" above the 0.6-mm diameter of the bare fiber.

Compared with using contact with the bare fiber, the use of the tips for transecting uterine septa has a theoretical advantage of reduced thermal damage to the myometrium. However, the tips are affected by the liquid distention media, resulting in higher power settings, poor cutting effect, and increased lateral coagulation of tissue. They can be used for this purpose but have no advantage. The bare fiber is easier to use and has the same thermal results.

Use of tips hysteroscopically has posed one major problem. The tips are generally used by attaching them directly to the coaxial fiberoptic cable. The coaxial cable has then been erroneously connected to air or high-flow CO_2. This erroneous connection has resulted in three unreported deaths and one near death due to air embolism. These procedures violated the basic principles of hysteroscopy. The hysteroscopic use of CO_2 flow greater than 100 ml/minute is contraindicated. Hysteroscopic use of air or high-flow CO_2 is lethal. These are hysteroscopic complications, not laser complications.

Laparotomy Use of Nd:YAG Contact Scalpels

No gynecological series have reported the use of contact scalpels during laparotomy. They can be used very effectively as a replacement for electrocautery in most laparotomies. Contact tips provide the same advantages in microsurgical laparotomies that they provide with advanced operative laparoscopy. They are excellent for hemostatic adhesiolysis. Myomectomies can be performed with less thermal effect in the surrounding myometrium. Ovarian cystectomies can be performed hemostatically with the contact scalpels. Laser scalpels have been used for these procedures, but no significant series have been reported.

Only Schultz and colleagues[14] have reported use of laser scalpels for gynecological indications in the general surgical literature. They used them to debulk tumors in advanced ovarian carcinoma, as well as in many other types of tumor debulking, including removal of large metastatic lesions from the liver. Joffe and associates[8] reported performing hepatectomies with laser scalpels. The literature in general surgery reports more investigative use of laser scalpels for intra-abdominal procedures than does the gynecological literature.

Advanced Operative Laparoscopic Uses

Endometriosis
The reported studies of the use of the Nd:YAG for advanced operative laparoscopy have mostly been concerned with the treatment of endometriosis. The advantage of

conservative surgical treatment by operative laparoscopic techniques has been established. The major advantages are (1) immediate treatment of the disease at the time of the diagnostic procedure and (2) avoidance or reduction of the trauma and complications of major surgery, both short and long term. The use of the Nd : YAG laser for treating endometriosis was initially reported by Lamono.[12] He described the use of the Nd : YAG using a non–contact treatment protocol. This technique is similar to those used with the blue-green lasers.[10,11] Lomono did show that the Nd : YAG laser was effective in treating endometriosis. Because it has a 4-mm depth of tissue coagulation, its use with this technique has many limitations. Its use close to vital structures has the same disadvantages experienced with the use of high-frequency electrocautery. Lysis of adhesions is not precise and results in unacceptable lateral thermal damage to tissue. It does have the advantage of a coagulative depth that is great enough to ensure complete treatment of most lesions. Because of the coagulation tissue effect and its ability to penetrate blood and body fluids, the Nd : YAG laser has excellent hemostatic abilities. It can be used laparoscopically for the treatment of endometriosis with this technique, but it has no distinct advantages over other systems.

Equipping the fiberoptic delivery system with a sapphire contact tip provides a delivery system with the ability to create various tissue effects, which are essential in meeting the surgical applications encountered during the treatment of endometriosis. The use of this system has been shown to be clinically safe and effective. The results of four recently published studies form the significant literature available for review.[1,2,15,16]

The results of any investigation of endometriosis have been judged by the reduction of pelvic pain, improvement of fecundity, and recurrence rates. Any conservative surgical treatment must be considered a debulking process, with the result being the reduction of disease volume to a minimum. This result may alleviate or reduce some of the symptoms but is not curative. Reduction of pelvic pain is the most common result desired by patients who seek relief of symptoms due to endometriosis. However, the mechanisms by which endometriosis causes pelvic pain are not well understood. The magnitude of the pelvic pain may not be related to the volume of the disease encountered. Treatment of macroscopic disease does reduce or relieve this symptom. In the study of 38 patients representing all four revised American Fertility Society (AFS) stages, Shirk[15] demonstrated a statistically significant improvement of pelvic pain by using the contact technique (Table 20–1). Complete relief of all symptoms is difficult to achieve, especially dysmenorrhea in AFS stage III or IV. The use of laser ultrasacral nerve ablation (LUNA) in this study does not suggest that it improves the outcome for dysmenorrhea. Corson and colleagues[2] allude to treatment of pelvic pain but give no detailed data of the outcome in 43 patients treated. However, the limited data presented suggest improvement.

The results of fecundity studies suggest treatment results similar to other operative laparoscopic studies using other thermal modalities.[13] Because the effect of endometriosis on fecundity is difficult to determine, the treatment success is likewise difficult to determine. In a study of 19 infertile patients, Shirk reported a 63% (12/19) pregnancy rate for all stages (Table 20–2). Most of these patients became pregnant within 6 months of treatment. Corson and associates treated 31 patients for infertility but only reported on pregnancies in a subgroup of 17 patients observed for

TABLE 20–1
Relief of Complaint After ND : YAG Laser/Sapphire Contact Tip Laparoscopy

INITIAL COMPLAINT	STAGE								TOTAL WITH COMPLAINT	
	I		II		III		IV			
	NC	PC	NC	PC	NC	PC	NC	PC	Number	%
Dysmenorrhea										
Postoperative	5	1	4	9	6	7	1	5	21	55
Preoperative	0	6	0	13	0	13	0	6	38	100
Significance	*		*		*		—			
Nodularity										
Postoperative	6	0	13	0	12	1	6	0	1	3
Preoperative	4	2	0	13	0	13	0	6	34	89
Significance	—		*		*		*			
Pelvic pain										
Postoperative	6	0	10	3	13	0	3	3	6	16
Preoperative	2	4	2	11	6	7	0	6	28	74
Significance	*		*		*		†			
Dyspareunia										
Postoperative	6	0	13	0	12	1	6	0	1	3
Preoperative	2	4	4	9	4	9	1	5	27	71
Significance	*		*		*		*			
Adnexal tenderness										
Postoperative	6	0	12	1	12	1	5	1	3	66
Preoperative	2	4	7	6	4	9	0	6	25	66
Significance	*		*		*		*			
Menstrual irregularity										
Postoperative	6	0	13	0	13	0	6	0	0	0
Preoperative	4	2	7	6	11	2	5	1	11	29
Significance	‡		*		*		‡			

NC, No complaint; PC, presenting complaint.
* $p < 0.05$.
† $p < 0.1$.
‡ No significant difference.

TABLE 20–2
Pregnancy and Stage of Endometriosis

AFS STAGE	NO. OF PATIENTS	PREGNANCY RATE (%)
I	3/3	100
II	3/3	100
III	6/10	60
IV	0/2	0
12/18		67

at least 6 months. In this group, eight patients achieved a pregnancy, with four of these being from the AFS stage IV group. These early studies were not well controlled and used limited numbers of cases. Because these studies are ongoing, significant data should substantiate the conclusion that Nd : YAG lasers with contact tips provide similar or better results than techniques now used.

The main advantage of using the contact technique for treating endometriosis is the ease of operating. Endometriosis presents various technical problems. The contact system provides a varied laser tissue reaction that is determined by the choice of the contact tip configuration. This choice can give surgeons the proper thermal tissue effect for treatment. Superficial peritoneal implants are the most commonly treated areas. Treatment can be accomplished using several techniques. The easiest is to completely ablate the lesion using the hemisphere tip (Fig. 20–8). The thermal lesion created has a central vaporization zone with a surrounding thermal coagulation zone. The depth of the thermal lesion is about 1 mm, exceeding the depth of the endometriotic lesion. Lateral coagulation ensures that lateral subperitoneal spread of endometriosis is effectively treated. This technique can be used safely in the anterior cul-de-sac, with the exception of deep penetrating lesions in the muscle of the urinary bladder.

A 0.2-mm cone tip can be used to excise or to create a vaporization ablation lesion, as with the CO_2 laser. The depth of penetration is less than 0.5 mm. This limited depth allows a surgeon to treat lesions superfically over the ureter and large bowel. The tips can be used to excise lesions if indicated. The advantage of using a tip for this technique is the excellent hemostasis achieved. This technique is generally

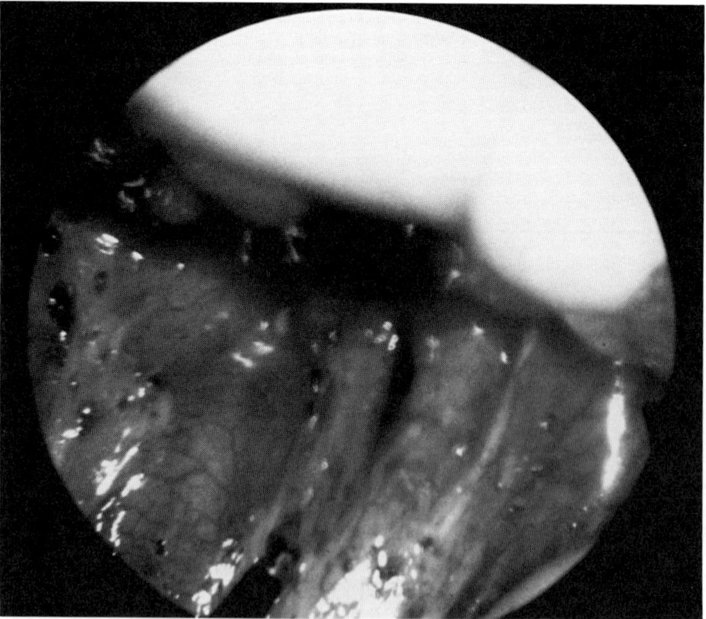

FIGURE 20–8. Laparoscopic treatment of endometriosis.

used in areas of deep penetration and high vascularity that would exceed the hemostatic abilities of a CO_2 laser.

Adhesions are a significant result of the inflammatory process from endometriosis. Release of these adhesive structures plays a significant part in the treatment of endometriosis. Distortion of the pelvic anatomy must be released to re-establish normal reproductive function and to reduce pelvic pain. Release of adhesions is also important to uncover underlying areas of endometriosis to complete effective treatment. The advantage of the contact technique is that no backstop for the laser beam is necessary. The cone tip can be used to lyse filmy or dense adhesions effectively and hemostatically. The release of adnexal adhesions provides minimal thermal damage to the ovaries and fallopian tubes. Dissection of a partially or completely obliterated cul-de-sac can be accomplished with care.

Laparoscopic operative techniques to treat endometriosis involving the ovary present some of the most difficult technical problems encountered. Treatment of endometriosis involving the ovary generally requires treatment of endometrial implants and destruction of adhesions formed from the inflammatory response of endometriosis. Endometriomas present the most difficult surgical problems, because these represent an involvement of the deep cortex and the medullary portions of the ovary. Treatment may result in a significant loss of cortical tissue and primary ova. It may also result in significant operative hemorrhage when the highly vascular medullary area is transgressed. Maintaining hemostasis may compromise the ovarian vascular system and may result in ovarian dysfunction or nonfunction. Laparoscopic use of the Nd:YAG laser with the new sapphire contact tips can successfully deal with most of the technical problems.

The most important step in deciding how to deal with an endometrioma is accurately assessing the extent and location of the structure. Endometriomas less than 2 cm generally involve only the cortex and superficial medullary areas. These small endometriomas may be treated in two ways. The capsule can be incised with the cone tip, the cyst lavaged and evacuated with lactated Ringer's solution, the lesion examined by biopsy, and the wall vaporized using the round tip. This is the simplest technique. Second, the endometrioma may be totally excised using the cone tip. It removes the entire lesion, avoiding incomplete treatment and providing for complete pathological inspection. Closure of these areas is unnecessary.

Endometriomas greater than 2 cm in diameter are treated with enucleation, if possible. If not possible, then an area is incised over a short length into the endometrioma. The contents are aspirated. This step is followed by lavage and aspiration of all wash solution from the peritoneal cavity. The cone contact tip is then used to complete the incision of the cyst wall. The cyst is examined for malignancy, as a biopsy is performed. The flat tip is used to paint the surface of the endometrioma. The result is that the cyst wall is released or "pops off" from underlying medullary structures. This technique provides good hemostasis with almost no medullary damage (Fig. 20–9).

Treatment of large endometriomas is facilitated by this technology. In a recent personal presentation, the results from an initial investigational study included the treatment of 13 endometriomas greater than 3 cm. The largest endometrioma treated measured 7 cm in diameter on ultrasonic evaluation. There have been no recurrences in this group, and second-look laparoscopic evaluation of six patients

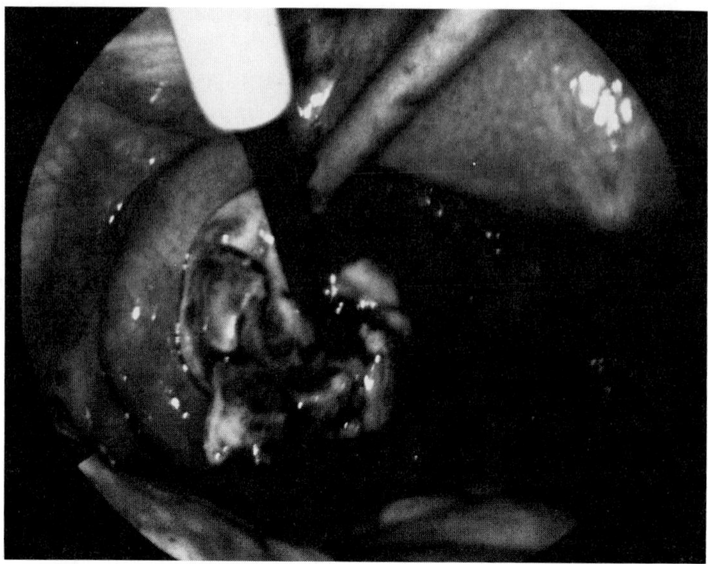

FIGURE 20–9. Treatment of endometriomas.

shows no significant periovarian adhesion formation from the procedure. All of these ovaries were allowed to heal by secondary intention.

Adhesiolysis

Treatment and lysis of adhesive disease are part of the treatment of any postinflammatory disease of the pelvis, including endometriosis, chronic pelvic inflammatory disease, and postoperative adhesion formation. Treatment of adhesions requires not only the ability to dissect tissue planes with minimal lateral damage, but also the ability to maintain maximal hemostasis during this process. Contact tips have provided an excellent tool for this process. The fine cone tips create minimal damage to surrounding normal tissue and if used correctly can help define tissue planes between two normal structures. Traction plays a significant part in this type of dissection. The other advantages are precise focal point, no need for a backstop, efficacy under body fluids, and minimal plume generation, even with fatty tissue. The ability to achieve hemostasis during the dissection is superior to that provided by any other laser. The cone tips can coagulate vessels to 2 mm in diameter. If large vessels are identified, an attempt to coagulate them before incision should be made by using the flat tip. Large, dense adhesions with significant vascularity can be released hemostatically without creating large areas of thermal necrosis or the need for suture material.

This technique was used in the treatment of endometriosis and in the treatment of pelvic adhesions in 97 patients. In this group, more than 50% had significant complaints of pelvic pain. Pelvic pain due to pelvic inflammatory disease and adhesions was significantly improved in all patients. There was no recurrence of symptoms or clinical findings. Because a second-look surgical re-evaluation protocol was not included in the investigation, it is impossible to determine the magnitude of recurrence of the lysed adhesions. The clinical improvement in this group suggests a reduction in anatomical distortion. This improvement was also true of the adhesions lysed during the procedures for endometriosis. In this group, some second-look procedures have been done and have shown excellent resolution of associated adhesive disease. The postoperative data from the hysterosalpingograms show excellent initial success with neosalpingostomy and improvement of adhesive disease.

Myomectomy

The use of operative laparoscopic techniques to perform myomectomies has been popularized by Semm. Contact tips can be used effectively to incise and achieve hemostasis. Pedunculated myomas are easily excised by transecting the connecting stalk. Subserosal myomas present more operative difficulties. A cone tip can be used to make a hemostatic incision over the serosal surface and subserosal myometrium. The myoma is then enucleated by blunt dissection to the vascular base. The tip is then used to transect across the vascular supply. The remaining hemostasis is achieved by using the flat contact tip or, if necessary, the non-contact coagulation technique. This technique has resulted in increased ease of operating and decreased operating time. In larger myomas, the technical problems associated with the removal of the mass from the abdominal cavity still remain.

DISCUSSION

Sapphire contact scalpels provide a laser delivery system that has a wide range of tissue effects that are important in most gynecological applications. The importance of exact control of thermal effect during a surgical procedure cannot be emphasized too strongly. Surgeons should be able to predict the incisional or coagulative depth. Lateral thermal effects on surrounding tissue should be limited but predictable.

High-frequency electrocautery has been used extensively as a thermal unit in surgery. This technique has been used mainly in a unipolar mode, which makes the patient one of the electrical poles. The isothermic effects of electrocautery in this mode are poorly understood by most surgeons. The lack of a predictable and sometimes limited tissue effect goes unappreciated. The use of bipolar electrocautery limits the isothermic effect but provides only coagulation of tissue.

The CO_2 laser is an efficient laser knife but provides very poor coagulative abilities. The many technical problems with the CO_2 laser have resulted in the proliferation of equipment to deal with these problems, especially during laparoscopic use. The plume from laser use may be biohazardous to operating room personnel and surgeons. The laser is still unmatched for fine incision/vaporization procedures, but it certainly has many limitations as a general-use laser.

Lasers in the blue-green spectrum have some advantages when there is a high hemoglobin concentration. They have a simple inexpensive fiberoptic delivery system. Their main drawback has been that they have been used with a non-contact technique. Although these lasers have a slightly shallower depth of penetration, the same disadvantages apply to the Nd:YAG laser using the same technique. The "near-contact" technique alluded to by blue-green laser users still creates by definition a non–contact effect. Contacting the bare fiberoptic cable limits some of the coagulative effect but is again variable. These lasers could use a contact scalpel for more exact control.

A combination of the Nd:YAG laser and the sapphire contact scalpels has provided a thermal unit for surgical use that yields the ability to choose tissue effect. If a surgeon understands the effects created by the different geometries of the contact scalpels, the exact thermal effect needed during a procedure can be created. The multiple applications of this system in gynecology have been discussed and demonstrated. Because of decreased technical difficulties, use of the contact scalpels requires less surgical skill.

There are still some limitations to their use, which can be affected by water and tissue buildup. If these are appreciated by the operator, they create minimal technical difficulties. In addition, the increasing use of advanced endoscopic gynecological surgery has placed greater demands on the use of surgical thermal units. They must provide hemostasis because of the limited ability to use suture. They must provide exact incisional abilities. They also must provide for limited use over vital structures. The endoscopic contact scalpels are ideal for this type of application.

Fiberoptic delivery systems and lasers will be used increasingly for gynecological surgical procedures. Understanding the effects of fiberoptics on the laser light energy delivered is important. If a surgeon wishes maximal performance from a laser, a surgeon must make the correct decision to use a non–contact technique, bare fiber contact, or contact scalpels. Each technique has important surgical applications. The Nd:YAG laser has the greatest possible variation of tissue effects when all three techniques are applied.

REFERENCES

1. Brumsted J, Shirk GJ: A second puncture probe for laparoscopic delivery of the Nd:YAG laser. Obstet Gynecol 73:672, 1989
2. Corson SL, Unger M, Kwa D et al: Laparoscopic laser treatment of endometriosis with the Nd:YAG sapphire probe. Am J Obstet Gynecol 160:718, 1989
3. Daikuzono N, Joffe SN: Artificial sapphire probe for contact photocoagulation and tissue vaporization with the Nd:YAG laser. Med Instrum 19:173, 1985
4. Doty JL, Auth DC: The laser photocoagulating dielectric wave guide scalpel. IEEE Trans Biomed Eng 28:1, 1981
5. Fuller TA: Operating characteristics of surgical lasers and delivery systems. In Surgical Lasers. New York, Macmillan, 1987.
6. Gimpelson RJ, Shirk GJ: Excisional conization of the cervix by Nd:YAG laser. Presented at the ASLMS (in press), 1989
7. Goldrath MH, Fuller TA, Segal S: Laser photovaporization of the endometrium for treatment of menorrhagia. Am J Obstet Gynecol 140:14, 1981
8. Joffe SN, Brackett KA, Sankar MY et al: Resection of the liver with the Nd:YAG laser. Surg Gynecol Obstet 163:437, 1986
9. Joffe SN, Schroder T: Lasers in general surgery. Adv Surg 20:125, 1987
10. Keye WR, Dixon J: Photocoagulation of endometriosis by the argon laser through the laparoscope. Obstet Gynecol 62:383, 1983
11. Keye WR, Hanson LW, Astin M et al: Argon laser therapy of endometriosis: A review of 92 consecutive patients. Fertil Steril 47:208, 1987
12. Lomano JM: Photocoagulation of early pelvic endometriosis with the Nd:YAG laser through the laparoscope. J Reprod Med 30:77, 1985
13. Martin DC, Diamond MP: Operative laparoscopy: Comparison of lasers with other techniques. Curr Probl Obstet Gynecol Fertil 9:564, 1986

14. Schultz LS, Hickock DF, Graber JN et al: Lasers in the treatment of advanced intraabdominal malignancy. Lasers Med Surg 5:5, 1989
15. Shirk GJ: Laparoscopic treatment of endometriosis by the use of the Nd : YAG laser sapphire contact tips. Am J Obstet Gynecol 160:1344, 1989
16. Shirk GJ, Brumsted JR, Gimpelson RJ et al: Operative laparoscopy using the Nd : YAG laser: An investigative study. Presented at the AAGL (in press), 1988
17. Totani R, Karasawa T, Suzucka Y: Application of newly developed contact type of surgical rod for Nd : YAG laser conization of uterine cervix. In: Lasers Opto-electronics in Medicine, pp. 495–501. New York, Springer Verlag, 1986
18. Zumwalt T, Wesseler T, Joffe SN: A comparison of artificial sapphire tip with the quartz tip: *In vitro* endometrial ablation. Colpo Gynecol Laser Surg 2:47, 1986

21

Laser, Cautery, or Scalpel: Which is Best?

Randle S. Corfman
Michael P. Diamond

"Certain knowledge is, however, equally beyond our reach in most departments of life. Oftener than not, we cannot wait for certain knowledge, but order our affairs in the light of probabilities."

—*Sir James Jeans*

New technologies are continually becoming available to physicians, providing new and innovative approaches to the diagnosis and treatment of disease entities that would have previously yielded poor prognosis. This fact is true for the field of pelvic reconstructive surgery, particularly infertility surgery.

The exchange of technologies between surgical specialties has never been more obvious than in the field of pelvic reconstructive surgery. The exchange of ideas and technologies within the gynecological community has been supplanted by information and technologies from various other surgical specialties, including general, plastic, urologic, and ophthalmic surgery. The new technology has been applied, tested, and modified, resulting in emergence of additional means of treating disease.

By the very nature of this process of exchange of new ideas, then, clinicians must keep in mind the history of the technology in question, including the effect of the modality on the system to which it has been applied. Extrapolation from one clinical scenario to another may or may not be warranted, making the need for adequate testing to avert poor clinical responses obvious.

The choice of laser, cautery, or scalpel is an excellent example of the need for surgeons to carefully weigh data from other surgical disciplines, involving a variety of tissues and organ systems, before choosing a particular modality. What follows is a description of factors that should bear consideration in choosing between these modalities.

FACTORS AFFECTING THE CHOICE OF MODALITY

The availability of only a single surgical modality might well make a discussion of options entirely academic. Certainly, every surgeon has access to a scalpel, and most probably a basic cautery unit. Access to the more advanced (or esoteric, depending on your perspective) laser modalities is usually inversely proportional to cost at many hospitals.

Access to a sophisticated electrocautery unit, capable of generating high electrical power by a microtip cautery, is quite variable. The optimal cautery delivery system must be able to generate a high power density in order to gain the desired tissue effect. The general bipolar unit, which is usually available, simply does not fit this requirement.

The least expensive and most commonly available laser is the carbon dioxide (CO_2) laser. The argon, neodymium : yttrium-aluminum-garnet (Nd : YAG), and potassium-titanyl-phosphate (KTP) lasers are more expensive, limiting the general availability of these to tertiary care facilities.

Access to the pelvic pathology also determines one's choice of therapeutic modalities. No longer is one limited to performing adhesiolysis or salpingostomy at laparotomy. Laparoscopic and pelviscopic surgery have emerged as, perhaps, the preferred *modus operandi* in treating many pelvic diseases, leading DeCherney[12] to eulogize "the obituary of laparotomy for pelvic reconstructive surgery has been written; it is only its publication that remains."

Traditionally, laparoscopic treatment of disease has used laparoscopic scissors for incising tissue and unipolar or bipolar cautery for tissue coagulation and ablation. The development of pelviscopic instrumentation has greatly expanded the potential endoscopic use of the scalpel and scissors. Additionally, virtually all forms of the laser can be delivered through the laparoscope, either through a series of mirrors in the articulating arm (CO_2 laser), or the fiber technology of the argon, KTP, or Nd : YAG lasers. All laser modalities may be used at laparotomy, and the CO_2 laser is adaptable to the operating microscope by a micromanipulator in order to achieve increased control of the delivered energy.

The importance and necessity of experienced operating room personnel in performing expedient and effective pelvic surgery, either at laparoscopy or laparotomy, cannot be overstated. Regardless of the modality chosen, support personnel can either make the surgery a pleasure or provide *tedium ad nauseam*. This is particularly true for microsurgical and laser techniques.

Safety standards, of utmost importance when using lasers, must be adhered to. Although a surgeon assumes responsibility for safety within the operating environment, it is most helpful for all involved to be familiar with safe operating procedures. If such support is not available, laser modalities cannot be used safely and should not be used at all.

At last, one must be honest about one's previous training and experience. Whether using a scalpel, cautery, or laser, one must not only be familiar with the instrument, but also be knowledgeable regarding the use of each modality.

DESIRED TISSUE EFFECT

In performing pelvic surgery, one or several of the following tissue effects are desired: (1) ablation, (2) vaporization, (3) coagulation, (4) incision, and (5) excision. It is difficult, if not impossible, to determine preoperatively exactly which of these effects one will require. Therefore, it is important either to have rapid access to several modalities to gain the desired effect or to have a single modality that may be used to achieve various effects. Obviously, the latter choice is preferable. Reality, unfortunately, lies somewhere short of ideality, and until such a modality is designed one must synthesize the best possible fit from existing options.

TISSUE EFFECT: THE ULTIMATE MEASURING STICK

In order to compare the tissue effects of each of the modalities, it is necessary to review the stages of wound healing in previously normal tissue. Masterson[32] has reviewed the literature on wound healing in skin and describes the response as consisting of three phases: the inflammatory phase, the fibroblastic phase, and the remodeling phase.

In the inflammatory phase, blood is released from small vessels in the area of injury, followed by vasoconstriction, for approximately 10 minutes. Vasodilation follows, and the cellular response immediately manifests with influx of leukocytes and platelets. Many proteinaceous and non-proteinaceous molecules are elaborated at the wound, including histamines, prostaglandins, and chemotactic agents, resulting in a gel-like substance. This phase varies in length of time, depending on the agent used to create the wound.

In the subsequent fibroblastic phase, collagen is deposited by fibroblasts that have been recruited to the site of injury. Optimal healing depends not only on good circulation to the site, but also on the adequacy of the cellular response. With capillary formation comes an increase in the local concentration of plasminogen activator, which catalyzes fibrinolysis of the fibrin component of the original clot. Subsequently, the resulting collagen fibrils cross-link, increasing the tensile strength of the wound to 30% of the original strength by day 21.

Finally, the remodeling phase consists of reconstruction of the previously laid collagen. This phase can vary in length of time for up to several months after the initial injury. The length and quality of this phase depend on various local and systemic factors, including nutrition, adequacy of blood supply, and oxygenation.

The mechanism by which peritoneum heals is less well-defined and has been reviewed elsewhere.[14] It was initially observed that within 5 days of injury, serosa on the small intestine of dogs was covered by a peritoneal membrane indistinguishable from surrounding peritoneum.[22,23] Early work was based on the hypothesis that this regeneration arose from transformation of peritoneal macrophages or by seeding of mesothelial cells from adjacent peritoneal surfaces.[16,17,24] Raftery,[34,35] however, in serial observations of peritoneal healing in rats using histochemical and electron microscopic techniques, found that peritoneal defects heal by the process of metaplasia of subperitoneal connective tissue. The resulting new peritoneum apparently arises by any of the following processes: (1) metaplasia of primitive mesenchymal cells present in the perivascular connective tissue; (2) indirectly, from primitive mesenchymal cells through fibroblasts; or (3) from subperitoneal fibroblasts, which arise, in turn, from differentiated, quiescent perivascular connective tissue fibroblasts.[14,15,17,35]

Considerable differences, then, are noted between the healing processes of skin and peritoneum. It is obvious that caution must be exercised in extrapolating not only the phases of the healing process from one epithelium type to another, but also in predicting healing responses in previously damaged or diseased tissue. Rarely does a pelvic surgeon deal with disease-free tissue. Rather, one or several pathologic processes has often influenced the pelvic milieu, predetermining the fate of surgical attempts to alter the natural history of the disease.

MODES OF ACTION OF SCALPEL, CAUTERY, AND LASERS

Each modality can be chosen to perform a specific function, either incision, coagulation, vaporization, or combinations thereof. We shall briefly discuss each modality, paying particular attention to capabilities and deficits of each.

Scalpel

The scalpel is used chiefly as an incising tool, exerting an effect precisely at the point of tissue incision. It simply incises the tissue to which it is applied and produces no direct effect on the surrounding tissue. As a result, one expects and sees no adverse effects in the surrounding tissues, thereby eliminating "field effects," such as thermal damage, seen with the other modalities to be discussed. The price to be paid for this benefit is, unfortunately, lack of hemostasis.

Before discussing the more technological oriented modalities, it is important to understand the difference between power and power density. Although not generally appreciated, power densities produced by both photons and electrons are approximated by the following equation:

$$Pd = \frac{watts \times 100}{d^2}$$

where Pd = power density, watts = power output, and d = spot diameter in millimeters. It follows that the power density is inversely proportional to the square of the spot size.

The theoretical work of McKenzie[33] predicts that the depth of thermal damage decreases as higher power densities are used and as short pulses of energy are chosen. The latter prediction theoretically occurs by allowing cooling of tissue between pulses. Although his work was directed toward the CO_2 laser, his predictions should hold true for electrocautery. As we shall see, the work of several authors supports predictions arising from his mathematical modeling.

Cautery

Cautery allows one either to incise or coagulate tissue, or both. The traditional cautery tip uses low power densities, providing coagulation of tissues. The advent of the microelectrode allows one to achieve power densities of 5000 watts/cm^2, transforming the modality into an incising device that acts very much like a CO_2 laser, in terms of tissue effect.

An understanding of cutting and coagulation electrocautery settings is necessary for surgeons to wisely adapt to various clinical situations.[36] If one considers that the cutting setting results in a waveform of constant oscillations, it follows that this undamped energy produces its effect secondary to intense heat generated within the tissue itself. The coagulation setting produces a highly damped energy form with bursts of rapidly decreasing current, causing cellular dehydration. It is useful to note obvious similarities between cutting and coagulation electrocautery settings, and continuous and pulsed laser waveforms, respectively.

Laser

Lasers can provide various functions including incision, coagulation, and vaporization. As has been described elsewhere in this text, each of the lasers used in surgical applications possesses inherent differences in the interaction of the delivered energy with the target tissue. Briefly, let us examine each laser in terms of its unique capabilities.

Carbon Dioxide Laser

The CO_2 laser beam impacts tissue and is absorbed by tissue water, resulting in vaporization, and the energy is transformed into heat. The cellular protein is incinerated to elemental carbon and smoke. There is very little scattering, and the radiation is completely absorbed in a relatively shallow layer of tissue. As a result, the CO_2 laser can be used to incise or vaporize tissue on which it impinges.

By altering the waveform of the CO_2 laser, one can vary the heating of the tissue surrounding the impact zone. For example, use of a continuous waveform provides higher average delivered energy, resulting in a greater temperature effect. This in turn seals vessels and favors hemostasis. In choosing a pulsed waveform, one can, by increasing the power, attain high power densities while decreasing the average delivered energy, resulting in lower tissue temperatures and less hemostatic effect.

It is important to note that the power density used determines the depth of thermal damage. This is demonstrated by the histologic findings of thermal damage extending 0.5 to 1.0 mm beyond the laser impact zone, using a power density of 700 watts/cm^2, as compared with the findings by Luciano and colleagues,[30] who report a depth of 0.16 mm at a power density of 58,946 watts/cm^2.

It should also be noted that the depth of thermal damage varies from one tissue to another at the same power density. For example, Luciano and colleagues[30] found a depth of thermal damage averaging about 0.04 mm in ovarian tissue, as compared with 0.16 mm in the uterus, perhaps reflecting differences in water content of the tissues.

It is of interest to note that the CO_2 laser has, until recently, required a set of well-aligned mirrors to direct the laser beam properly. Baggish and colleagues[6] reported clinical use of a flexible optic delivery system, providing up to 20 watts of power. Many believe that this technological advance will usher in increased safety and use of the CO_2 laser for intra-abdominal surgery.

Argon Laser

The argon laser beam, whose radiation lies between 488 and 515 mm, is selectively absorbed by pigmented tissues and is not absorbed by water. The beam is only slightly scattered on impact with pigmented tissue, resulting in photocoagulation to a tissue depth of 0.5 mm.

Frank and colleagues[20] described the immediate effect of the argon laser on rat bladder tissue, finding little difference from the effect of the Nd : YAG laser at scanning electron micrography. Light microscopy, however, revealed only a small coagulation necrosis with removal of overlying epithelium, thickening of collagen fibers, and interstitial edema. The deep effect is greater than that produced by the CO_2 laser, but not as great as that produced by the Nd : YAG laser. As we shall see, this deep effect can result in connective tissue alterations that may pose obstacles to regeneration of physiological function.

Neodymium : Yttrium-Aluminum-Garnet Laser

Like the argon laser, the Nd : YAG laser is passed through fiberoptics, permitting a surgeon considerable flexibility in accessing the pelvis. Operating at a wavelength of 1060 nm, it is transmitted through water and absorbed primarily by pigmented tissues. Scattering of radiation becomes important, leading to a homogeneous, uniform distribution, producing a deep thermal effect with relatively little damage to the surface of the tissue.

Frank and colleagues[20] demonstrated the utility of this laser in rats and rabbits, showing that necrosis in the bladder wall occurs up to 4 mm in depth, without producing defects in the tissue surface.

Potassium-Titanyl-Phosphate 532 Laser

The KTP/532 laser is the newest member of the fiberoptic lasers, in terms of tissue effects. At a wavelength of 532 nm, it is transmitted through water and produces coagulation to a depth of 0.5 mm. Like the argon and Nd : YAG lasers, it is color dependent, making it similar to those lasers in terms of tissue specificity. Very little attention has been paid toward this laser in the gynecological literature, owing to surgeons' limited access to this technology.

EFFECT OF MODALITIES ON WOUND HEALING AND ADHESION FORMATION

Having reviewed the normal healing process in previously disease-free tissue and the immediate tissue effects of each modality, let us now direct our attention to delayed sequelae of each. Precious little data exists on the peritoneal healing process, regardless of the mode of injury. As we have seen, much of what we know about normal wound healing is derived from skin and not from coelomic epithelium. With this in mind, let us examine data that might shed light on healing processes and their sequelae, adhesion formation and loss of physiological function.

Scalpel

The lack of a zone effect, if you will, around the site of scalpel-induced injury theoretically should result in minimal disruption of the blood supply and, perhaps more importantly, less cellular disruption and damage.

Fry and colleagues[21] reported the highest graft viability following scalpel excision of skin in pigs, in contrast to electrocautery and continuous-wave CO_2 laser using low power density. The most expedient wound healing, as indicated by graft viability and wound contracture, was noted in the scalpel group, followed by the electrocautery group and, lastly, the laser group. The significantly less wound contracture in the scalpel group was taken as evidence of greater secondary revascularization of the graft. Finsterbush and colleagues[19], working with rabbits, found less scarring and equal tensile strength when skin incisions were made with the scalpel, as compared with the low power density CO_2 laser. Histologically, they noted less inflammation and hyperemia in the scalpel group, but by 23 days both groups had equal histologic appearances. They also noted less thickening and fibrosis in the scalpel group.

Perhaps the best examination of the healing of peritoneal epithelium was that by Kott and associates.[26] They examined the effect of scalpel versus low power density CO_2 laser incisions on the healing of intestinal anastomosis in cats, describing histologic findings. At 24 hours, the anastomosis was filled with inflammatory infiltrate, and after 3 days, the acute inflammation progressed to include both epithelial and subepithelial layers. Fibroblasts and granulation tissue became evident, and by 4 days, immature collagen filled the anastomosis with partial covering of the surface by a single layer of cuboidal epithelium. After 6 days, there was incomplete fusion of young fibrous tissue, and after 11 days, the healing process was completed. This contrasted with the healing process of the laser group, with completion only on the 21st day.

It appears, in summary, that incision with the scalpel results in more rapid healing, both in skin and bowel. No differences in incision strengths are found. However, it must be kept in mind that these comparisons were made with a low power density laser.

Electrocautery

For reasons discussed earlier, high power densities, either with electrocautery or the laser, result in less thermal effect in tissues surrounding the injury site. The microelectrocautery has been used to optimize this modality, improving on macrocautery, as we have known it.

Fayez and colleagues[18] compared results of transection and microsurgical anastomosis of rabbit uterine horns, using microscissors, microelectrocautery, and low power density (900 watts/cm^2) continuous-wave CO_2 laser as the transecting modalities. Pregnancy rates were similar between the microscissor and microelectrocautery groups, with the laser group demonstrating a lower pregnancy rate and a higher rate of occlusion. Histologically, at the time of delivery, the microelectrocautery group demonstrated minimal fibrosis in the muscularis, without evidence of necrosis or coagulation, and with continuity of the mucosa. These findings compared favorably with the laser transection group, which manifested necrosis and coagulation of the mucosa at the anastomosis, even to the point of occlusion.

Pregnancy rates were found to be similar in groups of patients following salpingostomy, either with the high power density microelectrocautery (30%) or with a high power density (20,000 watts/cm^2) CO_2 laser (39.5%), in a study by Mage and Bruhat.[31] Second-look laparoscopy and evaluation of tubal patency were not available for both groups. The Intraabdominal Laser Study Group[11] evaluated terminal salpingostomy using the CO_2 laser, and as compared with non-laser modalities, laser treatment resulted in similar pregnancy rates, although it tended to reduce the mean time from surgery to pregnancy.

Diamond and colleagues,[13] in studying tubal patency and pelvic adhesions at early second-look laparoscopy, compared their results using the CO_2 laser with those of the Adhesion Study Group, which used non-laser modalities.[1] Although the laser group was found to have a higher rate of tubal patency, there was no significant difference in adhesion scores. They concluded that the laser "does not appear to be a panacea" as a modality in treating tuboperitoneal infertility,[13] a conclusion with which we heartily agree.

Luciano and associates[30] evaluated the healing patterns and postoperative adhesion formation following high power density (88,888 watts/cm^2) microelectrocautery and high power density (58,946 watts/cm^2) CO_2 laser incisions in rabbit uterine horns and ovaries. They found no difference in adhesion formation, nor in the width and extent of collagen deposition, in contrast to the findings by Bellina and colleagues,[8] who reported significantly less postoperative adhesion formation in CO_2 laser-treated animals.

In summary, it appears that at high power densities, electrocautery is comparable to the scalpel and high power density laser, in terms of postoperative histology, adhesion formation, and pregnancy rates when applied to salpingostomy and resection. It is superior to the scalpel in terms of providing hemostasis and, if used at high power densities, has minimal adverse tissue healing effects.

Laser

We have alluded to the concept that low power densities produce considerable field effects, principally by tissue heating. Negative effects of low power densities include burn injury to the skin and eyes[29] and impairment of skin graft viability after excision with the CO_2 laser in patients with melanoma.[28]

Positive effects of low power density laser radiation have been reported. Kana and associates,[25] using daily exposures to 45 mW/cm^2 of helium–neon laser to rat skin, showed a significant increase in collagen synthesis as well as an enhanced rate of wound closure over controls. Surinchak and colleagues,[37] however, subsequently found no significant differences in skin healing between rabbit skin wounds exposed to low-level helium-neon laser radiation and controls. Finally, Kovacs[27] reported an acceleration of ectropion regression with exposure to low power density helium-neon laser radiation; however, no controls were included, making interpretation difficult.

It can be concluded from this review of the literature[25,27–29,37] that low power density laser radiation results in no beneficial effects on the tissue to which it is applied; indeed, it clearly can have a negative effect on wound healing.

It is also clear, from our previous considerations of tissue effect, that high power density, whether with the cautery or the laser, results in less-adverse tissue effects relative to a low power density. Let us now address the issue of continuous- versus pulsed-wave lasers in surgery.

In an effort to decrease the heat effect of the laser modality, variations around the continuous-wave theme have been made. Basically, the waveform was altered to a pulsed mode, with a narrow pulse width, resulting in diminished "laser on" time and enhancing cooling of tissue between pulses. In theory, this would diminish necrosis and reduce thermal damage to the tissue. By increasing the amplitude (superpulsing), very high peak powers can result and very high power densities can be achieved.

Several studies have demonstrated less thermal damage and necrosis when comparing pulsed waveform with continuous waveform.[3,4,7] Acute and chronic evaluation of rat uterine horns transected with each waveform revealed less thermal effect and necrosis in the pulse-treated group relative to the continuous-wave group.[5] Inflammatory response and adhesion formation were also less with pulsed waveform. Badaway and colleagues,[4] comparing pulsed waveform and microscissor transection of rat uterine horns for anastomosis, found less fibrosis in the laser group; however, significant differences in adhesion formation and pregnancy rates were not noted. Using a similar experimental design, a comparison was made between continuous and pulsed waveforms for transection, and again no significant difference in pregnancy rates was noted.[3] Histologic evaluation did reveal less thinning of the muscularis and subserosal layers with the pulsed waveform.

The importance of power density also applies with this waveform, as demonstrated by Taylor and colleagues.[38] Using the skin model, they confirmed that the pulsed waveform produces less thermal coagulation than does continuous waveform. In addition, they found significantly greater depths of penetration at power densities of 2000 watts/cm^2 or higher for both waveforms. Power densities of 4750 watts/cm^2 and greater were necessary to optimize depth of coagulation. The advantages of a pulsed waveform and high power density are now obvious, in terms of both thermal effect and tissue necrosis. These may be particularly important for tasks requiring incision or transection.

Finally, it should be noted that approximation of severed tissue by laser "welding," using low power densities, has been attempted.[2,6,10] Results with laser anastomosis of rabbit and human fallopian tubes, using power densities of 700 watts/cm^2, have been extremely discouraging.[6,10] Ashworth and colleagues[2] had excellent results with laser anastomosis of carotid arteries in dogs, using power densities from 306 to 357 watts/cm^2. Application of such low power densities to tubal anastomosis might produce more favorable results.

SUMMARY

It is obvious that a great deal remains to be learned about each of the modalities discussed earlier. We are hampered, however, by lack of information in several crucial areas. Although a great deal is known about tissue effects of each modality on normal skin, it is perhaps ill advised to extrapolate data from squamous to coelomic epithelium. In addition, the effect of each modality on previously damaged or diseased tissue is virtually unexplored. Each of these deficits, in our understanding, might prove crucial in the clinical application of these and forthcoming technologies to reproductive surgery.

There certainly is no magic in any of the modalities we have examined. Rather, each is but a tool and not a therapeutic end in itself. By possessing an understanding of the limitations and effects of each modality, surgeons can best develop a therapeutic regimen that will serve patients most advantageously.

REFERENCES

1. Adhesion Study Group: Reduction of postoperative pelvic adhesions with intraperitoneal 32% dextran 70: A prospective, randomized clinical trial. Fertil Steril 40:612, 1983
2. Ashworth EM, Dalsing MC, Olson JF et al: Large-artery welding with a milliwatt carbon dioxide laser. Arch Surg 122:673, 1987
3. Badaway S, ElBakry MM, Baggish MS: Comparative study of continuous and pulsed CO_2 laser on tissue healing and fertility outcome in tubal anastomosis. Fertil Steril 47:843, 1987
4. Badaway S, ElBakry MM, Baggish MS et al: Pulsed CO_2 laser versus conventional microsurgical anastomosis of the rat uterine horn. Fertil Steril 46:127, 1986
5. Baggish MS, Baltoyannis P, Badawy S et al: Carbon dioxide laser laparoscopy performed with a flexible fiber in humans. Am J Obstet Gynecol 157:1129, 1987
6. Baggish MS, Chong AP: Carbon dioxide laser microsurgery of the uterine tube. Obstet Gynecol 58:111, 1981
7. Baggish MS and ElBakry MM: Comparison of electronically superpulsed and continuous-wave CO_2 laser on the rat uterine horn. Fertil Steril 45:120, 1986
8. Bellina JF, Hemmings R, Voros JI et al: Carbon dioxide laser and electrosurgical wound study with an animal model: A comparison of tissue damage and healing patterns in peritoneal tissue. Am J Obstet Gynecol 148:326, 1984
9. Bellina JH, Meandzija P, Schillt V et al: Analysis of electronically pulsed versus quasi-continuous wave carbon dioxide lasers in an animal model. Am J Obstet Gynecol 150:934, 1984
10. Choe JK, Dawood MY, Andrews AH: Conventional versus laser reanastomosis of rabbit ligated uterine horns. Obstet Gynecol 61:689, 1983
11. Daniell JF, Diamond MP, McLaughlin DS et al: Clinical results of terminal salpingostomy with the use of the CO_2 laser: Report of the Intraabdominal Laser Study Group. Fertil Steril 45:175, 1986
12. DeCherney AH: The leader of the band is tired. Fertil Steril 44:299, 1985
13. Diamond MP, Daniell JF, Martin DC et al: Tubal patency and pelvic adhesions at second-look laparoscopy following intraabdominal use of the carbon dioxide laser: Initial report of the intraabdominal laser study group. Fertil Steril 42:717, 1984
14. DiZerega GS: The cause and prevention of postsurgical adhesions. Bethesda, National Institute Child Health and Human Development, 1980
15. Ellis H, Harrison W, Hugh TB: The healing of peritoneum under normal and abnormal conditions. Br J Surg 52:471, 1965
16. Eskeland G: Prevention of experimental peritoneal adhesions in the rat by intraperitoneally administered corticosteroids. Acta Chir Scand 125:91, 1963
17. Eskeland G: Regeneration of parietal peritoneum. Acta Pathol Microbiol Scand 62:459, 1964
18. Fayez JA, McComb JS, Harper MA: Comparison of tubal surgery with the CO_2 laser and the unipolar microelectrode. Fertil Steril 40:476, 1983
19. Finsterbush A, Rousso M, Asher H: Healing and tensile strength of the CO_2 laser incisions and scalpel wounds in rabbits. Plast Reconstr Surg 70:360, 1982

20. Frank F, Keiditsch E, Hofstetter A et al: Various effects of the CO_2, the neodymium-YAG, and the argon laser irradiation on bladder tissue. Lasers Surg Med 2:89, 1982
21. Fry TL, Gerbe RW, Botros SB et al: Effects of laser, scalpel, and electrosurgical excision on wound contracture and graft "take." Plast Reconstr Surg 65:729, 1980
22. Glucksman DL: Serosal integrity and intestinal adhesions. Surgery 60:1009, 1966
23. Glucksman DL, Warren WD: The effect of topically applied corticosteroids in the prevention of peritoneal adhesions: An experimental approach with a review of the literature. Surgery 60:352, 1966
24. Johnson FR, Whitting HW: Repair of parietal peritoneum. Br J Surg 49:653, 1962
25. Kana JS, Hutschenreiter G, Haina D et al: Effect of low-power density laser radiation on healing of open skin wounds in rats. Arch Surg 116:293, 1981
26. Kott I, Gassner S, Mattos S et al: The surgical knife and the CO_2 laser beam. Am J Protocol Gastroenterol Colon Rectal Surg 27:27, 1976
27. Kovacs L: The stimulatory effect of laser on the physiological healing process of portio surface. Lasers Surg Med 1:241, 1981
28. Lejeune FJ, Van Hoof G, Gerard A: Impairment of skin graft take after CO_2 laser surgery in melanoma patients. Br J Surg 67:318, 1980
29. Litwin MS, Fine S, Klein E et al: Burn injury after carbon dioxide laser irradiation. Arch Surg 98:219, 1969
30. Luciano AA, Whitman G, Maier DB et al: A comparison of thermal injury, healing patterns, and postoperative adhesion formation following CO_2 laser and electrosurgery. Fertil Steril 48:1025, 1987
31. Mage G, Bruhat M: Pregnancy following salpingostomy: Comparison between CO_2 laser and electrosurgery procedures. Fertil Steril 40:472, 1983
32. Masterson BJ: Wound healing in gynecologic surgery. In Masterson BJ (ed): Manual of Gynecologic Surgery. New York, Springer-Verlag, 1979
33. McKenzie AL: How far does thermal damage extend beneath the surface of CO_2 laser incisions? Phys Med Biol 28:905, 1983
34. Raftery AT: Regeneration of parietal and visceral peritoneum: An electron microscopical study. J Anat 115:375, 1973
35. Raftery AT: Regeneration of parietal and visceral peritoneum: An enzyme histochemical study. J Anat 121:589, 1976
36. Rioux JE: Electrosurgery. In Hunt RB (ed): Atlas of Female Infertility Surgery. Chicago, Year Book Medical Publishers, 1986
37. Surinchak JS, Alago ML, Bellamy RF et al: Effects of low-level energy lasers on the healing of full-thickness skin defects. Lasers Surg Med 2:267, 1983
38. Taylor MV, Martin DC, Poston W et al: Effect of power density and carbonization on residual tissue coagulation using the continuous wave carbon dioxide laser. Colpos Gynecol Laser Surg 2:169, 1986

APPENDICES

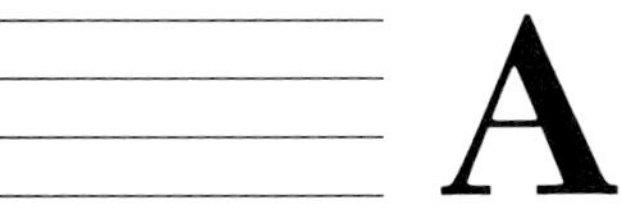# A

Appendix A

Advanced Laser Services Corp.
P.O. Box 99
Grove City, OH 43123
Phone: 614-228-0252

Coherent Medical Lasers
3270 W. Bayshore Road
P.O. Box 10122
Palo Alto, CA 94303
Phone: 415-858-2250

Gynecscope Corporation
36212 Euclid Avenue
Willoughby, OH 44094
Phone: 216-946-5659

Heraeus LaserSonics, Inc.
P.O. Box 58005
3420 Central Expressway
Santa Clara, CA 95052
Phone: 408-720-1100
Telex/FAX: 408-732-5259

HGM Medical Laser Systems, Inc.
3959 West 1820 South
Salt Lake City, UT 84104
Phone: 801-972-0500

Lase, Inc.
7209 E. Kemper Road
Cincinnati, OH 45249
Phone: 800-543-2070
Telex/FAX: 38-4288

Laserscope
3052 Orchard Drive
San Jose, CA 95134
Phone: 408-943-0636
Telex/FAX: 408-943-1051

Marlow Surgical Technologies
36212 Euclid Avenue
Willoughby, OH 44094
Phone: 216-946-2453
Telex/FAX: 216-946-1997

Olympus Corp., Medical Instruments
4 Nevada Drive
Lake Success, NY 11042
Phone: 516-488-3880

Sharplan Lasers, Inc.
1 Pearl Court
Allendale, NJ 07401
Phone: 201-327-1666
Telex/FAX: 201-445-4048

Stackhouse Associates, Inc.
150 Sierra Street
El Segundo, CA 90245
Phone: 213-322-6676
Telex/FAX: 213-414-0153

Storz Instrument Co.
3365 Tree Court Ind. Blvd.
St. Louis, MO 63122
Phone: 314-225-5051

Karl Storz Endoscopy-Americia, Inc.
10111 W. Jefferson Blvd.
Culver City, CA 90232
Phone: 213-558-1500

Surgical Laser Technologies
One Great Valley Pkwy.
Malvern, PA 19355
Phone: 800-772-5273
Telex/FAX: 215-647-8279

Surgilase, Inc.
I-95 Corporate Park
33 Plan Way
Warwick, RI 02886
Phone: 401-732-6440
Telex/FAX: 401-732-6445

Carl Zeiss, Inc.
One Zeiss Drive
Thornwood, NY 10594
Phone: 914-747-1800
Telex/FAX: 914-682-8296

B

Appendix B

Alphabetical Listing of Laser Types

MANUFACTURER	PRODUCT NAME/ MODEL NO.	OUTPUT POWER/ENERGY	COOLING SYSTEM	ELECTRICAL INPUT	WARRANTY	PRICE	SPECIAL FEATURES
Argon Lasers							
HGM Medical Laser Systems, Inc.	Model 20	0–16 watts, adjustable	Water	208–240 VAC 3 phase	1 year	See dealer	Portable, pulsed mode, large digital display, plug-in accessory.
HGM Medical Laser Systems, Inc.	Model 8	6 watts	Water	208–240 VAC	1 year	See dealer	Portable, pulsed modes, large digital display, plug-in accessories.
CO₂ Lasers							
Coherent Medical Lasers	Ambulase-15	Adjustable to 15 watts	Air	115 V	1 year parts and labor	Upon request	A microprocessor-controlled monitoring system continuously checks to help ensure safe and efficient operation.
Coherent Medical Lasers	Ambulase-20	Adjustable to 20 watts	Air	115 V	1 year parts and labor	Upon request	Start with the Ambulase-20 with continuous-wave mode and upgrade later, adding superpulse mode.
Coherent Medical Lasers	Ambulase-20 Superpulse	Adjustable to 20 watts	Air	115 V	1 year parts and labor	Upon request	Superpulse capability; 4 preselected settings.
Coherent Medical Lasers	XA-30 Superpulse	30 watts	Water	115 V/220 V/240 V	1 year parts and labor		Superpulse capability; 2 preselected settings.
Coherent Medical Lasers	XL-40 Superpulse	40 watts	Air	115 V	1 year		Superpulse capability; 3 preset modes, plus user-adjustable width and repetition rate.

Coherent Medical Lasers	XL-55 Superpulse	Adjustable to 55 watts	Air	115 V	1 year	Upon request	Superpulse capability; 3 preset modes, plus user-adjustable width and repetition rate.
Heraeus Laser-Sonics, Inc.	250Z Surgical Laser System	40 watts delivered to tissue	Self-contained	110–120 VAC, 220–240 VAC	1 year parts and labor	Ask for quote	Varipulse, digitally controlled.
Heraeus Laser-Sonics, Inc.	Illumina IL 25	25 watts delivered to tissue	Self-contained liquid to air	115 VAC, 50/60 Hz	1 year parts and labor	Ask for quote	Microprocessor control, internal diagnostics, sealed tube.
Heraeus Laser-Sonics, Inc.	Illumina IL 40	40 watts delivered to tissue	Self-contained liquid to air	115 VAC, 50/60 Hz, 6 A	1 year parts and labor	Ask for quote	Microprocessor control, internal diagnostics, sealed tube.
Heraeus Laser-Sonics, Inc.	Illumina IL 55	55 watts delivered to tissue	Self-contained liquid to air	115 VAC, 50/60 Hz, 7.5 A	1 year parts and labor	Ask for quote	Microprocessor control, internal diagnostics, sealed tube.
Heraeus Laser-Sonics, Inc.	LS 500	80 watts delivered to tissue	Closed-loop heat exchanger, air	200/220 VAC, 50/60 Hz	1 year parts and labor	Ask for quote	Microprocessor control, internal diagnostics, sealed tube.
Heraeus Laser-Sonics, Inc.	Model 860 Surgical Laser System	60 watts delivered to tissue	Self-contained closed loop, water	117 VAC, 240 VAC	1 year parts and labor	Ask for quote	Control/pulse, electronic pulsing.
Heraeus Laser-Sonics, Inc.	Model LS 880 Surgical Laser System	80 watts delivered to tissue	Self-contained, closed loop, water	117 VAC, 240 VAC	1 year parts and labor	Ask for quote	Control/pulse, electronic pulsing.

(continued)

Alphabetical Listing of Laser Types (Continued)

MANUFACTURER	PRODUCT NAME/ MODEL NO.	OUTPUT POWER/ENERGY	COOLING SYSTEM	ELECTRICAL INPUT	WARRANTY	PRICE	SPECIAL FEATURES
Sharplan Lasers, Inc.	Sharplan 1020	Adjustable 1–20 watts delivered to tissue	Air	115 VAC/4 A, 230 VAC/2 A	1 year		Small, compact; sealed-tube technology; microprocessor controlled; spring-balanced articulating arm.
Sharplan Lasers, Inc.	Sharplan 1040	High power 1–40 watts; low power 0.1–1 watt	Self-contained water to air heat exchanger	120 VAC/12 A; 230 VAC/6 A	1 year		Milliwatt and superpulse capability, TEM_{00} beam, spring balanced articulating arm.
Sharplan Lasers, Inc.	Sharplan 1060	High power 1–60 watts; low power 0.1–1 watt	Self-contained water to air heat exchanger	120 VAC/14 A; 230 VAC/7 A	1 year		Milliwatt and superpulse capability, TEM_{00} beam, spring balanced articulating arm.
Sharplan Lasers, Inc.	Sharplan 1100	1–100 watt high power; 0.1–.99 watt low power	Self-contained water to air heat exchanger	110 VAC/ 18 A; 220 VAC/9 A	1 year		Milliwatt and superpulse capability, TEM_{00} PD.
Surgilase, Inc.	Surgilase 25	25 watts	Closed liquid cooling system	110 V, 10 A	1 year parts and 3 on tube	$24,500 to 27,500	DC excited sealed free-space laser provides long-term reliability and easy use.

Surgilase, Inc.	Surgilase 40	40 watts	Closed liquid cooling system	110 V, 60 Hz	1 year parts and labor; 3 years on tube	$54,500	DC excited sealed free-space laser provides long-term reliability, easy use, and simple maintenance.
Surgilase, Inc.	Surgilase 55	55 watts	Closed liquid cooling system	110 V, 60 Hz	1 year parts and labor; 3 years on tube	$74,500	DC excited sealed free-space laser provides long-term reliability, easy use, and simple maintenance.
Surgilase, Inc.	Surgilase 80	80 watts	Self-contained liquid	110 V, 60 Hz, 12 A	1 year parts and 3 on tube	$90,000	DC excited sealed free-space laser provides long-term reliability, easy use, and simple maintenance.
Surgilase, Inc.	Surgilase 100	100 watts	Closed liquid cooling system	110 V, 60 Hz	1 year parts and labor; 3 years on tube	$115,000	DC excited sealed free-space laser provides long-term reliability, easy use, and simple maintenance.
KTP Lasers							
Laserscope	KTP/532* Model 501	Minimum 15 watts at head of laser	Water	208, single phase	1 year	$99,500	Microscopic or fiberoptic delivery.
Laserscope	KTP/532* Model 502	Minimum 15 watts at head of laser	Water	208, single phase	1 year	$79,500	Fiberoptic delivery.
YAG Lasers							
Heraeus Laser-Sonics Inc.	Model 4900	60 watts delivered to tissue	Self-contained air-cooling	200–240 VAC, single	1 year parts and labor	Ask for quote	UL approved, 400-micron fiber capabilities, variable repeat mode, autocalibrator, low-power stability.

(continued)

Alphabetical Listing of Laser Types (Continued)

MANUFACTURER	PRODUCT NAME/ MODEL NO.	OUTPUT POWER/ENERGY	COOLING SYSTEM	ELECTRICAL INPUT	WARRANTY	PRICE	SPECIAL FEATURES
Heraeus Laser-Sonics Inc.	Model 6000	100 watts delivered to tissue	External water	200–240 VAC, single	1 year parts and labor	Ask for quote	UL approved, variable repeat mode, autocalibration, excellent low-power stability.
Heraeus Laser-Sonics Inc.	Model 8900	Over 100 watts delivered to tissue	External water	208 VAC, 30 A, 3 phase	1 year parts and labor	Ask for quote	Built-in recirculating gas system, 5 color variable-intensity aiming beam, built-in printer.
Sharplan Lasers, Inc.	Medilas 2	3–100 watts	Water to water	3 phase 200–380 V	1 year		Long track record, small and portable.
Sharplan Lasers, Inc.	Sharplan 2100	5–100 watts to tissue	Water to water	3 phase 208 VAC; 380 VAC	1 year		Microprocessor control, portable, alpha numeric display, and error messages.
Sharplan Lasers, Inc.	Sharplan/Medilas 4060 N	1–60 watts delivered to tissue	Air or water	220 VAC, 16 A single	1 year		Air cooled, portable, compact, continuous or blinking helium-neon.

Sharplan Lasers, Inc.	Sharplan/Medilas 40 N	1–40 watts delivered to tissue	Air or water	220 VAC, 16 A single	1 year		Air cooled, portable, compact, continuous or blinking helium-neon.
Surgical Laser Technologies	CL60	1–60 watts	Internal, self-contained, air cooled	220 + or − 10%, 30 A	1 year—100%	$75,000	True portability, internal cooling system runs on available single-phase power.
Surgical Laser Technologies	CL100	1–100 watts	Internal, self-contained, air cooled	220 + or − 10%, 30 A	1 year—100%	$90,000	True portability, internal cooling system requires no external water source, runs on available single-phase power.
Surgilase, Inc.	Surgilase YAG 100	100 watts delivered to tissue	Liquid-to-liquid open system	208 volts, 60 Hz	1 year parts and labor	$84,900	Limited-duty cycle usage at lower powers without external cooling.

* The Laserscope KTP laser produces output at 532 nm and also has a 1064-nm YAG laser option.

Index

Page numbers in *italics* indicate figures;
those followed by *t* indicate tabular material.

D

E

G

H

W Y Z

ISBN 0-397-50986-3